AGING
Volume 12

The Aging Heart
Its Function and Response to Stress

Aging Series

Aging
Volume 12

The Aging Heart
Its Function and Response to Stress

Editor

Myron L. Weisfeldt, M.D.

Professor of Medicine
Director, Cardiology Division
The Johns Hopkins Medical Institutions
Baltimore, Maryland

Raven Press ■ New York

Raven Press, 1140 Avenue of the Americas, New York, New York 10036

Great care has been taken to maintain the accuracy of the information contained in the volume. However, Raven Press cannot be held responsible for errors or for any consequences arising from the use of the information contained herein.

Library of Congress Cataloging in Publication Data
Main entry under title:

The aging heart.

   (Aging; v. 12 ISSN 0160–2721)
   Includes index
   1. Heart—Aging. 2. Stress (Physiology)
I. Weisfeldt, Myron L. II. Series. [DNLM:
1. Heart—Physiopathology. 2. Stress. 3. Aging.
W1 AG342E v. 12 / WG200 H4366]
QP111.H42   612′.17   77–74615
ISBN 0–89004–307–8

To Nathan W. Shock, Ph.D.,
who touched nearly all of us as he pioneered
the study of aging changes in the cardiovascular system.

Preface

In recent years there has been a rapid acceleration of interest in characterizing the pathophysiological changes that occur in man over the course of the life span. Certainly a major impetus has come from knowledge of demographic characteristics of the American population. It is clear that there is an ever-increasing incidence of significant cardiac disease with advancing age, as well as increasing limitations in terms of exercise and general physical abilities. Many of these latter changes have been attributed to aging changes within the heart and the cardiovascular system.

I have selected the contributors to this volume on the basis of what I perceive as insight and commitment to the fundamental mechanisms and important clinical applications of pathophysiological data dealing with the aging cardiovascular system. In contrast to other works in this particular area, which are either accumulations of primary research information or sequential clinical observations, the present volume is an effort to place all available major scientific data into perspective. The authors concern themselves with the contractile and elastic properties of cardiac muscle, the heart as a single organ within the body, the integration of the cardiovascular system, and the response to pharmacological agents. In addition, important related areas including cardiac structure, the structure of the coronary vasculature, and the integrated response of the organism to exercise in the aging individual are reviewed. Each of us attempts not only to summarize the available data, but also to point out areas of inconsistency and to indicate areas for further research dealing with the cardiovascular system.

I am hopeful that this volume will provide a stimulus to many investigators to include the study of aging changes in their research efforts. It will provide the physician or investigator with an outline of current broad concepts with regard to cardiovascular aging. This volume will also be useful to clinicians and geriatricians who deal on a daily basis with the problems of the cardiovascular system in aged patients. They should find a framework for their day-to-day thinking in terms of those cardiovascular changes which can be attributed to the process of aging itself.

Myron L. Weisfeldt

Contents

Contributors

Bernard T. Engel, Ph.D., *Gerontology Research Center, National Institutes on Aging, Baltimore City Hospitals, Baltimore, Maryland 21224*

Gary Gerstenblith, M.D., *Department of Medicine, Johns Hopkins Medical Institutions, Baltimore, Maryland 21205*

Paula B. Goldberg, Ph.D., *Department of Pharmacology, Medical College of Pennsylvania, Philadelphia, Pennsylvania 19129*

Richard G. Hansford, Ph.D., *Gerontology Research Center, National Institues on Aging, Baltimore City Hospitals, Baltimore, Maryland 21224*

Grover Hutchins, M.D., *Department of Pathology, Johns Hopkins Hospital, Baltimore, Maryland 21205*

James A. Joseph, Ph.D., *Gerontology Research Center, National Institutes on Aging, Baltimore City Hospitals, Baltimore, Maryland 21224*

Edward Lakatta, M.D., *Cardiovascular Section, Gerontology Research Center, National Institutes on Aging, Baltimore City Hospitals, Baltimore, Maryland 21224*

Jere H. Mitchell, M.D., *Cardiopulmonary Division, University of Texas Southwestern Medical School at Dallas, Dallas, Texas 75235*

Peter B. Raven, Ph.D., *Department of Physiology, Texas College of Osteopathic Medicine, North Texas State University Health Science Center, Fort Worth, Texas 76107*

xi

Jay Roberts, Ph.D., *Department of Pharmacology, Medical College of Pennsylvania, Philadelphia, Pennsylvania 19129*

Robert J. Tomanek, Ph.D., *Department of Anatomy, University of Iowa College of Medicine, Iowa City, Iowa 52242*

Myron L. Weisfeldt, M.D., *Cardiology Division, Department of Medicine, Johns Hopkins Medical Institutions, Baltimore, Maryland 21205*

Frank C. P. Yin, M.D., Ph.D., *Cardiology Division, Department of Medicine, Johns Hopkins Medical Institutions, Baltimore, Maryland 21205*

The Aging Heart (Aging, Vol. 12),
edited by Myron L. Weisfeldt.
Raven Press, New York © 1980.

Chapter 1

Research on Aging

Myron L. Weisfeldt

*Cardiology Division, Department of Medicine, Johns Hopkins Medical
Institutions, Baltimore, Maryland 21205*

In this introductory chapter is a brief discussion of (a) the problems of differentiation of aging from disease; (b) the limitations and advantages of cross-sectional or longitudinal study design; (c) the importance of clear definition of the age range under study; and (d) a number of cautions in assessing the importance of specific, observed, age-associated changes.

AGING VERSUS DISEASE

The initial concern throughout all aging studies is the effectiveness of the differentiation between changes associated with specific pathological processes which may increase in frequency and severity with age versus changes related to the aging process itself. In attempting to differentiate aging from disease, it is clearly of primary importance to utilize the anatomical and pathological observations insofar as possible to identify the presence of specific disease states. It is reassuring when material studied for physiological aging change has been examined pathologically by other means to identify the presence of a disease or pathological process within a specific subset of the sample studied.

In addition to direct examination for the presence of disease, there are other types of evidence which would tend to support the notion that a specific change is an aging change rather than the result of the presence of disease. The first of these is the demonstration that the same age changes occur in multiple species rather than a single species. If one is able to demonstrate the presence of a specific aging change in myocardium or in the cardiovascular system of multiple species rather than in a single species, this would support the notion that the change is an aging change rather than one owing to a specific disease which was not identified in the single species under study. For example, as discussed in Chapters 4 and 11, there is evidence from a number of species including rats, guinea pigs, dogs, and man that prolonged cardiac muscle relaxation is present during the later portions of the life span. Although certainly there are various forms of cardiac disease described in rats, dogs, and humans (with increases in the frequency and severity of the disease in the older population), the frequent types of disease are not similar. For example, in the human atherosclerosis and ischemic heart disease might account for prolonged relaxation. In nonbreeder rats atherosclerosis is rare, and a nonspecific myocarditis is more commonly observed in pathological material. A second type of evidence supporting a given change as an aging- rather than a disease-related one is a longitudinal study of a large population. Here, reasonable uniformity in terms of a specific change occurring in all or nearly all subjects under study would support a change as being age related.

CROSS-SECTIONAL VERSUS LONGITUDINAL STUDIES: STUDY DESIGN

All cross-sectional studies have the clear disadvantage that one is dealing with a selected population. Clearly, in the older age groups one is studying only those animals that survive to that age. A characteristic difference between the two age groups may be an aging change or may be only a difference between survivors versus animals which succumb to disease or other causes of death at an earlier age.

Longitudinal studies avoid this pitfall and help in differentiating disease from aging, but difficulties of performing longitudinal studies are also easily identified. First, the methodology one uses to measure the variable under study cannot have a significant harmful effect on the organism and, of course, the organism cannot be sacrificed in order to make the measurement. Second, the research must continue over a time equal to the life span of the organism, which, even in the rat, would require several years for each study to be completed. Third, when organisms are studied over a longitudinal framework for a significant period of time, there is major concern about the adequacy of the methodology and the consistency of the methodology employed. Clearly, any change identified over a several year period, and particularly over a human life span, should be suspect in terms of representing evolutionary changes or consistent changes in the methodology utilized to make the measurement rather than longitudinal changes related to aging of the organism whose variables are being measured. Performance of studies on other younger controls along with the later studies after "aging" helps to overcome this problem, but tends to convert the study to cross-sectional design.

Although longitudinal study design has these major difficulties, it is certainly clear that the issue of disease versus aging and the magnitude of age changes will best be clarified by such longitudinal studies in multiple species. The magnitude of age change between adult and senescent populations may be overestimated in cross-sectional studies by selective loss of senescent animals with the least age-associated change in a given variable. For example, animals with greater age-related cardiac hypertrophy may live longer since this may serve as an effective compensatory mechanism. Also, the magnitude of an age-related change may be minimized by selective loss of animals with the greatest magnitude of age-related change in a specific variable from the population. Left ventricular hypertrophy may reflect more severe age-related changes in the peripheral vasculature, and animals exhibiting this might therefore die at a younger age. Cross-sectional data, which constitute the majority of the data presented in this volume, point mainly toward examination of variables in a longitudinal framework rather than providing a specific identification of physiologically important aspects or the quantitative extent of the aging process in the cardiovascular system.

DEFINITION OF AGE RANGE UNDER STUDY

A final general comment concerning experimental design and interpretation of aging studies is that there must be a clear identification of the portion of the life span which is under study in any specific investigation. It would not be surprising to find age-associated changes in the lattermost portion of the life span in one species and no age related changes in the same variable in an early portion of the life span in the same species or in another species. Also, maturational changes must be clearly differentiated from aging changes, although obviously both are governed by time as the critical variable. Maturational changes may continue beyond the point of sexual maturity. Thus, either longitudinal data must be obtained or significant groups of animals in a cross-sectional design study must be obtained at various points in the life span to eliminate the possibility that an apparent change related to senescence is not the end portion of a maturational change.

PHYSIOLOGICAL IMPORTANCE OF OBSERVED AGE CHANGES

There is a general impression that with aging there is a diffuse and general decline in all aspects of organ and integrated function. This conclusion results from the observation that there is a decline in most complex and multisystem integrated functions with age. One example is the age-associated decrease in maximal exercise ability (see Chapter 10). Since these integrated responses require performance of multiple organ systems, it is not surprising that highly integrated responses or parameters show some aging change as a result of critical decline in function or alteration in structure in one of the components. Understanding the mechanism of the decline in the integrated response requires the study of each specific organ and structure involved in the response. Clearly, in identifying the critically important mechanism of an age change it is as important to identify those aspects of organ structure and function that show no age change as it is to identify those aspects that show an age change. For example, if the inotropic response to catecholamines were shown to be unchanged with age, this would eliminate this specific aspect of sympathetic responsiveness from being accountable in the age-associated decrease in exercise ability or cardiac function. It would not eliminate the possibility of the sympathetic nervous system contributing to the age-associated decline as a result of decreased sympathetic stimulation either on the afferent or efferent side or a decrease in the ability of the efferent system to respond in terms of elaboration of neurotransmitter.

A final comment in terms of the issue of physiological importance of observed age changes is that an observed age change in a given parameter of structure or cellular function does not identify this age change as being physiologically important to organ function. For example, although the content or activity of a given enzyme system may show some decrease in the aged myocardium, this is not evidence that this age change is responsible for age associated alterations in contractile behavior and/or ability to respond to external stimuli or to resist damage. In terms of the investigator seeking to understand mechanisms of aging changes, this is a most difficult issue which is often overlooked. Often, investigators will attempt to relate specific variables measured in aging populations to one another (such as correlating activity of a specific enzyme with contractile function of the myocardium, taking individual data points from animals of multiple age groups). This is no better than correlating the number of gray hairs with recent memory in men of varying age. Clearly, there will be significant negative correlation between these two variables since both show a correlation or relationship to age. Such a correlation between gray hair and memory is of no interest. The change in the enzyme activity is not much more likely to be responsible for a change in contractile muscle behavior. More convincing evidence of a direct relationship between a change in an enzyme system and muscle function would come from demonstrating that the specific enzyme in question is a rate-limiting step in contractile behavior in the senescent group. Also, it would be more convincing to show that within an age group those animals showing the greatest age change in physiological function show the greatest age change in the enzyme system under question. Another approach would be to modify the enzyme change and then observe an increase or a reversal of the age change in organ function.

REFERENCE

1.   Rowe, J. W. (1977): Clinical research on aging: Strategies and directions. *N. Engl. J. Med.,* 297:1332–1336.

The Aging Heart (Aging, Vol. 12),
edited by Myron L. Weisfeldt.
Raven Press, New York © 1980.

Chapter 2

Structure of the Aging Heart

Grover M. Hutchins

*Department of Pathology, Johns Hopkins Medical Institutions,
Baltimore, Maryland 21205*

The experienced morphologist can estimate the age of a human heart with only limited success. There appear to be no objective morphologic characteristics of the heart which permit an accurate assessment of its age. It seems likely that it is the time-dependent accumulation of pathologic changes in the structures of the heart, rather than changes related to aging itself, which give the observer what limited success he enjoys. The discrimination of age-change from alterations induced by disease may be difficult and in some instances arbitrary in our present state of knowledge. For example, cardiac amyloidosis, mitral valve ring calcifications, basophilic degeneration of the myocardium, and coronary artery atherosclerosis are typically found in the elderly. However, not all old people develop these disorders nor are the abnormalities exclusively found in the aged. In the following sections we will consider several facets of the question of age-dependent morphologic changes in the heart.

HEART SIZE

Studies in large groups of patients at autopsy have shown in general an increase in average heart weight with age, except for a slight decline in the oldest groups. Linzbach and Akuoma-Boateng (24) reviewed the heart weights observed in 7,112 patients ranging from birth to 109 years. This group included hearts with a variety of diseases and a wide range of heart weights. Patient groups over the ninth decade had a decrease in the variability of heart size and average heart weight. In general, there was for the entire group of normal and abnormal hearts an increase of heart weight of 1 g/year for men and 1.5 g/year for women. The heart constituted from 0.55 to 0.8% of the total body.

A valuable study by Smith (46) of 1,000 autopsied patients without heart disease showed that heart weight correlated with body size but not with age. The mean heart weight of adult males was 294 g and of females 250 g. The ratio of heart to body weight was 0.43 for males and 0.40 for females, and this ratio would predict heart size with an error of 10% or less.

In a study (10) of 125 hearts, freed of all removable epicardial adipose tissue, from patients in the third through the ninth decades without cardiac hypertrophy or atrophy, it was shown that the remaining tissues showed little age-related weight difference. A similar result was obtained by Reiner and his associates (37) in a study of normal hearts, also freed of epicardial fat. Reiner (36) concluded that age probably does not influence myocardial weight and the apparent age-related increase in heart size is a function of the amount of epicardial fat.

The above studies also suggest that atrophy of the heart is not a simple function of age. The question of cardiac atrophy is a vexing one in that it is difficult to imagine a reduction of myocardial mass below that required for the maintenance of the circulation. Size reduction and disappearance of cardiac muscle cells has been described in atrophic hearts (18); and a greater proportionate loss of overall heart weight than body weight has been noted (11). Morphometric studies do not appear to have been made on such hearts, however. It seems probable that the myocardium of the "atrophic" heart may in fact be of the appropriate size for the functional demands of the individual patient who has usually died with starvation, carcinomatosis, or chronic infection. The relative loss of heart weight observed may be merely a consequence of serous atrophy of the epicardial fat.

Thus, it cannot be said that there is any relationship of age to altered heart size. The very largest hearts, 1,000 g and over (12), are not usually found in the elderly probably reflecting the decreased survival of a patient with any condition producing massive cardiac enlargement. On the other hand, it is conceivable that there is an inability of the aged heart to undergo such enlargement. It is also evident that cardiac weight must be interpreted in light of the heart disease present and the methods employed at autopsy to weigh the specimen.

MYOCARDIUM

Changes in the myocardium related to age have been described for both the cardiac muscle cells and for the interstitial connective tissues. Whether these alterations are age dependent or disease dependent remains unclear.

Cardiac Muscle Cells

Lipofuchsin accumulation at the poles of the nuclei of the cardiac muscle cells (Fig. 1) is a very common and perhaps invariable accompaniment of aging. Strehler et al. (48) performed histologic point count determinations of muscle cell pigment concentrations using fluorescence microscopy in 156 human hearts. Pigment was not found in patients from the first decade; thereafter, average concentrations increased linearly as a function of age and was present in all older hearts. No correlation was noted with disease state, heart size, sex, or race. However, low concentrations of lipofuchsin were observed in individual patients even in the ninth decade, and cases of brown atrophy of the heart do not appear to have been included in the study. The authors concluded that the pigment, which they found to occupy as much as 10% of the muscle cell volume, could probably interfere with

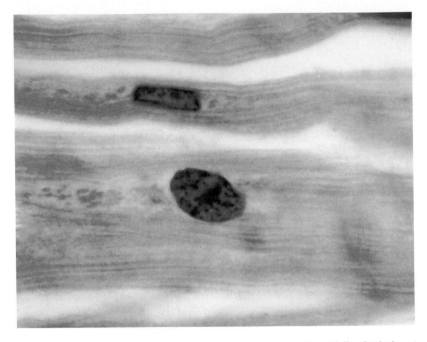

FIG. 1. Myocardial muscle cells showing accumulation of lipofuchsin at the poles of the nuclei. This change is present in the hearts of aged persons and the degree of accumulation tends to correlate with the patient's age. Hematoxylin and eosin, ×900.

cardiac function. Because no correlation was found with factors other than age, they regarded the lipofuchsin accumulation as a basic biological aging process.

Electron microscopic studies have demonstrated that lipofuchsin is a lipid containing material probably derived from breakdown of cytoplasmic constituents by lysosomes. Its exact precursor in the myocardium is unknown but may be mitochondria. Very large amounts of lipofuchsin may be observed in hearts with brown atrophy, the brown color being imparted by the pigment itself. Patients with brown atrophy generally have a severe chronic disease, most commonly a malignant tumor, and are generally malnourished and inactive (11). Malnutrition in otherwise healthy individuals may also lead to brown atrophy of the myocardium in association with a reduction in heart size (8). The implication of these observations may be that lipofuchsin accumulation is simply a function of reduced muscle cell size which in turn is a consequence of reduction of functional demands on the heart because of loss of body mass and decreased activity. Such an interpretation would be consistent with the absence of the pigment in children where cardiac muscle growth is occurring and its common occurrence in the elderly where episodic or sustained activity decrease may have led to lipofuchsin formation.

Basophilic degeneration of the myocardium is analogous to lipofuchsin accumulation in that it is a very common, if not universal, finding in the elderly and is accentuated in certain disease states. This material (Fig. 2), which is usually basophilic

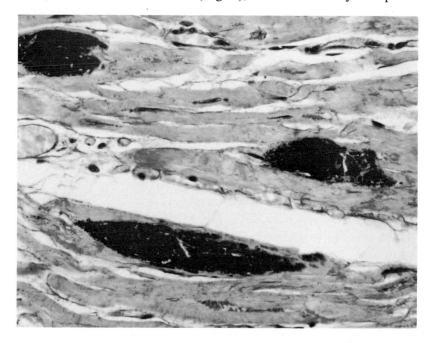

FIG. 2. Basophilic degeneration of myocardial muscle cells. The intrasarcoplasmic material is intensely positive by the periodic acid-Schiff reaction and is not removed by diastase treatment. Periodic acid-Schiff, ×225.

on hematoxylin and eosin staining and intensely positive by the periodic acid-Schiff reaction even after diastase digestion, is found within the sarcoplasm of the muscle cell as a sharply defined mass of variable density displacing the nucleus and separating or replacing the contractile elements. Ultrastructural, histochemical, and physiochemical characterization (40) of the material has suggested that it is a glucan representing a by-product of glycogen metabolism, possibly secondary to an enzymatic deficiency of the glycogenesis-glycogenolysis pathway. It is of interest that the material is present in large quantities in some muscle cells but completely undetectable in the majority. Patients with Lafora's disease (47), hypothyroidism (6), some instances of idiopathic myocardiopathy (9), and some with familial myocardiopathy (41), may have marked accentuation of myocardial basophilic degeneration. Even in these patients, however, the amount of material present seems insufficient to produce cardiac dysfunction. The focal accumulations of this nondegradable material suggest an acquired disease of individual muscle cells rather than an age-related process.

Myocardial Connective Tissue

The proportion of myocardium consisting of connective tissue or of collagen at various ages has been investigated in a number of studies. Connective tissue constitutes all that part of the myocardium consisting of nerves, fat cells, ground substance, and extracellular fibers including collagen. Histologic methods have shown that the ventricular myocardium consists of approximately 20 to 35% connective tissue and that this proportion either remains constant (31) or increases slightly (21) with advancing age. Chemical determinations of collagen only give values of about 1% of wet weight. The proportion of heart consisting of collagen has been found to remain unchanged with advancing age (3,32). Clausen (4) found a fall in the ratio of hexosamine to hydroxyproline occurred with advancing age. This change in the ratio, felt to reflect the proportion of ground substance to collagen content, was caused by significant decreases in hexosamine and increases of hydroxyproline content. This result was in contrast to that of Wegelius and von Knorring (56), who found no age-related change in myocardial hexosamine or hydroxyproline content.

Elastic tissue constitutes but a small proportion of the normal myocardium. Studies that have addressed the question of age-related changes in elastic content have described either no alteration (28) or an increase (29) with greater survival.

A very common finding in the myocardium in older patients, especially noticeable in the right ventricle but also present on the left, is the occurrence of adipose tissue between bundles of muscle cells. These fat cells may infiltrate the heart wall to produce a marbled appearance and may also be visible from the endocardial aspect. A similar process occurs in the interatrial septum and in its more advanced form constitutes lipomatous hypertrophy of the interatrial septum. This condition may be associated with disturbances of conduction (33).

Small foci of fibrosis in the myocardium, where connective tissues replace areas of lost muscle cells, also show an age-related increase.Mitchell and Schwartz (30) found two distinct size populations of myocardial lesions. The large lesions, all at least 3 cm in one or more dimensions, were infarcts and correlated with coronary artery disease. Small lesions averaged about 1 cm in diameter and correlated with the patient's age, but not with coronary artery disease or hypertension. The authors conclude that such lesions are probably the end result of a variety of causes of acute destruction of the myocardium. While their etiology could not be determined in most instances there was no reason to regard them as consequences of aging itself.

Amyloid deposition in the myocardium (Fig. 3) is a common finding in elderly patients. The material is found as a homogeneous deposit on the reticular framework surrounding the muscle cells or in the media of intramyocardial arteries. With large deposits, the muscle cells may become atrophic and disappear. Wright and his colleagues (59) have shown that when systematically searched for, cardiac amyloid may be found in up to 37% of

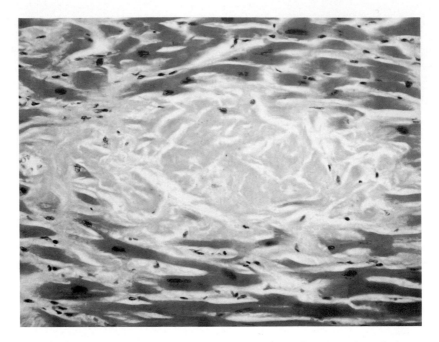

FIG. 3. Focus of intramyocardial amyloid deposition. The muscle cells have disappeared from the area occupied by the material. Hematoxylin and eosin, ×405.

elderly patients and that the incidence increases with age. Amyloid deposits are most frequently found in the atria. Despite its common occurrence in small amounts, clinically significant cardiac amyloidosis is uncommon (58).

Specialized Conduction Tissue

There appears to be general agreement (5,22,38) that loss of muscle cells from the sinoatrial node and a relative increase in connective tissue is a very common accompaniment of old age. The correlation of such relative fibrosis with conduction disturbances is poor (45,51). The etiology of the fibrosis is unclear. In a few patients vascular lesions have been implicated as the cause of muscle cell loss, but such an explanation does not appear tenable for most cases.

It is less clear if changes occurring in the atrial myocardium with age may contribute to interference with conduction along internodal pathways (17). The atrioventricular node and the His bundle show little change with age (7). Idiopathic atrophy and fibrosis of the left bundle branches are frequent abnormalities in elderly patients (23). The loss of continuity between proximal and distal portions of the left fascicles is probably the consequence of stretching of the tissues over the central fibrous body. The condition is more common in hearts enlarged as a consequence of hypertension or aortic stenosis.

Animal Studies

From an examination of the hearts of 487 rats who died after simply being maintained in the laboratory without any experimental manipulation, Wilens and Sproul (57) called attention to the high incidence of pathologic changes present. Myocardial fibrosis was present in almost 60% of the animals. Myocardial hypertrophy was also common and myocarditis, endocarditis, and pericarditis were each found in 2 to 4% of the animals. Simms and Berg (44) followed 1,410 rats until they became moribund and then examined them for the presence of lesions related to five diseases. It was found that the probability of the onset of any of the disorders, including myocardial degeneration, increased with age. There was, however, an age of maximum probability of onset and a limit to the percent of animals that would acquire each lesion. An increase in myocardial collagen concentration of the left ventricle of the rat with age has been confirmed by chemical determinations of hydroxyproline content (51). The degree of age-related collagen increase in these animals was unaffected by exercise.

Electron microscopic comparisons of myocardial ultrastructure in rats 3 to 6 months old have been made with senescent animals 27 to 28 months of age (52). The studies showed an increase in lipofuchsin, irregular myofibers, surface vesicles, and increased connective tissue cells in the older animals. The changes were felt to be unaccounted for by pathologic processes and therefore a likely consequence of aging. Similar observations on cardiac muscle cells were made by Travis and Travis (55) in rats ranging in age from 6 to 33 months. The origin of residual bodies (lipofuchsin) appeared to be from lysosomal degradation of mitochondria (54,55). This induction of lipofuchsin in cardiac muscle cells by hypoxia has been shown to occur more readily in old rats than in young ones (49). In mice age-related changes have been noted in cardiac muscle cell mitochondria consisting of a decrease of surface area of the cristae (50).

ENDOCARDIUM

The appearance of the endocardium varies between the cardiac chambers in the normal heart. It is thickest in the left atrium and thinnest in the ventricles (26). The histologic appearance of the mature endocardium is that of layers of elastic fibers, collagen, and mesenchymal cells (Fig. 4). Its appearance is very similar to the pathologic thickening of endocardial fibroelastosis which appears to be a nonspecific response to increase in the fluctuating tension applied to that portion of the heart wall (2,13,16). Causes of this increase in mural tension inducing fibroelastosis may be either dilatation of the cardiac chamber or increase in intracavitary pressure. The thickness and structure of the endocardium in the normal mature heart correlated well with the concept of tension-induced fibroelastotic proliferation. Localized areas of fibrosis on the endocardial surface are usually the end result of organization of mural thrombus (42).

VALVES

Changes in the cardiac valves after the heart has reached its maturity appear to be predominantly related to pathologic processes. In the absence of such abnormalities the valve leaflets

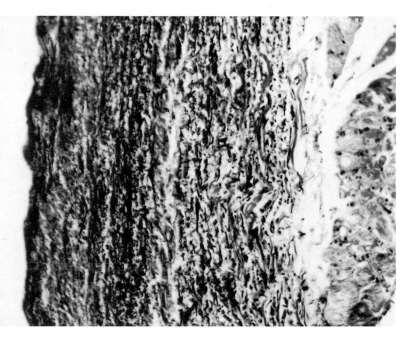

FIG. 4. Normal endocardium of tho loft atrium showing the parallel array of elastic lamellae. This structure resembles that found in the media of elastic arteries and in areas of endocardial fibroelastosis. Verhoeff-van Gieson elastic, ×180.

may remain thin and delicate into advanced age. McMillan and Lev (27) have described the changes seen with growth of the heart and reviewed earlier reports. The observations of Pomerance (34,35) are consistent with the interpretation that valve thickening is largely a function of cumulative injury and repair, a process accentuated by abnormal mechanics. One common result of minute valve injury is the deposition of thrombus on the line of closure of the valve. The subsequent conversion of this thrombus produces the Lambl's excrescences that are a virtually universal finding in the adult heart (42).

In contrast, Angrist (1) has called attention to the occurrence of sclerosis of the valve leaflets as a feature of aging. Age-related changes in 100 aortic and 200 mitral valves from patients ranging from infancy to the ninth decade were described by Sell and Scully (43). Both valves showed similar changes with advancing age, namely, reduction of size and number of nuclei in the leaflets, increase in fibrosis and fragmentation of collagen, and increased lipid accumulation and calcification. The fibrosa of the aortic valve tended to be involved by calcification, whereas in the mitral valve the annulus was more often affected. The authors suggest that the calcification, even when massive and leading to functionally significant alterations as sometimes observed in the mitral valve (19), is preceded by changes in collagen, ground substance, and lipid.

The caliber of the aortic valve has been shown to undergo a linear increase with age when its value is examined with respect to body surface area (20). It is probable that such continued dilatation of the aortic valve orifice is but a component of the age-related dilatation of the entire aorta, a phenomenon attributed to a relative loss of elastic tissue and increase in collagen in the aortic media.

EPICARDIUM AND MAJOR BLOOD VESSELS

A common observation is collagenous thickening of the most superficial layer of the epicardium, especially over the right ventricular outflow tract and over the course of the coronary arteries. The phenomenon may be particularly striking in dilated hearts but has also been considered to occur with advancing age.

Tortuosity of the epicardial coronary arteries is a very common finding in the elderly. Unlike the tortuosity of the aorta, it does not appear to be associated with dilatation of the vascular lumen (14). Studies of coronary artery collateral channels have suggested that tortuosity is an accompaniment of overall vascular growth induced by increased flow (15). The tortuosity of the larger nondilated coronary arteries of the aged may be the residue of previous periods of enlargement associated with high blood flow.

In general, coronary arteriosclerosis shows a correlation with increased age (25) as do the effects of other disease processes such as valve changes and amyloidosis. The thrombosis on ulcerated atherosclerotic plaques which produces coronary occlusion and subsequent myocardial infarction (39) may occur at any age. However, age alone does not appear to be the major factor leading to myocardial infarcts.

SUMMARY

Examination of the heart of an elderly patient requires that a distinction be made between those alterations which are simply the accumulated injuries of one or more disease processes and those changes which are an inevitable part of growing old. In the latter category are only a small number of changes which appear to develop without respect to disease, but are still variable in their intensity in individual patients. Lipofuchsin accumulation and basophilic degeneration in cardiac muscle cells and tortuosity of nonatherosclerotic epicardial coronary arteries are the best established alterations. Cardiac enlargement, atrophy, or fibrosis cannot be considered as universal or even common results of aging.

ACKNOWLEDGMENTS

Supported by Grant P50-HL-17655-04 from The National Institutes of Health, Public Health Service, Department of Health, Education and Welfare.

REFERENCES

1. Angrist, A. (1954): Ageing heart valves and a unitary pathological hypothesis for sclerosis. *J. Gerontol.,* 19:135–143.
2. Black-Shaffer, B. (1957): Infantile endocardial fibroelastosis: A suggested etiology. *Arch. Pathol.,* 63:281–306.
3. Blumgart, H. L., Gilligan, D. R., and Schlesinger, M. J. (1940): The degree of myocardial fibrosis in normal and pathological hearts as estimated chemically by the collagen content. *Trans. Assoc. Am. Physicians,* 55:313–315.
4. Clausen, B. (1962): Influence of age on connective tissue. Hexosamine

and hydroxyproline in human aorta, myocardium, and skin. *Lab. Invest.,* 11:229–234.

5. Davies, M. J., and Pomerance, A. (1972): Quantitative study of ageing changes in the human sinoatrial node and internodal tracts. *Br. Heart J.,* 34:150–152.

6. Douglas, R. C., and Jacobson, S. D. (1957): Pathologic changes in adult myxedema: a survey of 10 necropsies. *J. Clin. Endocrinol. Metab.,* 17:1354–1364.

7. Erickson, E. E., and Lev, M. (1952): Aging changes in the human atrioventricular node, bundle, and bundle branches. *J. Gerontol.,* 7:1–12.

8. Follis, R. H., Jr. (1958): *Deficiency Disease,* p. 557. Charles C Thomas, Springfield, Illinois.

9. Fowler, N. O., Gueron, M., and Rowlands, D. T., Jr. (1961): Primary myocardial disease. *Circulation,* 23:498–508.

10. Hegglin, R. (1934): Über Organvolumen und Organgewicht. Nebst Bemorkungen über die Gröbenbestimmungsmethoden. *Z. Konstitutionslehre,* 18:110–134.

11. Hellerstein, H. K., and Santiago-Stevenson, D. (1950): Atrophy of the heart: A correlative study of eighty-five proved cases. *Circulation,* 1:93–126.

12. Hutchins, G. M., and Anaya, O. A. (1973): Measurements of cardiac size, chamber volumes and valve orifices at autopsy. *Johns Hopkins Med. J.,* 133:96–106.

13. Hutchins, G. M., and Bannayan, G. A. (1971): Development of endocardial fibroelastosis following myocardial infarction. *Arch. Pathol.,* 91:113–118.

14. Hutchins, G. M., Bulkley, B. H., Miner, M. M., and Boitnott, J. K. (1977): Correlation of age and heart weight with tortuosity and caliber of normal human coronary arteries. *Am. Heart J.,* 94:196–202.

15. Hutchins, G. M., Miner, M. M., and Bulkley, B. H. (1978): Tortuosity as an index of the age and diameter increase of coronary collateral vessels in patients after acute myocardial infarction. *Am. J. Cardiol.,* 41:210–215.

16. Hutchins, G. M., and Vie, S. A. (1972): The progression of interstitial myocarditis to idiopathic endocardial fibroelastosis. *Am. J. Pathol.,* 66:483–496.

17. James, T. N. (1963): The connecting pathway between the sinus node and A–V node and between the right and left atrium in the human heart. *Am. Heart J.,* 66:498–508.

18. Karsner, H. T., Saphir, O., and Todd, T. W. (1925): The state of the cardiac muscle in hypertrophy and atrophy. *Am. J. Pathol.,* 1:351–371.

19. Korn, D., DeSanctis, R. W., and Sell, S. (1962): Massive calcification of the mitral annulus: A clinicopathological study of fourteen cases. *N. Engl. J. Med.,* 267:900–909.

20. Krovetz, L. J. (1975): Age-related changes in size of the aortic valve annulus in man. *Am. Heart J.,* 90:569–574.

21. Lenkiewicz, J. E., Davies, M. J., and Rosen, D. (1972): Collagen in human myocardium as a function of age. *Cardiovasc. Res.,* 6:549–555.

22. Lev, M. (1954): Aging changes in the human sinoatrial node. *J. Gerontol.,* 9:1–9.
23. Lev, M. (1964): The pathology of complete atrioventricular block. *Prog. Cardiovasc. Dis.,* 6:317–329.
24. Linzbach, A. J., and Akuomoa-Boateng, E. (1973): Die Alternsveränderungen des menschlichen Herzens. I. Das Herzgewicht im Alter. *Klin. Wochenschr.,* 51:156–163.
25. Linzbach, A. J., and Akuomoa-Boateng, E. (1973): Die Alternsveränderungen des menschlichen Herzens. II. Die Polypathie des Herzens im Alter. *Klin. Wochenschr.,* 51:164–175.
26. McMillan, J. B., and Lev, M. (1959): The aging heart. I. Endocardium. *J. Gerontol.,* 14:268–283.
27. McMillan, J. B., and Lev, M. (1964): The aging heart. II. The valves. *J. Gerontol.,* 19:1–14.
28. McMillan, J. B., and Lev, M. (1962): The aging heart: Myocardium and epicardium. In: *Biological Aspects of Ageing,* edited by N. W. Shock, pp. 163–173. Columbia University Press, New York.
29. Miller, A. M., and Perkins, O. C. (1927): Elastic tissue of the heart in advancing age. *Am. J. Anat.,* 39:205–217.
30. Mitchell, J. R. A., and Schwartz, C. J. (1965): *Arterial Disease.* F. A. Davis, Philadelphia.
31. Montford, I., and Pérez-Tamayo, R. (1962): The muscle–collagen ratio in normal and hypertrophic human hearts. *Lab. Invest.,* 11:463–470.
32. Oken, D. E., and Boucek, R. J. (1957): Quantitation of collagen in human myocardium. *Circ. Res.,* 5:357–361.
33. Page, D. L. (1970): Lipomatous hypertrophy of the cardiac interatrial septum: Its development and probable clinical significance. *Hum. Pathol.,* 1:151–163.
34. Pomerance, A. (1967): Ageing changes in human heart valves. *Br. Heart J.,* 29:222–231.
35. Pomerance, A. (1966): Pathogenesis of "senile" nodular sclerosis of atrioventricular valves. *Br. Heart J.,* 28:815–823.
36. Reiner, L. (1968): Gross examination of the heart. In: *Pathology of the Heart,* 3rd ed., edited by S. E. Gould, pp. 1111–1149. Charles C Thomas, Springfield, Illinois.
37. Reiner, L., Mazzoleni, A., Rodriguez, F. L., and Freudenthal, R. R. (1959): The weight of the human heart. I. "Normal" cases. *Arch. Pathol.,* 68:58–73.
38. Ridolfi, R. L., Bulkley, B. H., and Hutchins, G. M. (1977): The conduction system in cardiac amyloidosis: Clinical and pathological features of 23 patients. *Am. J. Med.,* 62:677–686.
39. Ridolfi, R. L., and Hutchins, G. M. (1977): The relationship between coronary artery lesions and myocardial infarcts. Ulceration of atherosclerotic plaques precipitating coronary thrombosis. *Am. Heart. J.,* 93:468–486.
40. Rosai, J., and Lascano, E. F. (1970): Basophilic (mucoid) degeneration of myocardium. A disorder of glycogen metabolism. *Am. J. Pathol.,* 61:99–116.

41. Ross, R. S., Bulkley, B. H., Hutchins, G. M., Harshey, J. S., Jones, R. A., Kraus, H., Liebman, J., Thorne, C. M., Weinberg, S. B., Weech, A. A., and Weech, A. A., Jr. (1978): Idiopathic familial myocardiopathy in three generations: A clinical and pathologic study. *Am. Heart J.*, 96:170–179.

42. Salyer, W. R., Page, D. L., and Hutchins, G. M. (1974): The development of cardiac myxomas and papillary endocardial lesions from mural thrombus. *Am. Heart J.*, 89:4–17.

43. Sell, S., and Scully, R. E. (1965): Aging changes in the aortic and mitral valves. Histologic and histochemical studies, with observations on the pathogenesis of calcific aortic stenosis and calcification of the mitral annulus. *Am. J. Pathol.*, 46:345–365.

44. Simms, H. S., and Berg, B. N. (1957): Longevity and the onset of lesions in male rats. *J. Gerontol.*, 12:244–252.

45. Sims, B. A. (1972): Pathogenesis of atrial arrhythmias. *Br. Heart J.*, 34:336–340.

46. Smith, H. L. (1928): The relation of the weight of the heart to the weight of the body and the weight of the heart to age. *Am. Heart J.*, 4:79–93.

47. Sokai, M., Austin, J., Witmer, F., and Trueb, L. (1970): Studies in myoclonus epilepsy (Lafora body form). II. Polyglucosans in the systemic deposits of mycoclonus epilepsy and in corpora amylacea. *Neurology*, 20:160–176.

48. Strehler, B. L., Mark, D. D., Mildvan, A. S., and Gee, M. V. (1959): Rate and magnitude of age pigment accumulation in the human myocardium. *J. Gerontol.*, 14:430–439.

49. Sulkin, N. M., and Sulkin, D. F. (1967): Age differences in response to chronic hypoxia on the fine structure of cardiac muscle and anatomic ganglion cells. *J. Gerontol.*, 22:485–501.

50. Tate, E. L., and Herbener, G. H. (1976): A morphometric study of the density of mitochondrial cristae in heart and liver of aging mice. *J. Gerontol.*, 31:129–134.

51. Thery, C., Gosselin, B., Lekieffre, J., and Warembourg, H. (1977): Pathology of sinoatrial node. Correlations with electrocardiographic findings in 111 patients. *Am. Heart J.*, 93:735–740.

52. Tomanek, R. J., and Karlsson, U. L. (1973): Myocardial ultrastructure of young and senescent rats. *J. Ultrastruct. Res.*, 42:201–220.

53. Tomanek, R. J., Taunton, C. A., and Liskop, K. S. (1972): Relationship between age, chronic exercise, and connective tissue of the heart. *J. Gerontol.*, 27:33–38.

54. Topping, T. M., and Travis, D. F. (1974): An electron cytochemical study of mechanisms of lysosomal activity in the rat left ventricular mural myocardium. *J. Ultrastruct. Res.*, 46:1–22.

55. Travis, D. F., and Travis, A. (1972): Ultrastructural changes in the left ventricular rat myocardial cells with age. *J. Ultrastruct. Res.*, 39:124–148.

56. Wegelius, O., and von Knorring, J. (1964): The hydroxyproline and hexosamine content in human myocardium at different ages. *Acta Med. Scand.*, 175(Suppl. 412):233–237.

57. Wilens, S. L., and Sproul, E. E. (1938): Spontaneous cardiovascular disease in the rat. I. Lesions of the heart. *Am. J. Pathol.,* 14:177–200.
58. Wright, J. R., and Calkins, E. (1975): Amyloid in the aged heart: Frequency and clinical significance. *J. Am. Geriatr. Soc.,* 23:97–103.
59. Wright, J. R., Calkins, E., Breen, W. J., Stolte, G., and Schultz, R. T. (1969): Relationship of amyloid to aging. Review of the literature and systematic study of 83 patients derived from a general hospital population. *Medicine (Baltimore),* 48:39–60.

The Aging Heart (Aging, Vol. 12),
edited by Myron L. Weisfeldt.
Raven Press, New York © 1980.

Chapter 3

Metabolism and Energy Production

Richard G. Hansford

*Gerontology Research Center, National Institute on Aging, Baltimore City
Hospitals, Baltimore, Maryland 21224*

There is a considerable body of experimental work on biological oxidations in tissues from aging animals. This follows from the fact that oxidative phosphorylation supplies the great majority of the energy required by most animal tissues and from the fact that the aged animal is often patently less "energetic." The heart in particular is dependent on oxidative metabolism, and because of its central role in the physiology of the animal the heart is an obvious organ in which to study effects of aging. However, because of the crucial importance of the major catabolic (i.e., energy-yielding) pathways in the heart to the life of the animal, it is unlikely that any major disturbance of these pathways can be tolerated. Thus, one should probably be skeptical of reports of large changes with age in the activity of, say, enzymes of the tricarboxylate cycle (35) or in the efficiency of coupling of oxidative phosphorylation (35). These may not be compatible with life. Instead, it is perhaps reasonable to look for rather modest decrease with age in the activities of enzymes which are rate limiting for obligatory pathways, like the tricarboxylate cycle. Another approach might be to look for shifts in the relative contributions of alternative energy sources, like the oxidations of carbohydrates and lipids, and one such study is discussed later in this chapter. Additionally, there may be changes with age in the modulation of energy metabolism by hormones and, for instance, a decreased inotropic response to catecholamines with age is described elsewhere in this volume (see Chapter 4).

SOME OBJECTIVES OF RESEARCH ON CARDIAC ENERGY-METABOLISM AND THE EFFECT OF AGE

This review will be from the perspective of a biochemist, but will deal with those changes in biochemistry which manifest themselves at the level of physiological performance. It is assumed that the two characteristics of a metabolic pathway which are important to the physiology of the animal are the flux through the pathway and the steady state concentrations of the intermediates that form branch-points. The latter may affect flux through other, derivative pathways. Flux may often be measured by the appearance of product or the disappearance of substrate, particularly where these are not recycled. Thus, the uptake of glucose from the medium plus the depletion (or minus the synthesis) of tissue glycogen would give a measure of the flux through glycolysis in the isolated perfused heart (see, e.g., 82,91). The accumulation of lactate, pyruvate, and alanine in the medium and the tissue, plus some determination of the oxidation of pyruvate (e.g., by release of $^{14}CO_2$), would give another measure of the same flux (see, e.g., ref. 82). Several such studies of flux have been made for the aging heart (1,4,35). The selection of methodology is crucial in this area; e.g., does one choose a tissue slice or an homogenate? This is dealt with below.

Failing the direct determination of flux through a metabolic pathway, it is possible to measure enzyme activities and make inferences about flux. This has perhaps been the most popular approach to the effect of age upon metabolism of the heart (see 113 for a current review in tabular form). It is the author's view that this approach is only meaningful if the enzyme selected for study catalyzes a nonequilibrium reaction. In this case, an altered catalytic activity with age will translate into an altered flux through the pathway and, eventually, altered availability of energy in the form of adenosine triphosphate (ATP). By contrast, a decrement in activity of any of the many enzymes which catalyze near-equilibrium reactions may have only a minimal impact on the operation of the pathway. The reactions which are far from equilibrium can be identified by analysis of tissue levels of reactants and products and the comparison of the mass–action ratio so obtained with the known K_{eq} for the reaction. A divergence of two orders of magnitude or more for these parameters may be taken, somewhat arbitrarily, to indicate a nonequilibrium reaction, and therefore one which limits flux through the pathway (see ref. 94 for a review). For the major catabolic pathways the nonequilibrium reactions are well known—for example, glycogen phosphorylase, hexokinase, phosphofructokinase, pyruvate kinase, and, possibly, triosephosphate dehydrogenase for the glycogenolytic and glycolytic sequences (see ref. 76 for a review).

For these reasons, this article will only present data on the change of enzyme activity with age when the enzyme has been shown to catalyze a nonequilibrium reaction. This means that excellent work on lactate dehydrogenase (98) or aldolase (40), etc., will not be described. This is not to denigrate such work; these enzymes may be an ideal choice of experimental material for the investigation of altered amino acid sequence or posttranslational modification since they are available in large amounts. Such studies may eventually bear on the mechanism of aging (39,40,84). However, for the description of enzyme changes which have an impact on the physiology of aging heart, it is maintained that the nonequilibrium enzymes are the appropriate ones to study, and these are often present in relatively small amounts and have complex molecular properties.

METHODOLOGY

For the measurement of fluxes, the isolated perfused heart is in many ways an ideal system. Some of the merits of the different methods of perfusion have been reviewed recently (76). One advantage, as mentioned above, is that substrate depletion and product formation can be monitored, mainly by assaying the perfusion fluid. Another is that an adequate supply of substrate and O_2 to the tissue can be guaranteed. Finally, and equally important, the work-performance of the heart can be maintained at a desired level by adjusting the hydrostatic pressure against which fluid is pumped, and, if necessary, pacing contractions electrically (see ref. 76 for a review). The imposition of an equal work-load is vital if comparisons are to be made between, for instance, hearts from young and old animals. Otherwise, findings of altered adenine nucleotide phosphorylation potential or creatine phosphate concentrations cannot be interpreted. The isolated perfused heart has been used surprisingly seldom in research on bioenergetics and aging, or development (1,93).

Metabolic studies involving slices or pieces of cardiac muscle (4,7) seem less well advised in that the access of substrate may be impeded by diffusion over relatively long distances. In addition, in most studies of this type the tissue is in a more or less quiescent state, with metabolic fluxes which are probably low and certainly ill defined. Thus the rate of O_2 uptake, and flux through catabolic metabolism, of an isolated piece of muscle might reflect the total adenosine triphosphatase (ATPase) activity stimulated by damage to the sarcolemma and mitochondrial membranes, with the resulting dissipation of ion gradients, as well as a contribution from actomyosin-ATPase. Under these circumstances it might be hard to establish differences due to the aging process. These criticisms would not apply to isolated muscle preparations which can be stimulated to contract and perform work, e.g., the trabeculae carneae preparation (107). However, one should probably be very critical about the level of work imposed, as some age-linked decrements may only appear when fluxes through the relevant pathways are near maximal.

Homogenates of heart muscle have been used for the determination of glycolytic activity, measured by lactate production (35), and for the determination of the oxidation of endogenous substrate (35), with respect to aging. It seems to the author that the degree of dilution involved in making an homogenate precludes the meaningful measurement of multistep pathways involving soluble enzymes, such as glycolysis. Even if substrate (e.g., glucose) is added, the substrates of the enzymes subsequent in the pathway will be greatly diluted, as will coenzymes and metal ions. By contrast, mitochondrial oxidations can often be measured in homogenates provided that mitochondrial structure is preserved by the use of an isotonic medium. This is because the mitochondrial matrix components presumably survive undiluted in the homogenate provided that the organelle does not undergo lysis. Thus, O_2 uptake owing to the oxidation of succinate can be accurately measured in an homogenate (6) and shows the same dependence upon adenosine diphosphate (ADP) availability that is shown by a suspension of mitochondria (see below).

A different use for tissue homogenates is the measurement of the activities of single enzymes. The advantage of the homogenate is that recovery is total; i.e., there is no fractionation process in which much of the activity is lost, as with a mitochondrial preparation. This may be particularly important in the comparison of young adult and aged tissue as there is some evidence that the progress of tissue fractionation is not the same for the two age groups (114). Care has to be taken in studies of this sort that there are no other interfering enzyme activities which might remove substrate or product. Sometimes these can be functionally removed by appropriate inhibitors. Thus, NADH-oxidase present in homogenates due to broken mitochondria interferes with all NAD-linked dehydrogenase assays, but can be 99% inhibited with rotenone (45). ATPase contributed by damaged mitochondria can likewise be inhibited with oligomycin (45). If mitochondrial enzymes are measured in homogenates, the permeability barrier of the inner mitochondrial membrane generally has to be removed and this can be done with low concentrations of nonionic detergents, usually without prejudice to the activity being measured. Some such studies are reported in Table 1.

Suspensions of isolated mitochondria have been used in many studies of oxidative metabolism of heart and aging (21,35,42,

TABLE 1. *Measurement of the activity of pyruvate dehydrogenase and of enzymes of the tricarboxylate cycle and of fatty acid oxidation in homogenates of whole hearts and preparations of mitochondria*

Activity measured	Enzyme activity[a]		Difference, 6–24 months, as % of 6-month value and significance, *p*
	6-month-old rat	24-month-old rat	
Homogenates of whole hearts (μmol/min/ g wet weight of heart)			
Citrate synthase	101 ± 4	82 ± 5	18%, 0.01–0.025
(E.C.4.1.3.7)	(6)	(6)	
NAD-isocitrate dehydrogenase	3.66 ± 0.18	3.09 ± 0.08	16%, 0.01–0.025
(E.C.1.1.1.41)	(6)	(6)	
α-ketoglutarate dehydrogenase	8.05 ± 0.46	6.52 ± 0.60	19%, NS
(E.C.1.2.4.2)	(6)	(5)	
Carnitine acetyltransferase	20.5 ± 1.5	10.0 ± 1.6	51%, 0.001–0.005
(E.C.2.3.1.7)	(5)	(4)	
3-Hydroxyacyl-CoA dehydrogenase	56 ± 3	41 ± 3	27%, 0.005–0.01
(E.C.1.1.1.35)	(4)	(3)	
Preparations of mitochondria (μmol/min/ mg mitochondrial protein)			
Pyruvate dehydrogenase complex	78 ± 1	82 ± 5	— NS
(E.C.1.2.4.1 + E.C.2.3.1.12 + 1.6.4.3)	(4)	(4)	
Acyl-CoA synthetase	2.68 ± 0.18	1.61 ± 0.15	40%, 0.001–0.005
(E.C.6.2.1.2 + E.C.6.2.1.3)	(9)	(8)	
Carnitine acetyltransferase	150 ± 6	98 ± 6	35%, 0.001
(E.C.2.3.1.7)	(5)	(6)	
Carnitine palmitoyltransferase	16.1 ± 0.8	15.8 ± 1.2	— NS
(E.C.2.3.1.21)	(4)	(5)	
Acyl-CoA dehydrogenase	7.73 ± 0.42	7.87 ± 0.84	— NS
(E.C.1.3.99.3)	(19)	(12)	
3-Hydroxyacyl-CoA dehydrogenase	687 ± 27	462 ± 31	33%, 0.001
(E.C.1.1.1.35)	(8)	(10)	

[a] Error is the SEM; number in parentheses is the number of preparations.
From Olewnik and Hansford *(unpublished)* and Hansford (45), with permission.

43,45). They offer the possibility of studying maximal fluxes through these pathways, if electron flow down the respiratory chain is facilitated by ADP and inorganic phosphate (P_i) (state 3 respiration) (16) or by an uncoupling agent such as dinitrophenol (DNP) or carbonyl cyanide *p*-trifluoromethoxyphenylhydrazone (FCCP). In heart, the rates of O_2 uptake thus obtained tend to be the same under these two conditions, with the flux being limited by the dehydrogenase involved or by the entry of substrate into the mitochondrion. In liver mitochondria, by contrast, ADP-phosphorylation generally gives rise to rates of O_2 uptake that are lower than those obtained with uncoupling agents (17). This reflects rate-limitation by the adenine nucleotide translocase responsible for allowing entry of ADP into the mitochondrion (see 59), or by the mitochondrial ATP-synthetase (also referred to as the F_1, or proton-translocating ATPase). Thus an age-linked decrement in the state 3 respiration of liver mitochondria will give information on one of these two activities, cf. heart. Clearly, the intact mitochondrion is an extremely complex system and results, though very informative, have to be interpreted with care. Mitochondrial preparations also allow the measurement of coupled, resting respiration obtained after the completion of ADP-phosphorylation (state 4) (16). The ratio of state 3 to state 4 is the respiratory control ratio (RCR) and has been advocated as the most sensitive index of coupling between oxidation and phosphorylation (see, for instance, ref. 19). There have been reports that the RCR is lower in mitochondria from aged tissue as compared to the young adult counterparts (80). This is possible, but it is disputed by other studies showing an unchanged and high RCR (42), at least with some respiratory substrates (21). Experimental artifacts tend to lower the ratios measured. For example, the almost unavoidable inclusion of some actomyosin-ATPase in preparations of mitochondria from muscle tissues will raise state 4 rates and thereby lower RCRs. Thus, the finding of a high, undiminished RCR in mitochondria from aged animals is probably the more credible result. This criticism would not apply, however, to cases in which the diminished RCR follows from a substrate-specific decline in the state 3 rate of respiration (21). Oxidative phosphorylation is discussed in more detail below.

Finally, work on aging may be carried out at the level of isolated, purified proteins. This would allow the determination of whether decreases of specific activity in whole tissues or homogenates are the result of a reduced concentration of active enzyme molecules or reflect an unchanged concentration of enzyme of impaired activity. The latter could follow from errors in primary structure or from modifications occurring after translation. The pioneering work of this nature has been done by Gershon and Gershon (39), but has used liver (39) or skeletal muscle (40) rather than cardiac muscle. This work has established quite clearly that tissues from aged animals may contain catalytically inactive material which crossreacts with an antibody raised against a purified enzyme protein and is clearly of fundamental importance to the question of the mechanism of aging. Whether such inactive molecules exist for any of the nonequilibrium enzymes of catabolic metabolism remains to be answered.

ENERGY-YIELDING METABOLIC PATHWAYS IN CARDIAC MUSCLE

The aim of the major portion of this article is to give a sketch of energy metabolism in heart and present what information there is about age-linked changes in activity of enzymes and processes selected by the criteria given above. For any one enzyme, information will be presented together, regardless of whether it emerges from studies of the whole heart or at the enzyme level. For another survey of energy-metabolism in heart, the reader is referred to a recent excellent review by Williamson (111).

Glycolysis and Glycogenolysis

Cardiac muscle is normally highly aerobic and derives the great majority of its energy from terminal oxidations, that is to say, from the complete oxidation of acetyl groups by the tricarboxylate cycle and from the oxidative phosphorylation that accompanies this. The preferred source of acetyl units is the β-oxidation of fatty acids, which in heart competes very effectively with carbohydrate oxidation (see ref. 76 for a review). Some index of the maximum fluxes through glycolysis and glycogenolysis can be derived from assays of the activities of the nonequilibrium enzymes involved, these being phosphofructokinase and glycogen phosphorylase, respectively. For rat heart at 25°C, Crabtree and Newsholme (23) found values of 12 μmol/min/g wet weight for glycogen phosphorylase and 10 for phosphofructokinase. The ratio of these values is near unity, as found in many other types of muscle (23). However, the activity of hexokinase is very high (6.1 μmol/min/g wet wt.) compared to other muscles (14,23), showing the extreme importance of glucose transport into the cell and phosphorylation in sustaining glycolytic flux in heart. As pointed out by Burleigh and Schimke (14), hexokinase activity essentially falls into a "constant proportion group" with tricarboxylate cycle enzymes, whereas glycogen phosphorylase tends to fall into a group with glycolytic enzymes, e.g., aldolase. The former group is relatively active in cardiac muscle, the latter in white, phasic muscles. Direct measurements of the contribution of glycogenolysis to glycolytic flux in isolated perfused hearts show that it depends on the presence or absence of insulin and of catecholamines (108; for a review, see ref. 76). The effect of catecholamines is discussed below.

Glycogen Phosphorylase (E.C.2.4.1.1) and Glycogen Synthetase (E.C.2.4.1.11)

Glycogen phosphorylase is subject to control by protein phosphorylation and dephosphorylation. The phosphorylated form *(a)* is active, while the dephosphorylated form *(b)* is inactive except in the presence of adenosine monophosphate (AMP). The amount of active enzyme at any one moment is determined by the relative activities of the phosphorylase kinase and phosphatase and is sensitive to modulation of either or both of these activities. The subject has been reviewed by Fischer et al. (31). Epinephrine increases phosphorylase *a* content via a cyclic AMP-dependent protein kinase which activates phosphorylase *b* kinase (for a review, see ref. 106). Muscular activity also leads to an increased content of phosphorylase *a* via an entirely separate mechanism, in that Ca^{2+} ions, present at higher concentration in the cytoplasm during contraction, have a direct activator effect upon the phosphorylase *b* kinase (13,61). In addition, increased muscular contraction increases phosphorylase activity, independently of enzyme interconversion, via an increase in AMP levels and an activation of the *b* form of the enzyme.

Glycogen synthetase is also regulated by covalent modification, with the phosphorylated form being inactive in the absence of glucose-6-phosphate and the dephosphorylated form being active. The phosphorylation is catalyzed by a cyclic AMP-dependent kinase, and the effect of epinephrine on glycogen synthetase activity is thus the converse of the effect on phosphorylase activity. This minimizes any "futile cycle" at the level of glycogen breakdown and synthesis. The control of glycogen synthetase has been reviewed by Larner and Villar-Palasi (67).

The total activity of phosphorylase ($a + b$) has been reported to be diminished 10% when measured in heart homogenates from 28- to 32-month-old rats as compared to young adult (8- to 12-month-old) rats (35). The same authors reported that the percentage of the enzyme in the *a* form was increased with age and linked this to a less aerobic metabolism in the aged animals. Judgment should perhaps be withheld on this latter finding in the absence of experimental details on how enzyme interconversion was prevented during tissue extraction. Equally critical would be the matter of whether or not the heart was contracting when extracted. To provide results capable of interpretation, the hearts would probably have to be perfused at a known work load in the presence or absence of epinephrine, quenched at the temperature of liquid N_2, and extracted in a buffer designed to prevent further interconversion. This does not seem to have been done (35). Phosphorylase ($a + b$) has also been measured in arterial tissue, although not in heart, with respect to aging in man (58). It was found that there was a statistically significant decrease in the aorta, with the group of 60- to 69-year-olds showing 72% of the activity of the 20- to 29-year-old group. The decline in activity in the coronary artery was larger, with only 32% of the 0- to 29-year-old activity remaining in the age bracket 60 to 79 years. There was no significant change in activity with age in the pulmonary artery (58).

Thus, there seems to be a modest decline in phosphorylase activity in the aged heart, with a more substantial decline in the aorta and coronary artery. Whether there is any shift with age in the balance between *a* and *b* forms under otherwise identical conditions remains to be elucidated. Equally, any age-linked changes in glycogen synthetase activity await examination.

Hexokinase (E.C.2.7.1.1)

As mentioned above, the activity of hexokinase is high in heart relative to other muscles (14,23). Flux through this step may be restrained first by the availability of glucose, reflecting glucose transport across the plasma membrane and the presence or absence of insulin (see 74), and second, by inhibition by the end product, glucose-6-phosphate. This allows the matching of fluxes through phosphofructokinase and hexokinase and the translation of an inhibition of the former by high adenine nucleotide phosphate potential or citrate concentration into an inhibition of the latter (see ref. 76 for a review). Frolkis and Bogatskaya (35) reported a decreased hexokinase activity in extracts of myocardium from aged rats (28- to 32-month-old) compared to young adult animals (8- to 12-month-old). The decrease was of the order of 50%. The experimental finding seems clear, but it is anomalous in the light of the authors' view that glycolysis becomes more important as a source of energy in the aged myocardium and the known dependence of glycolysis in heart on the phosphorylation of glucose. In addition, the result does not seem to be consistent with the finding of an undiminished rate of glycolysis, from exogenous glucose, in hearts isolated from aged rats and perfused under controlled conditions of work load (1).

In arterial tissue, Brandstrup et al. (11) found no decline in measured hexokinase activity in man over the age range 10 to 83 years. This was true for both the aorta and the pulmonary artery. The analytical method used may have minimized activity, as the accumulation of the product, glucose-6-phosphate, may have caused some inhibition. Probably this was not serious enough to vitiate the basic conclusion, as a more prolonged incubation period gave only a modest decline in activity (11).

In view of the unchanged flux through this reaction (1), one should probably be cautious about the decrease in hexokinase activity claimed to occur with age (35). However, it is not inconceivable that both findings are correct if, for instance, the steady state level of glucose in heart is higher in the old animal or the level of glucose-6-phosphate is lower. This is sheer speculation, however.

Phosphofructokinase (E.C.2.7.1.11)

The phosphofructokinase reaction is the primary site at which the flux through glycolysis is adjusted to the energy demands of the cell. The enzyme responds to the adenine nucleotide "energy-charge" (5) by virtue of the fact that ATP is an allosteric inhibitor and ADP and AMP are activators. The response to AMP makes for considerable sensitivity as this is the nucleotide that changes most in response to changes in workload (78,82; cf. 54). In addition, inorganic phosphate, which also increases substantially with increased workload (54,78), is an activator and creatine phosphate is an inhibitor. Creatine phosphate content falls considerably with increased workload (54). Thus, the response to the energy status of the myocardium is maximized. In addition, both the substrate fructose-6-phosphate and the product fructose-1,6-diphosphate are activators, and their effect depends critically on pH. These relationships are described in recent reviews (10,69). Finally, it is thought to be via the inhibitory effect of citrate on phosphofructokinase that fatty acid oxidation in heart acts to reduce flux through glycolysis (37), and this is an important element in the overall sparing of glucose by fatty acid availability.

The myocardial content of phosphofructokinase was shown to increase slightly with age (35) when senescent (28- to 32-month-old) rats were compared with young adults (8- to 12-month-old). It is not clear if the increase is statistically significant, but it is in accord with the authors' view of a less oxidative and more glycolytic metabolism with age (35). Ritz and Kirk (92) found no significant change in phosphofructokinase activity in arterial tissue over the age range of 20 to 87 years in man. However, one should probably be cautious in interpreting these data as the absolute activities recovered are less than 1% of those from cardiac muscle (on a specific activity basis). Moreover, the ratio of phosphorylase to phosphofructokinase activities reported in arterial tissue (58,92) is over 20, whereas in most muscles it is approximately 1 (23). This suggests that assay conditions may not have been optimal, possibly owing to the omission of the activator AMP (92).

It seems that there is scope for the further definition of whether the activity of this enzyme actually does increase with age; experiments must make allowance for its instability and complex kinetic properties (23).

Triosephosphate Dehydrogenase (E.C.1.2.1.12)

Although the activity of this enzyme measured in muscle tissue is very high (8,9), it nevertheless may not allow the attainment of near-equilibrium in heart muscle (109). This conclusion is based on a comparison of the measured mass–action ratio with the known equilibrium constant for the reaction. This apparent paradox may be reconciled by noting that *in vivo* the enzyme is far from its pH optimum and is also subject to inhibition by ATP (22,34,36). Physiologically, control of triosephosphate dehydrogenase activity is probably exerted by product inhibition (36). Inhibition by NADH may be of especial importance in anoxia or ischemia, when the cytosolic $NADH/NAD^+$ ratio will tend to rise owing to a failure of mitochondrial shuttle mechanisms to regenerate NAD^+. At the same time, phosphofructokinase may become activated by a fall in adenine nucleotide energy charge (110), shifting control from this step to the triosephosphate dehydrogenase.

Cardiac muscle triosephosphate dehydrogenase has not been investigated with respect to aging. However, Bass et al. (9) measured this enzyme activity as indicative of the glycolytic potential

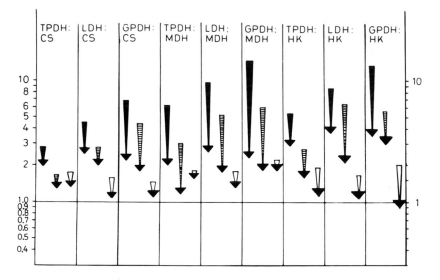

FIG. 1. The altered metabolic profile of three muscles in old age. The *arrows* indicate the direction and extent of changes with age in the relationship between muscles of certain enzyme activity ratios. The enzymes are TPDH, triosephosphate dehydrogenase; CS, citrate synthase; LDH, lactate dehydrogenase; GPDH, NAD-glycerol 3-phosphate dehydrogenase; MDH, malate dehydrogenase; HK, hexokinase. Enzymes expressed as numerators are members of the glycolytic sequence, whereas those expressed as denominators are considered members of the oxidative grouping. *Solid arrows* denote activities in the extensor digitorum longus/soleus; *hatched arrows,* diaphragm/soleus; *open arrows,* extensor digitorum longus/diaphragm. A value of unity on the graph would indicate that a particular ratio of activities, e.g., TPDH:CS, had the same magnitude in two different muscles. Thus the tendency towards unity in every case indicates a "dedifferentiation" of these three muscles with aging. (From Bass et al., ref. 9, with permission.)

of different types of muscle, with the age of the animals (rat) as a variable. They found a decrease with age in triosephosphate dehydrogenase activity in both fast (extensor digitorum longus, EDL) and slow (soleus) muscles, as well as an intermediate type (diaphragm). However, whereas the EDL muscle shows no loss in activity of enzymes characteristic of oxidative metabolism and thus shows a relative shift away from glycolysis in importance, the soleus loses oxidative capacity equally with glycolytic capacity. This is shown in Fig. 1, which reproduces this work because of its intrinsic interest, even though heart muscle is not directly involved. The figure clearly shows the "de-differentiation" in activity that occurs with aging, with a result of unity representing an identical metabolic profile for the three muscles. Of these muscles, the soleus most resembles cardiac muscle, with oxidative metabolism of great relative importance. By analogy with the soleus (9) and with another obligatorily aerobic muscle, i.e., fly-flight muscle (46), it seems quite likely that cardiac muscle triose-phosphate dehydrogenase may be diminished in activity with age. This would repay experimentation because of the possible rate-limiting role of this enzyme in ischemia mentioned above.

Pyruvate Kinase (E.C.2.7.1.40)

The pyruvate kinase reaction is displaced from equilibrium (109,110) and thus exerts some control over flux through glycolysis. The enzyme from muscle is inhibited by ATP competitively with respect to ADP, and thus will respond to the adenine nucleotide phosphate potential or to the "energy-charge" (5). Otherwise, the muscle enzyme appears to lack the control by fructose-1,6-diphosphate and by protein phosphorylation (see, e.g., ref. 55) which is shown by the liver enzyme. The latter has a more complex metabolic position in that it has to be inactivated under conditions requiring gluconeogenesis. The kinetics of pyruvate kinase are reviewed by Kayne (57). There appears to have been no study on the effect of age on pyruvate kinase activity in heart muscle.

Measurement of Glycolytic Flux in Heart Muscle from Young Adult and Aged Animals

When flux through the glycolytic pathway is measured as distinct from the activities of component enzymes, there is some suggestion that rates may be increased in the aging myocardium. Thus Frolkis and Bogatskaya (35) reported increased lactate production by homogenates from 28- to 32-month-old rats as compared to young adults (8 to 12 months), although the statistical significance of this finding is not clear. The authors (35) also cited a decreased glycogen content of the aging heart as proof of a more active glycolysis; this may not be permissible, as the glycogen content *in vivo* reflects both glycogenolysis and glycogen synthesis and does not give information on the maximum rate of either process. In addition, tissue extraction would have to be well controlled for the *in vivo* glycogen content to be preserved. Angelova-Gateva (4) also reported increased glycolysis in the aging rat myocardium, as measured by lactate production. Physical restraint of the animals (imposed hypodynamia) led to change in the same direction as for aging. One may question the biological significance of the results if the experiments really used 100-mg pieces of muscle, as implied in the methodology section. If homogenates were in fact used, the contribution of this paper becomes more clear and the stimulation by added glycogen comprehensible. The best-controlled of these studies was by Abu-Erreish et al. (1) and used isolated, perfused rat heart performing a defined amount of physical work. These authors found a slight, not statistically significant increase in glycolytic flux in the aging heart. Since on the same wet-weight basis oxygen consumption and palmitate oxidation decline with age, this slight increase in glycolysis becomes a provocative result.

On aggregate, therefore, there is tentative evidence that flux through the glycolytic pathway increases slightly with age in the rat myocardium with glucose (and possibly with glycogen) as substrate.

Pyruvate Oxidation

Pyruvate derived from glycolysis is oxidized to acetyl units in the form of acetyl coenzyme A [acetyl-(CoA)] by pyruvate dehydrogenase, this reaction being far from equilibrium. The acetyl groups are further oxidized to CO_2 in the tricarboxylate cycle, a pathway which will be described later as it is, of course, also the final process in the complete oxidation of fatty acids. The pyruvate dehydrogenase complex is subject to complicated metabolic control operating on two levels. On the first, the enzyme is interconverted between a phosphorylated (inactive) and dephosphorylated (active) form. Via differential effects on the kinase and the phosphatase enzymes catalyzing these reactions, decreases in ATP/ADP, NADH/NAD$^+$ and acetyl-CoA/CoA ratios favor an increase in the amount of active enzyme present. So do increases in the pyruvate and free Ca^{2+} ion concentrations. On the second level, the active (dephospho) enzyme is subject to end-product inhibition by acetyl-CoA and NADH. Thus, the acetyl-CoA/CoA and NADH/NAD$^+$ ratios modulate the activity of the enzyme by two different mechanisms. Together, these controls ensure that pyruvate dehydrogenase activity responds to both the energy-status of the cell (via ATP/ADP and NADH/NAD$^+$ ratios and Ca^{2+} ion concentration) and to the presence of fatty acids as an alternative substrate (via NADH/NAD$^+$ and acetyl-CoA/CoA ratios). This represents a second major site of action of fatty acids in the sparing of glucose. Many of these relationships have recently been reviewed (27,47).

Little attention has been paid to pyruvate dehydrogenase activity in aging studies with any tissue. This is surprising in view of its central role in metabolism and the clear nonequilibrium nature of the reaction. The information which is available is derived from studies with isolated rat heart mitochondria. These showed no change in O$_2$ uptake with pyruvate as substrate, when mitochondria from 6- and 24-month-old animals were compared (45). These data are reproduced as part of Table 2. Under these conditions, O$_2$ uptake reflects not only the functioning of pyruvate dehydrogenase but also that of dehydrogenases in the tricarboxylate cycle. However, direct measurement of pyruvate dehydrogenase activity, after conversion of all of the enzyme into the active (dephospho) form, also showed an unchanged activity in heart mitochondria from aged rats (44). These data are included in Table 1.

This unchanged pyruvate dehydrogenase activity of isolated mitochondria is in marked contrast to the decreases in the ability

TABLE 2. *Rate of O_2 consumption by mitochondria isolated from the hearts of young adult and senescent rats[a]*

Substrate (mM)	Rate of O_2 consumption (ng-atoms of O/min/mg protein)		Significance of difference (6-month versus 24-month)
	6 month	24 month	*p*
Pyruvate (2.5) +L-malate (0.5)	613 ± 26 (6)	593 ± 11 (5)	NS
Palmitoyl-L-carnitine (0.05) + L-malate (0.5) + albumin (0.04)	534 ± 15 (5)	398 ± 23 (5)	<0.001
Palmitoyl-CoA (0.02) +L-malate (0.5) +albumin (0.04) +DL-carnitine (5)	483 ± 5 (4)	424 ± 15 (4)	0.005–0.01
Octanoate (0.1) +L-malate (0.5)	427 ± 18 (5)	239 ± 30 (4)	<0.001
Acetyl-L-carnitine (5) +L-malate (0.5)	489 ± 33 (4)	397 ± 9 (4)	0.025–0.05
Pyruvate (2.5) + malonate (2.5) + DL-carnitine (10)	178 ± 2 (4)	139 ± 5 (5)	<0.001
L-Glutamate (5) +L-malate (5)	462 ± 18 (5)	444 ± 4 (5)	NS
L-Malate (0.5)	10	9	

[a] Experiments were carried out at 37°C, with other experimental conditions as given in ref. 45. Results are presented as the mean ± SEM, with the number of mitochondrial preparations given in parentheses. From Hansford (45), with permission.

to oxidize fatty acids (see below). These findings can only be related to the physiology of the whole organ if the mitochondrial content of the heart is known. However, there is some reason to believe that this may not change with aging (2).

β-Oxidation of Fatty Acids

A discussion of fatty acid oxidation is central to any survey of energy yielding pathways in cardiac muscle, because of the quantitative significance of this process (77). Fatty acid oxidation and its control in heart are the subject of an excellent review by Neely and Morgan (76), and this section will give only a brief description plus some details on carnitine translocation which have appeared very recently. The question of rate-limiting steps in fatty acid oxidation has been debated at length (see, e.g., refs. 33,48,76,86), and yields a series of different answers depending on experimental system (intact heart versus mitochondria) and flux (high work load versus low).

In the intact heart, uptake of fatty acid from plasma triglyceride requires the action of lipoprotein lipase, which is hormonally sensitive and may be rate limiting (see ref. 76). Uptake of albumin-bound fatty acid is dependent on concentration and again may be rate-limiting at high work loads (76). Once within the cell, the fatty acid is activated by an acyl-CoA synthetase in a reaction which is probably nonequilibrium *in vivo* owing to the removal of the product pyrophosphate (see ref. 68). Flux through this step is inhibited by high fatty acyl-CoA/CoA ratios; this inhibition is relieved in the response to high work load when cytosolic fatty acyl-CoA content probably falls and cytosolic CoA content probably rises. These statements are based on whole-tissue assays (77) and should be cautious. However, in general, an increase in intramitochondrial CoA content, as seen on the addition of ADP to heart mitochondria (48), would be expected to give some increase in cytosolic CoA concentration via the action of the carnitine acyltransferases discussed below. The addition of ADP to mitochondria is in many ways the counterpart of the transition of low to high work load for the heart.

Our understanding of the mitochondrial metabolism of the long-chain acyl-CoA compounds, formed as described above, has changed somewhat since the review by Neely and Morgan (76). It is now thought that the palmitoylcarnitine (taking the palmitoyl group as a physiologically important example) formed from palmitoyl-CoA and carnitine by carnitine palmitoyltransferase I (CPT I) actually enters the mitochondrion, in exchange for carnitine (45,87,88,89,90). Inside the mitochondrion, the reverse reaction occurs, catalyzed by CPT II, giving rise to palmitoyl-CoA as a substrate for the β-oxidation spiral. Thus, to the participation of two acyltransferases (see ref. 76) has been added that of a membrane carrier which is designated the carnitine:acylcarnitine translocase in this article. These relationships are depicted in Fig. 2. The importance of these reactions is that one or more

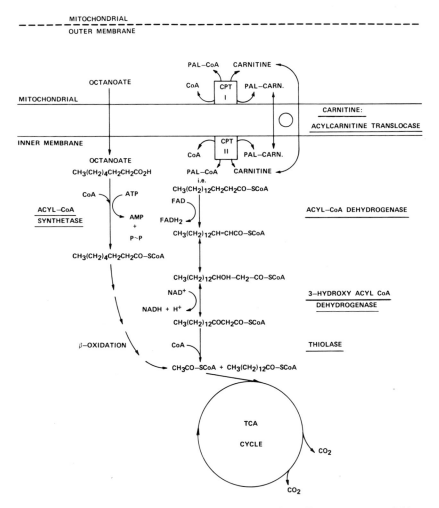

FIG. 2. An outline of mitochondrial lipid oxidation. Enzymes or activities discussed in the text are underlined.

of them may be rate limiting under conditions of high work load. The basis for this statement is that perfusion of an isolated rat heart with octanoate leads to the maintenance of acetyl-CoA levels during a transition from a low to a high work load, whereas perfusion with palmitate does not (77). Both of course share the β-oxidation pathway, but the oxidation of octanoate does not require the participation of the two carnitine acyltransferase enzymes or the carnitine:acylcarnitine translocase described above. When the substrate is palmitate, an increase in work load leads to an increase in tissue palmitoylcarnitine content and a decrease in palmitoyl-CoA content (77). Since most heart CoA (and CoA thioester) is mitochondrial (53) and most carnitine (and carnitine ester) is cytosolic (53), these changes indicate a rate limitation by the translocase or the inner carnitine palmitoyltransferase, i.e., CPT II (see Fig. 2).

When the oxidation of fatty acids is studied instead with isolated mitochondria, different activities may become rate limiting. Thus, the fatty acid activation and outer carnitine palmitoyltransferase (I) reactions are not involved, as the substrate is usually supplied in the form of palmitoylcarnitine. Moreover, concentrations of palmitoylcarnitine that generate maximal rates of respiration are usually used, and under these conditions the carnitine:acylcarnitine translocase and the inner carnitine palmitoyltransferase are active enough to generate high levels of intramitochondrial palmitoyl-CoA in experiments with rabbit heart mitochondria (48). Thus, under these experimental conditions, rate limitation of the overall process of fatty acid oxidation shifts to reactions "beyond" palmitoyl-CoA, when not exercised by the respiratory chain itself. The most obvious rate-limiting step within the β-oxidation spiral is that catalyzed by the first enzyme, the acyl-CoA dehydrogenase (see Fig. 2). The basis of this statement is the accumulation of substrate (palmitoyl-CoA) in mitochondria, but the failure to find significant amounts of product or of subsequent intermediates in the pathway (38,101). One would expect the activity of the acyl-CoA dehydrogenase to be controlled by substrate availability (48) and by competition with other dehydrogenases, acting via the redox poise of mitochondrial flavin and of the coenzyme Q pool. The other dehydrogenase in the pathway of β-oxidation, the β-hydroxyacyl-CoA dehydrogenase, is NAD linked and will be affected by the mitochrondrial NADH/NAD$^+$ ratio. To what extent this reaction limits flux through the whole pathway is not clear, however, as the absolute activity of this enzyme is high (see below) and β-hydroxyacyl-CoA does not accumulate in the mitochondrion, except when the NADH/NAD$^+$ ratio is unphysiologically high (101). The final reaction in the β-oxidation sequence, that catalyzed by thiolase, is nonequilibrium (105) and represents a site where the availability of free CoA could possibly increase the rate of fatty acid metabolism.

Finally, in the whole organ, or indeed in the intact mitochondrion, the overriding influence on the rate of fatty acid oxidation, or the oxidation of any other substrate, is the activity of oxidative phosphorylation. Increased contractile activity of the myocardium leads to the increased availability of ADP and P$_i$ to the heart mitochondrion, increased electron flow down the respiratory chain and, typically, a decrease in the mitochondrial NADH/NAD$^+$ ratio. This will affect β-oxidation directly, as mentioned above, but probably more important is the activation of the tricarboxylate cycle oxidations that occurs. This is described below. Increased citrate synthase activity leads to a fall in acetyl-CoA content, with a concomitant rise in free CoA content (48). This favors fatty acid activation and, via the related rise in free carnitine content, acylcarnitine formation and translocation. Once the palmitoylcarnitine is within the mitochondrion, the increased content of free CoA favors the formation of palmitoyl-CoA, the substrate for β-oxidation. In turn, β-oxidation is active because of the more oxidized coenzyme Q pool found with the increased availability of ADP (62). It is noted that we do not know of any very specific control of fatty acid oxidation and that control seems to be secondary to the modulation of the tricarboxylate cycle. It may be that when other dehydrogenase systems have been adjusted in activity by more delicate control mechanisms (see, for example, the discussion of the pyruvate dehydrogenase complex above), β-oxidation simply picks up the slack in the supply of reducing equivalents to the respiratory chain.

The reason for this preamble is that fatty acid oxidation is of pre-eminent importance in heart muscle (77) and has been studied to some extent in senescence. At the mitochondrial level, Chen et al. (21) showed that there was an age-linked decrement in the rate of palmitoylcarnitine oxidation, the largest decline occurring in the age range of 16 to 20 months (male Fisher rats). The decrease becomes the more credible in light of unchanged rates of succinate and ascorbate oxidation by mitochondria from the senescent rats. These data, together with a differential effect of senescence on the oxidation of various NAD-linked substrates, suggested that respiratory chain activity was unimpaired and that one should look instead at particular dehydrogenases or ancillary enzymes, e.g., acyltransferases, for any age-linked lesion. Subsequently, Hansford (45) confirmed the diminished rate of palmitoylcarnitine oxidation by heart mitochondria from aged Wistar rats and went on to search for the enzymatic locus of this decrement.

As well as the decrease in the rate of palmitoylcarnitine oxidation, decreases were also noted with acetylcarnitine and with pyruvate plus malonate plus carnitine as substrates (reproduced in Table 2). These processes have in common the operation of the carnitine:acylcarnitine translocase, and directed attention to this transport process as a possible site of the age-linked decrement. Direct measurement of transport activity by the rate of displacement of ^{3}H-carnitine from the mitochondrial matrix by external carnitine or acylcarnitine produced the data shown in Table 3. It is seen that when a saturating concentration of translocated acylcarnitine (20 mM acetyl-L-carnitine) is present outside the mitochondria, rates of egress of matrix ^{3}H-carnitine are significantly less in the mitochondria from the older animals. However, measurement of the exchangeable matrix carnitine pool, reflected by the total mitochondrial content of ^{3}H-carnitine when all of the endogenous carnitine and acylcarnitine has been exchanged,

TABLE 3. *Measurement of carnitine:acylcarnitine translocase activity in heart mitochondria from adult and senescent rats*[a]

Parameter measured or calculated	6-month-old rat	24-month old rat	Significance of difference (6-month versus 24-month), p
Total exchangeable mitochondrial carnitine pool (nmol/mg of protein)	1.05 ± 0.03 (5)	0.82 ± 0.02 (5)	<0.001
$V_{max.(apparent)}$ at 5°C, $= K_t \times$ [carnitine]$_{in}$ (nmol/min/mg protein)	0.71 ± 0.03 (7)	0.46 ± 0.04 (5)	<0.001
Mitochondrial carnitine at time of measurement of $V_{max.(apparent)} =$ [carnitine]$_{in}$ (nmol/mg of protein)	0.57 ± 0.03 (7)	0.37 ± 0.03 (5)	
First-order rate constant for exchange $= K_t$ (min^{-1})	1.24 ± 0.03 (7)	1.24 ± 0.04 (5)	NS

[a] Translocation was measured by the rate of displacement of internal ^{3}H-carnitine (with which the mitochondria were preloaded) upon the addition of 20 mM acetyl-L-carnitine, at 5°C. This concentration of substrate saturated the translocase on the outside face of the membrane and gave velocities of exchange referred to as $V_{max\ (apparent)}$. Results are presented as mean values $\pm$ SEM, with the number of mitochondrial preparations in parentheses. For experimental details, the reader is referred to the original paper. From Hansford (45), with permission.

reveals that this is diminished in mitochondria from the aged rats. Calculation of a first-order rate constant (Table 3) shows that this parameter is unchanged with age. Thus, there is no evidence for a change with age in the properties of the translocase protein per se; rather, the mitochondria from the old animals retain less carnitine and this limits the rate of translocation. The effect may well be physiologically important as the whole-heart content of carnitine and acylcarnitine is much diminished with age (1), as reproduced in Table 4, and the mitochondrial results are therefore not merely an artifact of preparation. Moreover, the K_m for the transport process is high (90) as compared to the whole-tissue concentration of carnitine (1), so that a decreased

TABLE 4. Tissue metabolite contents after the 30 min perfusion, at 175 mm Hg aortic peak systolic pressure, of hearts from young adult and senescent rats[a]

Age (months)	No. of rats	CoASH	Acetyl-CoA	Fatty acyl-CoA	Free carnitine[b]	Acetyl carnitine[c]	Fatty acyl carnitine[b]	Lactate	ATP	ADP	AMP	CP
7	7	180 ± 7	18 ± 5	136 ± 11	3,333 ± 173	415 ± 43	540 ± 13	5.7 ± 1.0	17.4 ± 0.5	2.98 ± 0.1	0.25 ± 0.03	22.9 ± 1.2
27–28	6	176 ± 10	19 ± 4	136 ± 12	2,038 ± 169	292 ± 27	355 ± 12	6.2 ± 1.3	15.3 ± 0.6	3.14 ± 0.1	0.39 ± 0.04	18.0 ± 0.30

[a] Metabolites (nmol/g dry tissue) were estimated in perchloric acid extracts made after quenching metabolism by freezing the beating hearts at the temperature of liquid N_2. Values are means ± SE.
[b] Free carnitine and long-chain fatty acyl carnitine are significantly lowered in the hearts of old animals, $p < 0.005$.
[c] Acetyl carnitine is lowered in the hearts of old rats, $p < 0.025$.
From Abu-Erreish et al. (1), with permission.

tissue content with age may be expected to translate into a decreased activity of transport. Whether this in turn limits the rate of O_2 uptake was debated for the substrates acetylcarnitine and pyruvate plus malonate plus carnitine in the original paper (45), to which the reader is referred. At first sight, transport into the mitochondrion seems unlikely to limit the oxidation of palmitoylcarnitine, as the process is almost as active as the transport of acetylcarnitine (88) and leads to more than 10 times as much O_2 uptake per mole. However, the activity of the carrier towards palmitoylcarnitine *in vivo* will be much diminished by other acylcarnitine species present at higher concentrations and by futile exchanges [i.e., palmitoylcarnitine (in) for palmitoylcarnitine (out)]. Thus, membrane transport remains a plausible site of the age-linked decrement in palmitoylcarnitine oxidation. The process deserves further study.

No decrease in activity was shown in other enzymes identified above as potentially rate limiting for the mitochondrial oxidation of palmitoylcarnitine (45). Thus, carnitine palmitoyltransferase (sum of I and II) was undiminished, as was the activity of acyl-CoA dehydrogenase. The β-hydroxyacyl-CoA dehydrogenase did show diminished activity, but this is of questionable biological significance in view of the high absolute activity and other reasons given above. These results for individual mitochondrial enzyme are presented in Table 1, together with unpublished measurements from whole-heart homogenates.

The decreased rate of acetylcarnitine oxidation with senescence noted in Table 2 may be attributed either to decreased rates of substrate translocation (Table 3) or to a reduced carnitine acetyltransferase activity (Table 1). The biological significance of the carnitine acetyltransferases (unlike the palmitoyltransferases) is not clear. It has been surmised (83) that the system serves to communicate between mitochondrial and cytosolic pools of CoA, which otherwise are segregated, such that a highly acetylated mitochondrial CoA pool leads to an acetylation of the cytosolic CoA, which is necessary to restrain the process of fatty acid activation. If so, it is not clear that the acetyltransferases have to be of high activity and the age-linked decrement may not be incapacitating.

The decreased rate of octanoate oxidation noted in Table 2 may probably be attributed to the much diminished activity of the activating enzyme, the acyl-CoA synthetase (Table 1). The basis for this is that the oxidation of palmitoyl moieties shares the same (β-oxidative) pathway and shows a rate that is higher. Thus, it is unlikely that the β-oxidation process limits the oxidation of octanoate. The biological significance of this decrement is not clear, because mid-chain length fatty acids are probably not a big contributor to total energy needs.

These cautions notwithstanding, it is clear that the whole-heart concentration of carnitine and the activities of at least three enzymes involved in fatty acid oxidation are all materially diminished (30–40%) with age. This suggests an orchestrated decline in the ability to handle fatty acids and perhaps an increased reliance on carbohydrate oxidation for energy. Interestingly, the neonatal heart is very inactive in fatty acid oxidation and has diminished carnitine palmitoyltransferase activity and a diminished tissue carnitine content, all relative to the young adult (115). By contrast with the situation in old age, the oxidation of mid-chain length fatty acids is unimpaired in neonatal heart (115). Perhaps also relevant to the discussion is the finding that the treatment of guinea pigs with thyroxine increases the ability of heart muscle homogenates to oxidize palmitate and, interestingly, increases both carnitine palmitoyltransferase activity and tissue carnitine content (12). The effect may be mediated via the release of fatty acids from adipose tissue. This finding raises questions about the thyroid status and plasma free fatty acid concentration of the aged animal.

Despite the clearcut decrease in the activity of fatty acid oxidation seen with heart mitochondria (21,45), senescence has little effect on palmitate oxidation by the perfused rat heart (1). Essentially, palmitate oxidation per heart was found to be unchanged, whereas there was a slight decrease in activity on the basis of heart weight. These results are shown in Fig. 3. Hearts from

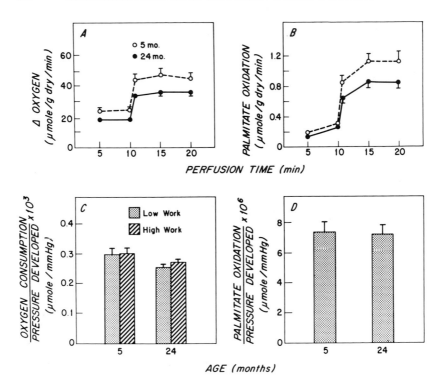

FIG. 3. Effects of ventricular pressure development on rate of O_2 consumption and palmitate oxidation. Hearts were removed from 5- and 24-month-old male Fisher 344 rats. The parameters measured are shown in the figure. Total pressure developed was calculated as the product of the peak systolic pressure and the heart rate and is a measure of work performed. For experimental details, see the original work. (From Abu-Erreish et al., ref. 1, with permission.)

both young and old animals were capable of sustaining a high work output and maintaining high ATP/ADP ratios and creatine phosphate levels, as discussed in the section on oxidative phosphorylation. One way of reconciling these results with the mitochondrial study is to say that the enzyme measurements express the maximum potential flux through the pathways, being $V_{\max}$ measurements, and that maximal fluxes were not achieved in the perfusion study. However, in defense of the latter, it is noted that the hearts developed systolic pressure of 180 mm Hg and were stimulated to beat at 240 beats/min (1). Alternatively, one could emphasize the fact that the glycolytic flux was not diminished with senescence in the perfusion study (on the basis of heart weight) and so carbohydrate metabolism may in fact be more important relative to fatty acid oxidation in the aging heart.

The Tricarboxylate Cycle

The tricarboxylate cycle functions in heart to catalyze the complete oxidation of acetyl groups derived from pyruvate, ketones, and fatty acids. Because of the unimportance of synthetic reactions in heart, the cycle operates with a minimal loss of intermediates to other pathways in contrast to the situation, for instance, in liver. Equally, the repletion of the cycle intermediates is also of very modest activity (see 24,25). A case can be made for the division of the cycle into three functional segments (see 111), that from oxaloacetate to α-ketoglutarate, that from α-ketoglutarate to malate, and that from malate to oxaloacetate. The functional division exists because of the ready transport of α-ketoglutarate and of malate across the mitochondrial membrane. The first segment is controlled in activity by an interaction between NAD-isocitrate dehydrogenase and citrate synthase, both catalyzing nonequilibrium reactions, and this will be described below. The second segment is controlled at the level of the α-ketoglutarate dehydrogenase, which is again a nonequilibrium step, and the third consists solely in the malate dehydrogenase reaction. Although Safer and Williamson (96) have emphasized unequal fluxes through segments 1 and 2 in response to changed substrate availability in the perfused heart, in the steady state these fluxes must be the same. The response of the tricarboxylate cycle to substrate-transition of this sort has been modelled very recently by Achs and Garfinkel (3). By contrast, the flux through the malate dehydrogenase in the steady state must equal that through the remainder of the cycle plus the flux through the malate–aspartate shuttle (18) which is responsible in the heart for the reoxidation of glycolytically derived reducing equivalents (95).

The control of tricarboxylate cycle activity has been the subject of two recent reviews (47,111) and will only be discussed briefly here. When respiratory chain activity is limited by the availability of ADP, the mitochondrial $NADH/NAD^+$ ratio is high (16,65). This restrains citrate synthase activity in two ways. First, at a given malate concentration, it reduces the amount of oxaloacetate available as a substrate via a direct effect on the malate dehydrogenase reaction. Second, a high $NADH/NAD^+$ ratio inhibits NAD-isocitrate dehydrogenase (20,41,48,64) causing tricarboxylates to accumulate and limiting the formation of dicarboxylates, including malate. Finally, the binding of the diminished amount of oxaloacetate which is available to citrate synthase is inhibited by citrate present at high concentration (100). When the mitochondrial $NADH/NAD^+$ ratio falls, more oxaloacetate is made available to citrate synthase, and what there is binds more effectively.

A high $NADH/NAD^+$ ratio also inhibits flux through the α-ketoglutarate dehydrogenase, which responds in addition to the ATP/ADP ratio. This affects the enzyme directly (70) and also through linkage to the succinyl-CoA/CoA ratio (66,99). In the low-work case (or in the controlled respiration of a mitochondrial suspension), ATP/ADP, $NADH/NAD^+$ and succinyl CoA/CoA ratios will be high and activity will be restrained accordingly. Finally, flux through the third segment of the cycle depends on both the $NADH/NAD^+$ ratio and the supply of malate, reflecting the activity of the two previous segments discussed above.

To this picture of control by the ATP/ADP ratio and (more importantly) $NADH/NAD^+$ ratio of the mitochondrion must be added the intriguing finding that micromolar levels of free Ca^{2+} ions activate both NAD-isocitrate dehydrogenase (28) and α-ketoglutarate dehydrogenase (70). This raises the possibility that Ca^{2+} ions act as a direct messenger between energy dissipation of muscle contraction and the most important pathway of energy generation in heart muscle.

Much of our knowledge of age-linked changes in the activity of the tricarboxylate cycle has come from studies with isolated rat heart mitochondria. The oxidation of pyruvate in the presence of malate requires the activity of pyruvate dehydrogenase, malate dehydrogenase, citrate synthase, aconitase, and NAD-isocitrate dehydrogenase, as well as transport processes for pyruvate and for malate. It thus provides a measure of the activity of the first segment of the tricarboxylate cycle as defined above. The α-ketoglutarate formed may leave the mitochondrion in short term experiments; in the long term, a steady state is reached in which the efflux of α-ketoglutarate to the medium becomes balanced by an equal rate of influx (48,64,65). Under these conditions, pyruvate is oxidized to completion, requiring the participation of the whole cycle. Measurements of O_2 uptake with pyruvate plus malate as substrate provide no evidence for any impairment of this first segment of the tricarboxylate cycle with aging (21,45). This is particularly clear in the studies of Hansford (45), where the rates achieved are higher than with any other NAD-linked substrate.

Studies with added α-ketoglutarate should provide evidence on the activity of the second segment of the cycle. Results are equivocal, as Chen et al. (21) showed no decrement with age, whereas Frolkis and Bogatskaya (35) showed a decrease in activity of approximately 20% (28- to 32-month-old versus 8- to 12-month-old rats). Absolute rates were low in the first study (21), possibly owing to the omission of malate which is required for the penetration of α-ketoglutarate into the mitochondrion (see ref. 18). P:O ratios were low for mitochondria from the young adults in the second study (35), raising doubts about the intactness of the mitochondria. Thus, there is scope for further study on this point.

The oxidation of exogenous succinate by mitochondria involves just the transport of succinate, succinate dehydrogenase, and fumarase and the transport of the product, malate, and is a frequently measured parameter. Evidence for an age-linked decrement is equivocal, with Nohl et al. (80) reporting a small (approximately 12%) decline at 24 months relative to oxidation at 3 months in rats of unstated strain, while Chen et al. (21) report no change from 9 to 24 months in male Fisher rats. The reports are equally convincing in that they both involve rates of respiration which are high in absolute terms.

The third segment of the cycle, the malate dehydrogenase reaction, is measured in experiments with glutamate plus malate as substrate. These show a decrement in rate of approximately 18% in preparations from aged rats (21). However, aspartate aminotransferase and membrane components catalyzing the transport of glutamate in exchange for aspartate and malate in exchange for α-ketoglutarate are also necessary for O_2 uptake in these experiments. Thus, there may or may not be a decrement in malate dehydrogenase activity per se. One direct measurement of the enzyme in a mitochondrial fraction from rat heart (97) indicated a 12% decrease in activity with age (96 versus 22 weeks); the validity of this finding rests on the assumption (of the reviewer) that the hypotonic buffer used was sufficient to release the latency of this activity.

The activity of tricarboxylate cycle dehydrogenases, freed from the restraints of mitochondrial permeability, can be measured directly in heart muscle homogenates provided that care is taken to disrupt the mitochondrial membrane. This was the approach in a recent study in which the activities of citrate synthase, NAD-isocitrate dehydrogenase, and α-ketoglutarate dehydrogenase were measured with respect to age (Table 1). These are the non-equilibrium enzymes of the cycle and provide loci at which decrements in enzyme activity with age could have a dramatic effect on metabolism (see above). It is seen that each activity is diminished between 15 and 20% in the heart from the aged animal when expressed on a weight basis. The decrease in cytochrome oxidase activity in the same homogenates was 24% (not shown). These decrements are modest and could reflect a diminished mitochondrial content of the aged heart; this is challenged by data on the specific activity of cytochrome oxidase, however, and this will be presented in the section on oxidative phosphorylation.

By contrast, the decrease in two enzymes involved in fatty acid oxidation is much greater, when measured in the same homogenates (Table 1).

Finally, tricarboxylate cycle flux in intact heart can be approximated from the studies of Abu-Erreish et al. (1) on the grounds that approximately 70% of the O_2 uptake in their experiments may be attributed to the operation of the tricarboxylate cycle. There is a modest decrease in O_2 uptake by hearts from the aged animals, especially at high work loads, when expressed on the basis of weight (see Fig. 3).

It might be reasonable to conclude that studies with isolated mitochondria provide no good evidence for a decline with age in the functioning of the tricarboxylate cycle, in contrast to some rather marked decreases in the ability to catabolize fatty acids. On the other hand, studies with the whole heart and with homogenates identify some modest decrements, when expressed on a protein basis. Taken together, these might suggest a slightly lowered content of mitochondria in the aging heart.

Oxidative Phosphorylation

The NADH and reduced flavine adenine dinucleotide ($FADH_2$) generated by the β-oxidation of fatty acids, the pyruvate dehydrogenase reaction, and the operation of the tricarboxylate cycle are reoxidized by the process of respiratory chain phosphorylation, with the concomitant phosphorylation of ADP. Oxidative phosphorylation in heart muscle and its control is the subject of two recent reviews (47,111), and the discussion here is intended merely to put age-linked changes in perspective.

Increased muscular work leads to a minimal increase in cytosolic ADP concentration and a rather large increase in creatine concentration (50,54,78). By virtue of the location of an isozyme of creatine kinase on the outer surface of the inner mitochondrial membrane (56), the latter change leads to an increased availability of ADP in the immediate vicinity of the adenine nucleotide translocase. This catalyzes the movement of ADP into the mitochondrion in exchange for ATP and is the subject of a recent review by Klingenberg (59). The intramitochondrial ADP, plus P_i which enters the mitochondrion on another carrier protein (see 18), serves as the substrate for phosphorylation, which is catalyzed by the oligomycin-sensitive ATPase (or F_1-ATPase), which is perhaps better known as an ATP-synthetase. The mitochondrial ATP-synthetase also serves to conduct protons across the mitochondrial membrane and it is the electrochemical proton gradient across the membrane that provides the driving force for phosphorylation (see 73). This gradient is formed by the functioning of the respiratory chain which is so arranged in the membrane that hydrogen flow from substrate to O_2 leads to the expulsion of protons from the mitochondrion. In the steady state there is, therefore, a continuous proton circuit with exit occuring via respiration, and entry via ATP synthesis. This view of the coupling between redox events and phosphorylation is known as the chemiosmotic mechanism, and is owing to the work of Mitchell (71,72).

On this view, increased availablility of ADP and P_i within the mitochondrion leads to a decrease in the extent of the proton electrochemical gradient, which normally restrains the rate of hydrogen flow down the respiratory chain. Thus, respiratory rate increases in response to ADP and P_i, this being a recent explanation of the well-known phenomenon of respiratory control (16). In heart muscle, it is unlikely that mitochondria are ever exposed to the extremely low ATP/ADP ratios which are used in *in vitro,* state 3 (16) studies of mitochondria (see refs. 50,54,78 for whole-tissue ATP/ADP ratios). Instead, respiration is probably always limited by the availability of ADP (26) and, possibly, also by P_i (51). In these respiratory states it seems likely that the energy of oxido-reductions corresponding to the first two spans of the respiratory chain from the $NAD^+/NADH$ couple to the cytochrome c Fe^{3+}/Fe^{2+} couple) comes into near-equilibrium with the free energy of synthesis of cytosolic ATP (51,85). This near-equilibrium probably also extends to the third span of the respiratory chain (cytochrome a Fe^{3+}/Fe^{2+} to cytochrome a_3 Fe^{3+}/Fe^{2+}) but certainly does not include the transfer of electrons from cytochrome a_3 to O_2, which is nonequilibrium and exerts rate control over the whole process (29). The phosphorylation potential of adenine nucleotides in the cytosol directly affects the flux through the terminal step, by determining the concentration of reduced cytochrome c (and presumably a_3) available as a substrate, owing to the near-equilibrium between phosphorylation and redox events, as outlined above. Normally, in the mitochondrion flux through cytochrome oxidase (i.e., cytochrome a plus a_3) is a small fraction of that which can be measured using artificial electron donors (2,112). The reason for this is that the activity of the remainder of the respiratory chain is not great enough to keep cytochrome a plus a_3 as highly reduced as in the artificial system and that flux is limited by the steady state level of reduced cytochrome a_3. Thus, an apparent excess of cytochrome oxidase activity, measured with artificial donors, should not be taken to mean that age-linked decrements (2) are without physiological importance.

The effect of aging on the ability of the myocardium or of isolated myocardial mitochondria to carry out oxidative phosphorylation has been probed in a number of ways. First, the concentrations of the cytochromes have been determined spectroscopically. This approach revealed that mitochondria from the hearts of 26-month-old rats contain less cytochrome b, c plus c_1 and a plus a_3 than those from 15-month-old animals (2). The contents were, respectively, 0.56 versus 0.74, 0.26 versus 0.47, and 0.39 versus 0.48 nmol/mg of mitochondrial protein, with the senescent result being the first of each pair. For errors, the reader is referred to the original paper (2). The activity of cytochrome c oxidase was found to be decreased in parallel with the content of cytochrome $a + a_3$ in suspensions of mitochrondria, giving an unchanged turnover number for this activity. Moreover, study of cytochrome c oxidase activity in whole heart homogenates revealed a decrease with the age of the animal, results being 3.26, 2.87, and 2.37 μatoms of O_2/min/mg of protein for 5-, 15-, and 26- to 29-month-old animals, respectively (2). Comparison of specific activities in homogenates and isolated mitochondria allows the statement that the mitochondrial content of the myocardium is the same at 5 and 26 months of age, although it is somewhat elevated at an intermediate age (14 months). The authors conclude from the altered specific activity of cytochrome oxidase in mitochondrial preparations that the composition of the inner mitochondrial membrane (of which cytochrome oxidase forms a part) changes with age. It should be noted that Gold et al. (42) also reported a decreased specific activity of cytochrome oxidase with age in mitochondria prepared from rat heart. However, Farmer et al. (30), in a study primarily concerned with spontaneous hypertension, found quite different results, with an unchanged cytochrome oxidase activity per milligram of mitochondrial protein, leading to the conclusion that the mitochondrial content of the myocardium declines from 6 to 17 months of age in the normotensive rat. There is no obvious way of resolving this difference.

Of the other enzyme activities mentioned in the introductory comments on oxidative phosphorylation, the mitochondrial ATPase has been found to be unchanged with age in homogenates (52). However, this activity is latent in intact mitochondria and is only expressed when the proton electrochemical gradient (see above) is collapsed by an uncoupling agent like dinitrophenol or by the dissolution of the membrane with detergents. It is not clear that the latency of this enzyme was adequately relieved in this study or that discrimination from other cellular ATPases was complete. In an isotonic homogenate the mitochondrial ATPase should not require added Mg^{2+} ions, owing to the preservation of mitochondrial structure. Under these conditions, inclusion of ethylene diaminetetraacetic acid (EDTA) would minimize the contribution of other ATPases and a useful measurement of the mitochondrial activity might be possible on the addition of an uncoupling agent. Specificity could then be established by the use of the inhibitor oligomycin.

In isolated mitochondria, Farmer et al. (30) reported no change in the specific activity of ATPase, whereas Nohl et al. (80) reported a decrease for mitochondria from 23-month-old rats compared to 3-month-old animals (strain not stated). Moreover, the latter paper showed that the discontinuity in the Arrhenius plot shifted from 19.3° for mitochondria from the young animal to 22.3° for the senescent animal. This was part of a general trend and taken as indicative of a decrease in the fluidity of the inner mitochondrial membrane during senescence. These data are presented as part of Fig. 4 and will be discussed further below in connection with ADP:O and RCRs. Again, measures were not taken to collapse the mitochondrial proton electrochemical gradient and so the data on ATPase presented by Nohl et al. (80) are hard to interpret; in fact, a measure of the degree to which ATPase activity was masked can be gained by reference to another paper (79) in which activities in the presence of the detergent Triton X-100 are also presented. There is a substantial gain in activity of ATPase in the presence of detergent and a disappearance of the age-related difference. The author concludes that senescence affects lipid–protein interactions and links this to an increased peroxidation of membrane lipid and an attendant loss in fluidity. This is plausible and very interesting, but the alternative explanation that ATPase activity in the intact mitochondrion was limited by substrate translocation or proton permeability remains to be answered. Perhaps one could investigate ATPase in uncoupling agent-treated submitochondrial particles; this would preserve protein–lipid interactions while removing permeability barriers.

The other major approach to the study of oxidative phosphorylation during aging has been to measure the uptake of O_2 and the phosphorylation of ADP by suspensions of isolated mitochondria. As outlined in the section on methodology, the rate of O_2 uptake in the presence of ADP (state 3) gives information (in heart mitochondria) on rates of substrate transport and dehydrogenase activity; rates in the absence of ADP reveal the rate at which the mitochondrial proton gradient is dissipated by ion cycling, [e.g., of Ca^{2+} ions (102)] and by any intrinsic leakiness, whereas rates of O_2 uptake after the completion of ADP-phosphorylation (state 4) reflect both these dissipative processes and

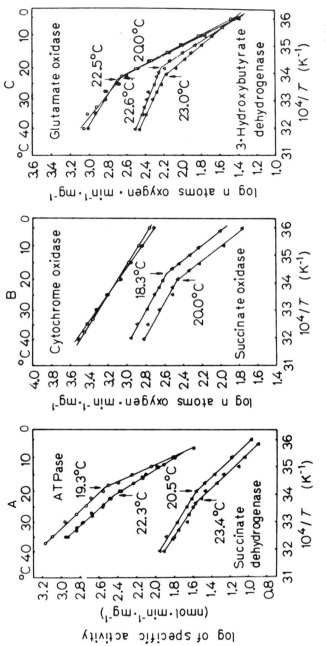

FIG. 4. Arrhenius plots of enzyme activities in heart mitochondria of young and old rats. The enzyme activities measured are given in the figures. *Open symbols* give results from 3-month-old rats, *filled symbols* those from 23-month-old rats. (From Nohl et al., ref. 80, with permission.)

any extramitochondrial ATPase in the preparation. The contribution of extramitochondrial ATPase to the state 4 rate can be assessed by preventing entry of ADP into the mitochondrion with the inhibitor atractyloside (see ref. 59 for a review). Typically, this causes a substantial decrement in the rate of O_2 uptake with heart muscle preparations. The ratio of state 3 to state 4 rates of O_2 uptake is the RCR and is a good criterion of mitochondrial integrity. The ratio of ADP-phosphorylated (moles) to O_2 consumed (atoms) during stimulated respiration (the ADP:O or P:O ratio) is another such criterion, but is a less sensitive indicator in the sense that finite (although diminished) P:O ratios can be measured in the absence of respiratory control (RCR $= 1$).

Until very recently, there was good agreement that perfectly intact mitochondria with undiminished P:O and RC ratios could be isolated from aging myocardium. Thus Gold ct al. (42) prepared mitochondria from 24- to 27-month-old Wistar rats that oxidized β-hydroxybutyrate with a P:O ratio of 2.85 and an RCR of 6.3, essentially unchanged from the young values. Equally, Chen et al. (21), in another convincing study, showed undiminished P:O ratios with glutamate plus malate, pyruvate plus malate, β-hydroxybutyrate, α-ketoglutarate, and succinate as substrates when mitochondria from 24-month-old Fisher rats were compared with those of 8- to 9-month-old animals. Respiratory control ratios were only diminished with age to the extent that there was a substrate-specific decline in state 3 rates; that is, there was no evidence of a deterioration of mitochondrial structure in that state 4 rates were unchanged (21). Against this background is set the recent work by Nohl et al. (80), which does show a decrease with senescence (24- versus 3-month-old rats) in P:O and RCRs with β-hydroxybutyrate, succinate, or glutamate plus malate as substrate. State 3 rates were also diminished with the two former substrates, but not with the latter. These data, together with those on ATPase mentioned above, are reproduced in Figs. 4 and 5. They are presented because they show age-linked changes, not because they are typical of findings in the literature. In particular, the relatively large de-

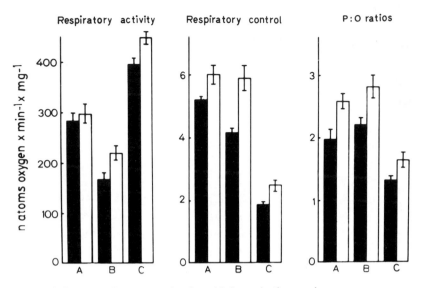

FIG. 5. Influence of age on mitochondrial respiration and energy conservation. Substrate was (A) glutamate plus malate, (B) 3-hydroxybutyrate, and (C) succinate. The *shaded bars* express results from aged (24-month-old) rats, the *open bars* those from young (3-month-old) rats. (From Nohl et al., ref. 80, with permission.)

creases in P:O ratio in the presence of modest changes in RCR (especially for glutamate plus malate) are notable. Nohl et al. (80) link this decreased efficiency of energy coupling to a change in structure of the inner mitochondrial membrane, which is evidenced both by the shifts in the breaks in the Arrhenius plots for several membrane-associated activities (Fig. 4) and by the results of spin-label studies. This change in structure is suggested to follow from increased peroxidation of membrane lipid, a consequence of increased rates of radical production from O_2 in mitochondria from the aged tissue. This theory is greatly strengthened by the finding that the generation of radicals in an *in vitro* system involving xanthine, xanthine oxidase, and isolated mitochondria leads to decrements in the performance of mitochondrial oxidations similar to those associated with aging (80). Added superoxide dismutase and catalase have a protective effect, indicative of a role for O_2^- radicals and H_2O_2 in the functional changes. Furthermore, a previous paper (81) showed that both intact heart mitochondria and submitochondrial particles from aged rats do in fact produce O_2^- radicals more actively than preparations from young animals. At the same time, their membranes contain a higher organic peroxide content. Quantitative aspects of this suggested mechanism of age-linked deterioration are not good, however, with a greater degree of lipid oxidation necessary to give the functional change when radicals are generated *in vitro* rather than *in vivo* (80). This discrepancy notwithstanding, this work is provocative and serves to direct attention to the lipid environment of membrane-bound enzymes as the site of a major age-linked lesion. In fact, Nohl (79) reports no age-dependent differences which can be attributed to proteins, as differences in activity disappear when the mitochondria are solubilized with detergent. The reviewer feels that the detergent-solubilized mitochondria deserve further study, as the finding of Nohl (79) that detergent treatment does not affect glutamate plus malate oxidation is inconsistent with his own (unpublished) experiments, in which it is greatly diminished. In this context, there is no reason why the oxidation of glutamate plus malate should necessarily be exempt from age-linked changes at the level of membrane lipid, as implied by Nohl (79), as it may be limited by glutamate/aspartate exchange across the mitochondrial membrane (63) or, in state 3, by the adenine nucleotide translocase or the ATP-synthetase, both proteins intimately associated with membrane lipid.

The discrepancy between Nohl et al. (80) on the one hand and Chen et al. (21) and Gold et al. (42) on the other concerning age-linked changes in P:O ratios may possibly be resolved by a recent finding by Murfitt and Sanadi (75) that isolated heart mitochondria may be separated into two fractions on the grounds of density, with one fraction showing far larger changes in respiratory properties including an age-linked decrement in RCR. The authors speculate that the fraction which shows the marked age-linked changes may consist of mitochondria which were being degraded *in vivo* as part of the normal turnover process. Conceivably, loss of this fraction during the isolation procedure of Chen et al. (21) and Gold et al. (42), which, incidentally, involved proteolysis, might have minimized age-linked changes in their preparations. This is speculation, however.

Finally, the flux through oxidative phosphorylation can be assessed indirectly in experiments involving whole hearts. A modest decrease with age in the rate of work performance (on a weight basis), as seen by Abu-Erreish et al. (1), implies an equally modest decrease in the rate of ATP-generation, which is dominated by the process of oxidative phosphorylation. In this study (1), moreover, the ratio of O_2 uptake to pressure development was unchanged with age, as shown in Fig. 3. This indicates no decrease with aging in the efficiency of energy coupling, a finding apparently at odds with the decreased $P:O$ ratios found for isolated mitochondria (80). In addition, ATP/ADP ratios and creatine phosphate content are well maintained in the aging heart (1), with just the hint of a decrease after a 30 min perfusion at high systolic pressure (175 mm Hg). These results are given in Table 4. They should help to dispense with the notion that there are major decreases in ATP/ADP ratio (35) or creatine phosphate content (15) with age, the absolute values of these parameters being so low in the earlier work as to question the procedures used for quenching metabolism.

Mitochondrial Structure and the Tissue Content of Mitochondria During Aging

Electron microscopic examination of tissue allows the definition of age-linked changes in size, structure, and tissue content of mitochondria, as well as possibly identifying subpopulations of the organelles, which may differ in properties and, conceivably, be lost during tissue fractionation (see ref. 114 for a description of this phenomenon in liver). Histochemistry adds another dimension, allowing the localization of functional changes.

There is an apparent discrepancy between results on the effect of aging on mitochondrial size and number in heart muscle. Thus, Von Kment et al. (60) reported a significant increase in the number of mitochondria per unit of cell area in hearts from 20-month-old rats compared to those from young adults (5 months old). The individual sectional area of the mitochondria was significantly decreased with age, resulting in an unchanged contribution of the mitochondrial compartment to the total volume of the cell. Similar results have been reported recently (32) for left ventricular muscle taken from man (5 to 15 years old compared to 42 to 78 years old).

On the other hand, Herbener et al. (49) showed a decreased number of mitochondria per unit of cellular volume in left ventricular muscle from senescent (43- to 44-month-old) mice compared to young adults (8 months old). The volume of the average mitochondrion was unchanged with age, giving rise to a 16% decrease in the fraction of total cell volume occupied by mitochondria. A subsequent paper (103) extended these findings and showed that because the area of the cristael (inner) mitochondrial membrane was unchanged with age per volume of mitochondria, the total area of cristael membrane of left ventricular muscle decreased by 35% over the age range 9 to 36 months, reflecting the decreased number of mitochondria. One would expect the total area of inner mitochondrial membrane of a tissue to correlate with the capacity for oxidative phosphorylation, owing to the siting of the respiratory chain and ATP-synthetase in this membrane.

There is no evidence in aging heart of a subpopulation of swollen and distorted mitochondria analogous to those found by Wilson and Franks (114) in liver from senescent animals. There is evidence (104) for increased numbers of residual bodies and primary lyosomes in close proximity to mitochondria in the aging heart (33-month-old compared to 6-month-old rat). A role of primary lyosomes in the degradation of mitochondria to residual bodies was inferred, and the rate of this process was suggested on the grounds of the increased numbers of lyosomes and residual bodies visible to be greater with age. This may be true, but the conclusion depends on assumptions about the rate of export of material from the cell.

CONCLUDING REMARKS

Despite uncertainties inherent in the comparison of results obtained on different animals and in different laboratories, it seems fairly clear that many of the enzymes involved in fatty acid oxidation(21,45), the tricarboxylate cycle (Table 1), and oxidative phosphorylation (2) show a decreased specific activity in the aging heart. These are all mitochondrial activities, and one view of the changes that occur in old age would be that the number of mitochondria is reduced on the basis of tissue weight or volume. This is consistent with at least a portion of the morphological evidence (49,103). However, it is certainly not the whole answer, as there are differential losses in activity among mitochondrial enzymes in homogenates (Table 1; cf. citrate synthase and carnitine acetyltransferase) and there are appreciable decrements in the activities of some enzymes in suspensions of mitochondria (Table 1). In fact, direct comparisons of specific activities of cytochrome oxidase (2) and β-hydroxyacyl-CoA dehydrogenase (Table 1) in mitochondrial preparations and homogenates indicate no decrease in the tissue content of mitochondria with age. Comparisons based on carnitine acetyltransferase indicate a slight decrement (Table 1). Since other enzyme systems in the mitochondrion, e.g., pyruvate oxidation, are unchanged with age (Table 2), it is clear that the balance of enzymic activities of the organelle shifts and a part of this is the trend away from active fatty acid oxidation (Table 2). This is a topic which should reward further investigation.

To what extent are these diminished enzyme activities significant at the physiological level? The study by Abu-Erreish et al. (1) with perfused rat hearts suggests that O_2 uptake and palmitate oxidation are diminished between 12 and 23%, on a weight basis, in the older heart. Equally, work output, as measured by the product of heart rate and peak systolic pressure, decreases by 11% at high work loads (see Fig. 3). These differences disappear when expressed on a per-heart basis, owing to hypertrophy in the aged, but it is not clear that this is a more valid basis of comparison. It seems, therefore, that the decrement in enzymatic machinery leads to a modest impairment in work performance in the intact heart. Equally clear, however, is that the aging heart can respond to demands to increase work with an unchanged efficiency (1; see Fig. 3) and with the maintenance of a high energy state, as evidenced by adenine nucleotide and phosphagen contents (1; see Table 4). This limits the extent to which mitochondria *in situ* can display the diminished $P:O$ ratios which were determined with isolated mitochondria from aging heart in a recent study (80). Such a diminution would lead to an increased ratio of O_2 uptake to work performed and, possibly, a failure to maintain phosphagen levels and perform work for extended periods at the higher systolic pressures.

REFERENCES

1. Abu-Erreish, G. M., Neely, J. R., Whitmer, J. T., Whitman, V., and Sanadi, D. R. (1977): Fatty acid oxidation by isolated perfused working hearts of aged rats. *Am. J. Physiol.,* 232:E258–262.
2. Abu-Erreish, G. M., and Sanadi, D. R. (1978): Age-related changes in cytochrome concentration of myocardial mitochondria. *Mech. Ageing Dev.* 7:425–432.
3. Achs, M. J., and Garfinkel, D. (1977): Computer simulation of rat heart metabolism after adding glucose to the perfusate. *Am. J. Physiol.,* 232:R175–R184.
4. Angelova-Gateva, P. (1969): Tissue respiration and glycolysis in quadriceps femoris and heart of rats of different ages during hypodynamia. *Exp. Gerontol.* 4:177–187.
5. Atkinson, D. E. (1968): The energy charge of the adenylate pool as a regulatory parameter. Interaction with feedback modifiers. *Biochemistry,* 7:4030–4034.
6. Barrows, C. H., Jr., Falzone, J. A., Jr., and Shock, N. W. (1960): Age differences in the succinoxidase activity of homogenates and mitochondria from the livers and kidneys of rats. *J. Gerontol.* 15:130–133.
7. Barrows, C. H., Jr., Yiengst, M. J., and Shock, N. W. (1958): Senescence and the metabolism of various tissues of rats. *J. Gerontol.,* 13:351–355.

8. Bass, A., Brdiczka, D., Eyer, P., Hofer, S., and Pette, D. (1969): Metabolic differentiation of distinct muscle types at the level of enzymatic organization. *Eur. J. Biochem.,* 10:198–206.

9. Bass, A., Gutmann, E., and Hanzlíková, V. (1975): Biochemical and histochemical changes in energy supply–enzyme pattern of muscles of the rat during old age. *Gerontologia,* 21:31–45.

10. Bloxham, D. P., and Lardy, H. A. (1973): Phosphofructokinase. *Enzymes,* 8:239–278.

11. Brandstrup, N., Kirk, J. E., and Bruni, C. (1957): The hexokinase and phosphoglucoisomerase activities of aortic and pulmonary artery tissue in individuals of various ages. *J. Gerontol.,* 12:166–171.

12. Bressler, R., and Wittels, B. (1966): The effect of thyroxine on lipid and carbohydrate metabolism in the heart. *J. Clin. Invest.,* 45:1326–1333.

13. Brostrom, C. O., Hunkeler, F. L., and Krebs, E. G. (1971): The regulation of skeletal muscle phosphorylase kinase by Ca^{2+}. *J. Biol. Chem.,* 246:1961–1967.

14. Burleigh, I. G., and Schimke, R. T. (1969): The activities of some enzymes concerned with energy metabolism in mammalian muscles of differing pigmentation. *Biochem. J.,* 113:157–166.

15. Casten, G. G. (1950): Effects of aging process on acid-soluble phosphorus compounds in myocardium of rats. *Am. Heart J.,* 39:353–360.

16. Chance, B., and Williams, G. R. (1956): The respiratory chain and oxidative phosphorylation. *Adv. Enzymol.,* 17:65–134.

17. Chappell, J. B. (1964): The effects of 2,4-dinitrophenol on mitochondrial oxidations. *Biochem. J.,* 90:237–248.

18. Chappell, J. B. (1968): Systems used for the transport of substrates into mitochondria *Br. Med. Bull.,* 24:150–157.

19. Chappell, J. B., and Hansford, R. G. (1972): Preparation of mitochondria from animal tissues and yeasts. In: *Subcellular Components,* edited by G. D. Birnie, pp. 77–91. Butterworth, London.

20. Chen, R. F., and Plaut, G. W. E. (1963): Activation and inhibition of DPN-linked isocitrate dehydrogenase of heart by certain nucleotides. *Biochemisty,* 2:1023–1032.

21. Chen, J. C., Warshaw, J. B., and Sanadi, D. R. (1972): Regulation of mitochondrial respiration in senescence. *J. Cell. Physiol.,* 80:141–148.

22. Constantinides, S. M., and Deal, W. C., Jr. (1969): Reversible dissociation of tetrameric rabbit muscle glyceraldehyde-3-phosphate dehydrogenase into dimers or monomers by adenosine triphosphate. *J. Biol. Chem.,* 244:5695–5702.

23. Crabtree, B., and Newsholme, E. A. (1972): The activities of phosphorylase, hexokinase, phosphofructokinase, lactate dehydrogenase and the glycerol 3-phosphate dehydrogenases in muscles from vertebrates and invertebrates. *Biochem. J.,* 126:49–58.

24. Davis, E. J., and Bremer, J. (1973): Studies with isolated surviving rat hearts. Interdependence of free amino acids and citric-acid-cycle intermediates. *Eur. J. Biochem.,* 38:86–97.

25. Davis, E. J., Lin, R. C., and Chao, D. L.-S. (1972): Sources and disposition

of aerobically-generated intermediates in heart muscle. In: *Energy Metabolism and the Regulation of Metabolic Processes in Mitochondria,* edited by M. A. Mehlman and R. W. Hanson, pp. 211–238. Academic Press, New York.

26. Davis, E. J., and Lumeng, L. (1975): Relationships between the phosphorylation potentials generated by liver mitochondria and respiratory state under conditions of adenosine diphosphate control. *J. Biol. Chem.,* 250:2275–2282.

27. Denton, R. M., Randle, P. J., Bridges, B. J., Cooper, R. H., Kerbey, A. L., Pask, H. T., Severson, D. L., Stansbie, D., and Whitehouse, S. (1975): Regulation of mammalian pyruvate dehydrogenase. *Mol. Cell. Biochem.,* 9:27–52.

28. Denton, R. M., Richards, D. A., and Chin, J. G. (1978): Calcium ions and the regulation of NAD^+ linked isocitrate dehydrogenase from the mitochondria of rat heart and other tissues. *Biochem. J.,* 176:899–906.

29. Erecínska, M., Wilson, D. F., and Nishiki, K. (1978): Homeostatic regulation of cellular energy metabolism: experimental characterization in vivo and fit to a model. *Am. J. Physiol.,* 234:C82–C89.

30. Farmer, B. B., Harris, R. A., Jolly, W. W., and Vail, W. J. (1974): Studies on the cardiomegaly of the spontaneously hypertensive rat. *Circ. Res.,* 35:102–110.

31. Fischer, E. H., Heilmeyer, L. M. G., Jr., and Haschke, R. H. (1971): Phosphorylase and the control of glycogen degradation. *Curr. Top. Cell. Regul.,* 4:211–251.

32. Fleischer, M., Warmuth, H., Backwinkel, K. P., and Themann, H. (1978): Ultrastructural morphometric analysis of normally loaded human myocardial left ventricles from young and old patients. *Virchows Arch.* [*Pathol. Anat.*], 380:123–133.

33. Fong, J. C., and Schulz, H. (1978): On the rate-determining step of fatty acid oxidation in heart. Inhibition of fatty acid oxidation by 4-pentenoic acid. *J. Biol. Chem.,* 253:6917–6922.

34. Francis, S. H., Meriwether, B. P., and Park, J. H. (1971): Interaction between adenine nucleotides and 3-phosphoglyceraldehyde dehydrogenase. II. A study of the mechanism of catalysis and metabolic control of the multifunctional enzyme. *J. Biol. Chem.,* 246:5433–5441.

35. Frolkis, V. V., and Bogatskaya, L. N. (1968): The energy metabolism of myocardium and its regulation in animals of various age. *Exp. Gerontol.,* 3:199–210.

36. Furfine, C. S., and Velick, S. F. (1965): The acyl-enzyme intermediate and kinetic mechanism of the glyceraldehyde-3-phosphate dehydrogenase reaction. *J. Biol. Chem.,* 240:844–855.

37. Garland, P. B., Randle, P. J., and Newsholme, E. A. (1963): Citrate as an intermediary in the inhibition of phosphofructokinase in rat heart muscle by fatty acids, ketone bodies, pyruvate, diabetes and starvation. *Nature,* 200:169–170.

38. Garland, P. B., Shepherd, D., and Yates, D. W. (1965): Steady-state concentrations of coenzyme A, acetyl-coenzyme A and long-chain fatty

acyl-coenzyme A in rat-liver mitochondria oxidizing palmitate. *Biochem. J.,* 97:587–594.

39. Gershon, H., and Gershon, D. (1973): Inactive enzyme molecules in aging mice: liver aldolase. *Proc. Natl. Acad. Sci. USA,* 70:909–913.

40. Gershon, H., and Gershon, D. (1973): Altered enzyme molecules in senescent organisms: Mouse muscle aldolase. *Mech. Ageing Dev.,* 2:33–41.

41. Goebell, H., and Klingenberg, M. (1964): NAD-specific isocitrate dehydrogenase in mitochondria. *Biochem. Z.,* 340:441–464.

42. Gold, P. H., Gee, M. V., and Strehler, B. L. (1968): Effect of age on oxidative phosphorylation in the rat. *J. Gerontol.,* 23:509–512.

43. Grinna, L. S., and Barber, A. A. (1972): Age-related changes in membrane lipid content and enzyme activities. *Biochim. Biophys. Acta,* 288:347–353.

44. Hansford, R. G. (1977): Studies on inactivation of pyruvate dehydrogenase by palmitoylcarnitine oxidation in isolated rat heart mitochondria. *J. Biol. Chem.,* 252:1552–1560.

45. Hansford, R. G. (1978): Lipid oxidation by heart mitochondria from young adult and senescent rats. *Biochem. J.,* 170:285–295.

46. Hansford, R. G. (1978): A comparison of energy-yielding reactions in the flight muscle of young adult and senescent blowflies. *Comp. Biochem. Physiol.,* 59B:37–46.

47. Hansford, R. G. (1980): Control of mitochondrial substrate oxidation. *Curr. Top. Bioenerg.,* 10*(in press).*

48. Hansford, R. G., and Johnson, R. N. (1975): The steady state concentrations of coenzyme A-SH and coenzyme A thioester, citrate and isocitrate during tricarboxylate cycle oxidations in rabbit heart mitochondria. *J. Biol. Chem.,* 250:8361–8375.

49. Herbener, G. H. (1976): A morphometric study of age-dependent changes in mitochondrial population of mouse liver and heart. *J. Gerontol.,* 31:8–12.

50. Hiltunen, J. K., and Hassinen, I. E. (1976): Energy-linked regulation of glucose and pyruvate oxidation in isolated perfused rat heart: Role of pyruvate dehydrogenase. *Biochim. Biophys. Acta,* 440:377–390.

51. Holian, A., Owen, C. S., and Wilson, D. F. (1977): Control of respiration in isolated mitochondria: Quantitative evaluation of the dependence of respiratory rates on [ATP], [ADP], and [P_i]. *Arch. Biochem. Biophys.,* 181:164–171.

52. Honorati, M. C., and Ermini, M. (1974): Myofibrillar and mitochondrial ATP-ase activity of red, white, diaphragmatic and cardiac muscle of young and old rats. *Experientia,* 30:215–216.

53. Idell-Wenger, J. A., Grotyohann, L. W., and Neely, J. R. (1978): Coenzyme A and carnitine distribution in normal and ischemic hearts. *J. Biol. Chem.,* 253:4310–4318.

54. Illingworth, J. A., Ford, W. C. L., Kobayashi, K., and Williamson, J. R. (1975): Regulation of myocardial energy metabolism. In: *Recent Advances in Studies on Cardiac Structure and Metabolism, Vol. 8,* edited

by P.-E. Roy and P. Harris, pp. 271–290. University Park Press, Baltimore.

55. Ishibashi, H., and Cottam, G. L. (1978): Glucagon-stimulated phosphorylation of pyruvate kinase in hepatocytes. *J. Biol. Chem.,* 253:8767–8771.
56. Jacobus, W. E., and Lehninger, A. L. (1973): Creatine kinase of rat heart mitochondria: Coupling of creatine phosphorylation to electron transport. *J. Biol. Chem.,* 248:4803–4810.
57. Kayne, F. J. (1973): Pyruvate kinase. *Enzymes,* 8:353–382.
58. Kirk, J. E. (1962): The glycogen phosphorylase activity of arterial tissue in individuals of various ages. *J. Gerontol.,* 17:154–157.
59. Klingenberg, M. (1976): The ADP-ATP carrier in mitochondrial membranes. In: *The Enzymes of Biological Membranes, Vol. 3,* edited by A. Martonosi, pp. 383–438. Plenum Press, New York.
60. Kment, Von A., Leibetseder, J., and Burger, H. (1966): Gerontologische Untersuchungen an Rattenherzmitochondrien. *Gerontologia,* 12:193–199.
61. Krebs, E. G., Huston, R. B., and Hunkeler, F. L. (1968): Properties of phosphorylase kinase and its control in skeletal muscle. *Adv. Enzyme Regul.,* 6:245–255.
62. Kröger, A., and Klingenberg, M. (1967): On the role of ubiquinone. *Curr. Top. Bioenerg.,* 2:152–190.
63. LaNoue, K. F., Bryla, J., and Bassett, D. J. P. (1974): Energy-driven aspartate efflux from heart and liver mitochondria. *J. Biol. Chem.,* 249:7514–7521.
64. LaNoue, K. F., Bryla, J., and Williamson, J. R. (1972): Feedback interactions in the control of citric acid cycle activity in rat heart mitochondria. *J. Biol. Chem.,* 247:667–679.
65. LaNoue, K., Nicklas, W. J., and Williamson, J. R. (1970): Control of citric acid cycle activity in rat heart mitochondria. *J. Biol. Chem.,* 245:102–111.
66. LaNoue, K. F., Walajtys, E. I., and Williamson, J. R. (1973): Regulation of glutamate metabolism and interactions with the citric acid cycle in rat heart mitochondria. *J. Biol. Chem.,* 248:7171–7183.
67. Larner, J., and Villar-Palasi, C. (1971): Glycogen synthase and its control. *Curr. Top. Cell. Regul.,* 3:195–236.
68. Lehninger, A. L. (1975): *Biochemistry,* 2nd ed. Worth Publishers, New York.
69. Mansour, T. E. (1972): Phosphofructokinase. *Curr. Top. Cell. Regul.,* 5:1–46.
70. McCormack, J. G., and Denton, R. M. (1979): The effects of calcium ions and adenine nucleotides on the activity of pig heart 2-oxoglutarate dehydrogenase complex. *Biochem. J.,* 180:533–544.
71. Mitchell, P. (1961): Coupling of phosphorylation to electron and hydrogen transfer by a chemi-osmotic type of mechanism. *Nature,* 191:144–148.
72. Mitchell, P. (1966): *Chemiosmotic coupling in oxidative and photosynthetic phosphorylation.* Glynn Research Ltd., Bodmin.

73. Mitchell, P. (1979): The Ninth Sir Hans Krebs Lecture. Compartmentation and communication in living systems. Ligand conduction: A general catalytic principle in chemical, osmotic and chemiosmotic reaction systems. *Eur. J. Biochem.,* 95:1–20.

74. Morgan, H. E., and Neely, J. R. (1972): Insulin and membrane transport. In: *Handbook of Physiology,* edited by D. F. Steiner, and N. Freinkel, pp. 323–331. American Physiological Society, Washington, D.C.

75. Murfitt, R. R., and Sanadi, D. R. (1978): Evidence for increased degeneration of mitochondria in old rats. A brief note. *Mech. Ageing Dev.,* 8:197–201.

76. Neely, J. R., and Morgan, H. E. (1974): Relationship between carbohydrate and lipid metabolism and the energy balance of heart muscle. *Annu. Rev. Physiol.,* 36:413–459.

77. Neely, J. R., Rovetto, M. J., and Oram, J. F. (1972): Myocardial utilization of carbohydrate and lipids. *Prog. Cardiovasc. Dis.,* 15:289–329.

78. Nishiki, K., Erecínska, M., and Wilson, D. F. (1978): Energy relationships between cytosolic metabolism and mitochondrial respiration in rat heart. *Am. J. Physiol.,* 234:C73–81.

79. Nohl, H. (1979): Influence of age on thermotropic kinetics of enzymes involved in mitochondrial energy-metabolism. *Z. Gerontologie,* 12:9–18.

80. Nohl, H., Breuninger, V., and Hegner, D. (1978): Influence of mitochondrial radical formation on energy-linked respiration. *Eur. J. Biochem.,* 90:385–390.

81. Nohl, H., and Hegner, D. (1978): Do mitochondria produce oxygen radicals *in vivo? Eur. J. Biochem.,* 82:563–567.

82. Opie, L. H., Mansford, K. R. L., and Owen, P. (1971): Effects of increased heart work on glycolysis and adenine nucleotides in the perfused heart of normal and diabetic rats. *Biochem. J.,* 124:475–490.

83. Oram. J. F., Bennetch, S. L., and Neely, J. R. (1973): Regulation of fatty acid utilization in isolated perfused rat hearts. *J. Biol. Chem.,* 248:5299–5309.

84. Orgel, L. E. (1963): The maintenance of the accuracy of protein synthesis and its relevance to aging. *Proc. Natl. Acad. Sci. USA,* 49:517–521.

85. Owen, C. S., and Wilson, D. F. (1974): Control of respiration by the mitochondrial phosphorylation state. *Arch. Biochem. Biophys.,* 161:581–591.

86. Pande, S. V. (1971): On rate-controlling factors of long chain fatty acid oxidation. *J. Biol. Chem.,* 246:5384–5390.

87. Pande, S. V. (1975): A mitochondrial carnitine acylcarnitine translocase system. *Proc. Natl. Acad. Sci. USA,* 72:883–887.

88. Pande, S. V., and Parvin, R. (1976): Characterization of carnitine acylcarnitine translocase system of heart mitochondria. *J. Biol. Chem.,* 251:6683–6691.

89. Parvin, R., and Pande, S. V. (1978): Carnitine-acylcarnitine translocase. Inhibition by α-cyano-4-hydroxycinnamate and evidence for separate identity from the pyruvate transporting system of mitochondria. *J. Biol. Chem.,* 253:1944–1946.

90. Ramsay, R. R., and Tubbs, P. K. (1976): The effects of temperature and some inhibitors on the carnitine exchange system of heart mitochondria. *Eur. J. Biochem.,* 69:299–303.

91. Randle, P. J., Newsholme, E. A., and Garland, P. B. (1964): Regulation of glucose uptake by muscle. *Biochem. J.,* 93:652–665.

92. Ritz, E., and Kirk, J. E. (1967): The phosphofructokinase and sorbitol dehydrogenase activities of arterial tissue in individuals of various ages. *J. Gerontol.,* 22:433–438.

93. Rodis, S. L., and Vahouny, G. V. (1970): Uptake and oxidation of fatty acids and glucose by perfused hearts from young and mature rats. *Biochim. Biophys. Acta,* 208:153–155.

94. Rolleston, F. S. (1972): A theoretical background to the use of measured concentrations of intermediates in study of the control of intermediary metabolism. *Curr. Top. Cell. Regul.,* 5:47–75.

95. Safer, B., Smith, C. M., and Williamson, J. R. (1971): Control of the transport of reducing equivalents across the mitochondrial membrane in perfused rat heart. *J. Mol. Cell. Cardiol.,* 2:111–124.

96. Safer, B., and Williamson, J. R. (1973): Mitochondrial-cytosolic interactions in perfused rat heart. Role of coupled transamination in repletion of citric acid cycle intermediates. *J. Biol. Chem.,* 248:2570–2579.

97. Singh, S. N. (1973): Effect of age on the activity and citrate inhibition of malate dehydrogenase of the brain and heart of rats. *Experientia,* 29:42–43.

98. Singh, S. N., and Kanungo, M. S. (1968): Alterations in lactate dehydrogenase of the brain, heart, skeletal muscle and liver of rats of various ages. *J. Biol. Chem.,* 243:4526–4529.

99. Smith, C. M., Bryla, J., and Williamson, J. R. (1974): Regulation of mitochondrial α-ketoglutarate metabolism by product inhibition of α-ketoglutarate dehydrogenase. *J. Biol. Chem.,* 249:1497–1505.

100. Smith, C. M., and Williamson, J. R. (1971): Inhibition of citrate synthase by succinyl CoA and other metabolites. *FEBS Lett.,* 18:35–38.

101. Stanley, K. K., and Tubbs, P. K. (1974): The occurrence of intermediates in mitochondrial fatty acid oxidation. *FEBS Lett.,* 39:325–328.

102. Stucki, J. W., and Ineichen, E. A. (1974): Energy dissipation by calcium recycling and the efficiency of calcium transport in rat liver mitochondria. *Eur. J. Biochem.,* 48:365–375.

103. Tate, E. L., and Herbener, G. H. (1976): A morphometric study of the density of mitochondrial cristae in heart and liver of aging mice. *J. Gerontol.,* 31:129–134.

104. Travis, D. F., and Travis, A. (1972): Ultrastructural changes in the left ventricular rat myocardial cells with age. *J. Ultrastruct. Res.,* 39:124–148.

105. Wakil, S. J. (1970): Fatty acid metabolism. In: *Lipid Metabolism,* edited by S. J. Wakil, pp. 1–49. Academic Press, New York.

106. Walsh, D. A., and Krebs, E. G. (1973): Protein kinases. *Enzymes,* 8A:555–581.

107. Weisfeldt, M. L., Loeven, W. A., and Shock, N. W. (1971): Resting

and active mechanical properties of trabeculae carneae from aged male rats. *Am. J. Physiol.,* 220:1921–1927.

108. Williamson, J. R. (1964): Metabolic effects of epinephrine in the isolated, perfused rat heart. I. Dissociation of the glycogenolytic from the metabolic stimulatory effect. *J. Biol. Chem.,* 239:2721–2728.

109. Williamson, J. R. (1965): Glycolytic control mechanisms. I. Inhibition of glycolysis by acetate and pyruvate in the isolated perfused rat heart. *J. Biol. Chem.,* 240:2308–2321.

110. Williamson, J. R. (1966): Glycolytic control mechanisms. II. Kinetics of intermediate changes during the aerobic–anoxic transition in perfused rat heart. *J. Biol. Chem.,* 241:5026–5036.

111. Williamson, J. R. (1979): Mitochondrial function in the heart. *Annu. Rev. Physiol.,* 41:485–506.

112. Wilson, D. F., Owen, C. S., and Holian, A. (1977): Control of mitochondrial respiration: A quantitative evaluation of the roles of cytochrome *c* and oxygen. *Arch. Biochem. Biophys.,* 182:749–762.

113. Wilson, P. D. (1980): Enzyme levels in animals of various ages. In: *CRC Handbook Series in Aging, Sect. D, Vol. 1,* edited by J. R. Florini. CRC Press, Boca Raton, Florida *(in press).*

114. Wilson, P. D., and Franks, L. M. (1975): The effect of age on mitochondrial ultrastructure. *Gerontologia,* 21:81–94.

115. Wittels, B., and Bressler, R. (1965): Lipid metabolism in the newborn heart. *J. Clin. Invest.,* 44:1639–1646.

The Aging Heart (Aging, Vol. 12),
edited by Myron L. Weisfeldt.
Raven Press, New York © 1980.

Chapter 4

Excitation–Contraction

Edward G. Lakatta

*Cardiovascular Section, Gerontology Research Center, National Institute on
Aging, Baltimore City Hospitals, Baltimore, Maryland 21224*

To determine if the age-associated alterations in myocardial
ultrastructure and metabolism delineated in the previous chapters
are of functional significance, it is necessary to examine the performance of cardiac muscle isolated from adult and aged animals.
The scope of this chapter will include a review of the experimental
studies that have compared functional aspects of cardiac muscle
isolated from adult and aged animals and an interpretation of
these data in the context of a general model of the excitation–
contraction (E-C) process. The majority of such investigation
to date has utilized the laboratory rat which is considered to
reach adulthood at 6 to 12 months of age and to be senescent
or aged at or after 25 months of age, at which time approximately
50% colony mortality occurs (41).

A General Model of the Excitation–Contraction–Relaxation Cycle

There are several detailed models of E-C coupling in cardiac
muscle (3,21,28,29,51,54), all of which share several common
features. A simplified version of such a model (Fig. 1) is useful
to integrate and interpret the age-related changes that have been

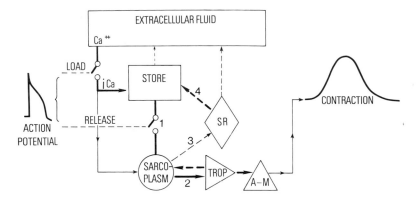

FIG. 1. Excitation–contraction–relaxation in cardiac muscle. See text for details. (Modified from Jewell, ref. 21.)

demonstrated in the excitation, contraction, and relaxation of cardiac muscle. In a resting muscle, the process begins with the initiation of action potential which excites the cell by eliciting the release of Ca^{2+} from a storage site (Store) into the sarcoplasm (step 1 in the model). Sarcoplasmic Ca^{2+} binds to troponin (Trop, step 2), a protein intimately associated with tropomyosin and actin, actin-myosin interaction occurs (A-M), and contraction ensues. The extent to which Trop binds Ca^{2+} regulates the degree of interaction of A-M and represents the "level of activation" of the contractile protein (in approximate terms, also referred to as inotropic or contractile state). Following excitation, the sarcoplasmic $[Ca^{2+}]$ falls as a result of sequestration by the sarcoplasmic reticulum (SR, step 3 in Fig. 1), Ca^{2+} disassociates from Trop, the A-M interaction ceases, and contractile force dissipates.

Activation and force production vary with the level of free Ca^{2+} surrounding the myofibrils as determined in single cardiac cells (9) or bundles of cells (4) from which the sarcolemma has been removed or disrupted (Fig. 2). It should be noted (Fig. 2A) that small alterations in pCa result in marked changes in relative force. Force production also requires adenosine triphosphate (ATP) and an ATPase that are intimately related to the myofilaments. Although the level of activation may vary with the number and/or affinity of Ca^{2+} binding sites, the acute experi-

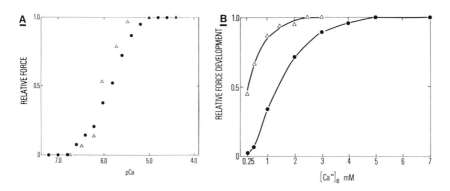

FIG. 2. A: Relative force in mechanically skinned single cardiac cells (△) (9) and in chemically skinned kitten cardiac cell bundles (●) (4) as a function of pCA. These curves were derived under similar but not identical conditions of temperature and ATP, and Mg²⁺ concentrations. **B:** Typical examples of relative force as a function of bathing fluid calcium concentration [Ca²⁺]ₑ in a right ventricular papillary muscle of a rat (△) and kitten (●) stimulated via field stimulation at a rate of 24 min⁻¹ at 29°C in Krebs-Ringer bicarbonate solution (28). Similar results were obtained for dT/dt. In each muscle when maximum force was achieved by elevation of [Ca]ₑ, neither paired stimulation nor isoproterenol (1 × 10⁻⁸ to 5 × 10⁻⁵ M) increased DT or dT/dt.

mental perturbations of the activation process in cardiac muscle with intact sarcolemmae, which will be discussed, appear to operate by effecting a change in the sarcoplasmic free [Ca²⁺] in response to excitation. This results from a change in Ca²⁺ release from the Store which can occur from either a change in the extent to which the Store is loaded and/or a change in the proportion of stored Ca²⁺ that is released. Loading of the Store is regulated by many factors including the slow inward current associated with each action potential, by electroneutral exchange with the extracellular space, and by exchange with other intracellular organelles, i.e., by transfer from the SR (step 4 in the model).[1]

---

[1] In the present scheme, the storage site may be considered to represent the terminal cisternae of the sarcoplasmic reticulum. In other models of E-C coupling (30) the storage site is depicted as a negatively charged mucopolysaccharide layer of the sarcolemma. In such a scheme, there is no intracellular recycling of Ca²⁺ from the relaxing apparatus to the release site, and the storage site is not loaded via slow inward current.

In muscles with intact sarcolemmae, the load of the Store is highly dependent on extracellular calcium concentration, $[Ca^{2+}]_e$, and force development (DT) and maximum rate of force development (dT/dt) vary with $[Ca^{2+}]_e$ as demonstrated in Fig. 2B. When the Store is loaded by increasing $[Ca^{2+}]_e$ to that level which produces maximal contraction, other perturbations that increase activation via enhanced loading of the Store (e.g., a change in the pattern of stimulation or exposure to catecholamines or cardiac glycosides) do not result in an appreciable increase in DT or dT/dt (E. G. Lakatta and H. A. Spurgeon, *in preparation;* 1,7, 10,17,34,35,45). It is noteworthy that in rat myocardium (Fig. 2B), DT and dT/dt are maximal at a $[Ca^{2+}]_e$ of 2.5 mM, and that 50% of maximal DT occurs in the rat at a $[Ca^{2+}]_e$ of less than 0.5 mM. In the absence of major differences in the pCa-force relationship (Fig. 2A) the species difference in Fig. 2B may be related to a difference in the capacity of the Store and/or its loading and release characteristics (8). The implications of the species difference noted in Fig. 2B are that (a) comparison of E-C coupling in the rat to other species should be made at similar levels of relative DT (and therefore similar loading conditions of the Store, in the context of the model in Fig. 1); and (b) perturbations that enhance DT in the intact rat cardiac muscle need to be studied with $[Ca^{2+}]_e$ at relatively low levels.

Action Potential and Excitation in Cardiac Muscle Isolated from Adult and Aged Rats

Studies in paced atria (6,38) and ventricular trabeculae (26) indicate that no significant differences occur in the transmembrane action potential when hearts from adult and senescent animals are compared. The parameters measured included resting membrane potential, maximum rate of rise, plateau duration, repolarization time, and effective electrical refractory period. These measurements were made in the absence of force production, at a single frequency of stimulation and a single $[Ca^{2+}]_e$, each of which significantly alter these actions potential parameters.[2] These experiments, although serving to characterize the transmembrane action potential as it may vary with age, do not provide information regarding possible age changes in the major functions of the action potential in terms of the model in Fig. 1: to excite the cell and to load the Ca^{2+} Store. The action potential, either as a result of depolarization itself, or as a result of a small rise in intracellular $[Ca^{2+}]$ secondary to the slow inward current, triggers the release of Ca^{2+} from the Store. In situations in which the Store is depleted of Ca^{2+}, e.g., following removal of Ca^{2+} from the bathing fluid, or in the presence of pharmacological and ionic inhibitors of slow inward current, the action potential persists on stimulation, but no contraction ensues. This results in electromechanical dissociation (EMD). It has been demonstrated in the rat that EMD can occur when a second stimulus is administered early in the contraction, usually during the rising phase of the twitch, without employing "zero" $[Ca^{2+}]_e$ or slow channel inhibitors (30). One reason why this is possible in the rat is that the action potential is of relatively short duration, and the cell is not electrically refractory at these early intervals.

Muscles isolated from hearts of senescent animals, when compared to those from hearts of adult animals fail to generate a mechanical response to very early premature stimuli (Fig. 3). This age difference is unlikely to be the result of an age difference in the electrical refractory period, as this is nearly identical under similar experimental conditions in both age groups (see Fig. 3 legend). However, the electrical and mechanical refractory peri-

---

[2] In guinea pig papillary muscles, contracting isometrically at optimal preload, the action potential duration is greater in muscles isolated from 36- to 40-month-old animals compared to those from 3- to 4-month-old animals. This 20 to 35% difference in action potential duration persisted over a simulation frequency range of 30 to 420 min^{-1} (40). It has not been ascertained, however, if the 3- to 4-month-old guinea pig is considered as adult or the 36- to 40-month-old animals can be considered senescent. The extreme difference in heart rate and heart weight may indicate that the 3- to 4-month-old guinea pig has not yet reached adult status. Significant changes in action potential configuration has been demonstrated in the rat when atria from animals of developmental age are compared to those of adult animals (38).

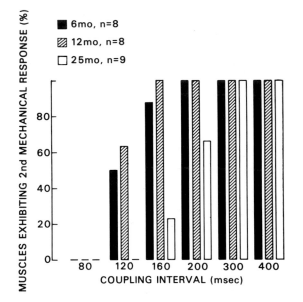

FIG. 3. Effect of age on the ability of muscles to respond to a second stimulus during paired pacing at varied coupling intervals. The muscles were maintained at the length at which DT was maximal, and were stimulated via plate electrodes at a rate of 24 min^{-1} at 29°C in Krebs-Ringer bicarbonate solution, with $[Ca^{2+}]_e$ of 1.0 mM and glucose of 16 mM. During the regular stimulation pattern premature stimuli were inserted at varying coupling intervals. As the coupling interval shortens, fewer muscles in the 25 month group exhibit a second mechanical response when compared to the other two age groups ($p < 0.01$ X^2). The electrical effective refractory period in other muscles under similar conditions was 83.3 ± 5.6 msec in the 6-month-old group ($n = 9$) and 86.5 ± 5.4 msec in the 25-month-old group ($n = 10$, N.S.). Failure of all muscles to respond at a coupling interval of 80 msec likely results from electrical refractoriness. (From Lakatta et al., ref. 26, with permission of the *Journal of Clinical Investigation.*)

ods, as a function of age, have not been measured simultaneously in the same muscle and under varying $[Ca^{2+}]_e$. Interpreted in terms of the E-C coupling model in Fig. 1, the apparent EMD results from an insufficient release of Ca^{2+} from the Store upon excitation. One possibility for the mechanical failure may result from insufficient time for replenishment of the Store by the relaxing apparatus (step 4). However, a reasonable alternative is that, although the cell is depolarized at early intervals, the early action potential is not effective in its ability to trigger the release of Ca^{2+} from the Store. The loading and trigger functions of the myocardial action potential may be intimately related. In the rat myocardium Ca^{2+} release from the internal Store can be induced by a small amount of Ca^{2+} (9) (which may be provided by the slow inward current). Perturbation of slow inward current (measured via voltage clamp technique) by increasing $[Ca^{2+}]_e$ or by the addition of catecholamines results in characteristic alterations in the plateau amplitude and duration of the simultaneously measured transmembrane action potential (37).

Similar changes can be demonstrated in rat cardiac muscle in response to these perturbations and are associated with a marked increase in DT (Fig. 4). Measurements of this type may be useful in characterizing the trigger and loading functions of the action potential in rat myocardium as they may vary with age, and may be particularly useful in elucidating the mechanism for the apparent EMD in muscles from senescent rats.

Contraction and Relaxation in Cardiac Muscle from Adult and Aged Rats

Contraction and relaxation have been studied as a function of age and to some extent can be interpreted in the context of the model in Fig. 1. Various parameters of contraction have been correlated to the activity of an ATPase associated with the contractile proteins (2,16,18,44,47). It has been reported that the activity of cardiac A-M ATPase at varying concentrations of CA^{2+}, ATP, K^+, and myofibrillar ATPase are diminished with age from 100 to 1,000 days in the Simonsen strain rat (2). While peak isometric force was unaltered with age in columnae carneae from these hearts, an age-related progressive decline in shortening velocity at light loads was observed. The age-dependent decrease in isotonic velocity and extent of shortening, especially at light preloads and a decline in myosin B ATPase activity has been confirmed over the range of 3 to 12 months of age (16). Since

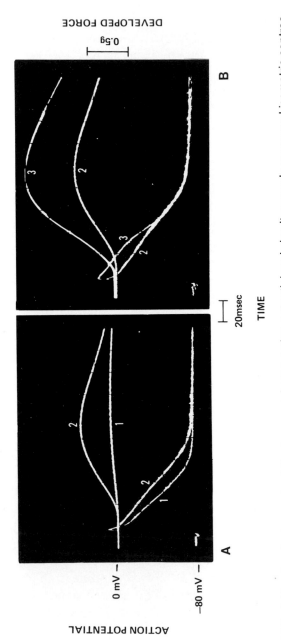

FIG. 4. Unretouched records of the transmembrane action potential and simultaneously measured isometric contraction in a rat right ventricular papillary muscle (28). **A:** (1) Action potential and force of contraction in $[Ca^{2+}]_e$ of 0.20mM, at 29°C, stimulated at 24 min^{-1}. (2) Action potential and force at a new steady state during infusion of Isoproterenol (1×10^{-6}M). **B:** (2) as in **A**; (3) A new steady state after an increase in $[Ca^{2+}]_e$ to 2.5 mM in the presence of isoproterenol. The microelectrode remained impaled in a single cell throughout the experiment. (From Lakatta and Spurgeon, *in preparation*.)

ATPase activity appears to be linked to the activation process, these data may indicate that the extent of activation diminished with age. However, myofibrillar ATPase activity measured in rat hearts from animals 4 to 6 and 20 months old showed no age dependency (19).[3] Further characterization of cardiac myofibrillar, A-M, and myosin ATPase activity, and their functional correlates in adult and aged rats of a single species strain would likely clarify this apparent discrepancy.

Another approach toward characterizing the activation process in adult and aged myocardium is to compare the change in the force of contraction over a range of loading levels of the Store by modification of $[Ca^{2+}]_e$. When $[Ca^{2+}]_e$ is increased from 0.5 to 2.5 mM (that at which contraction in rat cardiac muscle is maximal) in trabeculae from adult and aged hearts, there is no age difference in the increase in DT (25). In addition, at all $[Ca^{2+}]_e$ from 0.5 to 2.5 mM the absolute DT is not age related. The response of dT/dt to a change in $[Ca^{2+}]_e$ is also not age related (Fig. 5).

Another method potentiating the force of contraction is to alter the rate and/or pattern of stimulation at a given $[Ca^{2+}]_e$. The latter has been performed as continual paired stimulation in adult and aged myocardium. Figure 6 demonstrates that there is no age difference in the potentiation of dT/dt over a wide range of pairing intervals. Similar results were obtained in the response of DT.

Since paired stimulation or a change in $[Ca^{2+}]_e$ would not be expected to modify the purely passive properties of muscle (*vide infra*), the change in DT and dT/dt in response to these perturbations likely reflects a change in the extent of activation. That no age difference in the change of DT or dT/dt occurs in response to these interventions and that the absolute value of DT and dT/dt at all levels of potentiation is not age related may be inter-

---

[3] In dog myocardium, myosin ATPase is unaltered over the age range of 2 months to 10 years (32); myosin ATPase, measured in hearts of humans aged 6 to 90 does not vary with age (33).

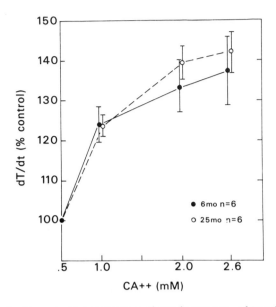

FIG. 5. Effect of age on the response of maximum rate of tension development (dT/dt) to increasing concentration of $[Ca^{2+}]_e$. Means ± SE are shown; n = number of rats tested. Control dT/dt at Ca 0.5 mM was 21.2 ± 2.4 g/mm²/sec in the 6-month-old group and 22.0 ± 3.1 g/mm²/sec in the 25-month age group. (From Lakatta et al., ref. 25, with permission of the American Heart Association.)

preted to indicate that the activation process or contractility is unaltered in aged myocardium. Both alterations in $[Ca^{2+}]_e$ and paired stimulation are gross perturbations of the entire E-C system, and the effects on DT or dT/dt represent a net effect of responses in many parameters that are depicted in the scheme in Fig. 1. Additional studies designed to measure a specific component of the model are needed to determine to what extent, if any, those individual components may be altered in hearts from animals of advanced age.

Pharmacologic intervention may provide some additional information on the effect of advanced age on various components of the activation process. Two such agents, ouabain and catecholamines, have been investigated in cardiac muscle isolated from adult and aged rats. Figure 7 demonstrates the response to incremental concentrations of norepinephrine and indicates that the change in dT/dt induced by this agent is greater in myocardium of adult compared to that of aged animals. Similar results were obtained for DT (25). An age difference was also found after a single high concentration of isoproterenol a relatively pure beta agonist (25). The response of dT/dt to ouabain is also markedly reduced in muscles from aged hearts compared to those from young hearts as indicated in Fig. 8. Similar results were obtained for DT and total tension.

In terms of the model in Fig. 1, both catecholamines and ouabain enhance DT and dT/dt via increased loading of the calcium Store resulting in an increase in the extent of activation upon stimulation. Figures 5 and 6 indicate that no age difference in DT or dT/dt is observed when activation is enhanced by increased loading to similar or greater extent by changes in $[Ca^{2+}]_e$ or

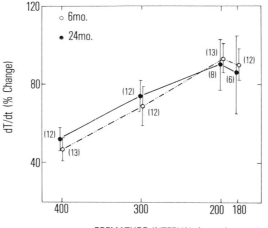

PREMATURE INTERVAL (msec.)

FIG. 6. The effect of age on the potentiation of dT/dt in response to paired stimulation at varying premature intervals. Means ± SE are shown; n = number of muscles tested. Temperature and stimulation pattern and muscle length are identical to those in Fig. 3; $[Ca^{2+}]_e = 0.25$mM. Control values for dT/dt were not different between age groups. (Redrawn from Gerstenblith et al., ref. 13.)

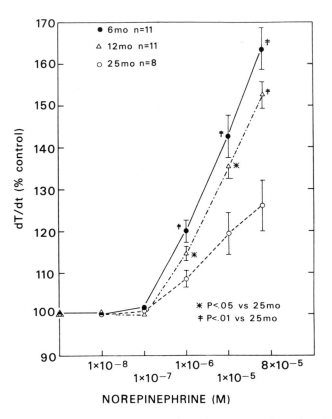

FIG. 7. Effect of age on the response of maximum rate of tension development (dT/dt) to increasing concentrations of norepinephrine. Means ± SE are shown; n = number of rats tested. Control values of dT/dt at a $[Ca^{2+}]_e$ of 1.0 mM were 33 ± 3, 35 ± 2, and 34 ± 4 g/mm²/sec respectively in the 6-, 12-, and 25-month groups. (From Lakatta et al., ref. 25, by permission of the American Heart Association.)

paired stimulation. These data may be interpreted to indicate that the age difference in response to ouabain and catecholamines results from an age difference in the mechanisms by which the Store is loaded. Both agents are mediated via protein receptor binding at the sarcolemmal surface and require intermediate steps which link receptor binding and increased Ca^{2+} loading of the Stores. Additional studies investigating the purported mechanisms of enhanced Ca^{2+} transport into the cell by these agents may identify age-related changes in these systems in the myocardium.

The perturbation of the E-C process discussed thus far have been performed at a single resting muscle length, L_{max}, or that length at which DT and dT/dt are maximal. The length–developed tension relationship at a single $[Ca^{2+}]_e$ is not significantly different in cardiac muscle isolated from adult and aged animals (Fig. 9). As a change in muscle length not only alters the geometrical relationship of the myofilaments, but also alters activation as well (21,27), it would be of interest to compare the length–tension relationship in muscles from adult and aged animals at varying levels of activation, e.g., at widely varying $[Ca^{2+}]_e$ (Fig. 10). Interventions that modify the loading of the Store might

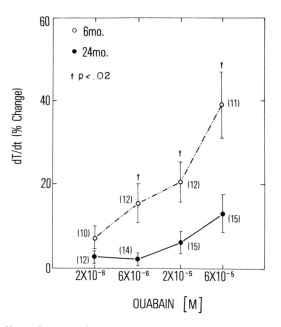

FIG. 8. The effect of age on the response of dT/dt to incremental concentrations of ouabain. Conditions and control values are as in Fig. 6. (Redrawn from Gerstenblith et al., ref. 13.)

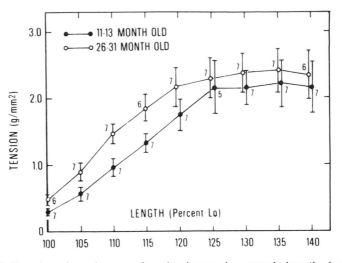

FIG. 9. Developed tension as a function increasing muscle lengths in trabe-culae carneae from (●) 11- to 13- and (○) 26- to 31-month-old rats. Values are means ± SE. Tension is expressed per unit cross-sectional area. Num-bers next to points are number of muscles. Lo is shortest length at which a distinct resting tension was noted. The muscles were stimulated at a rate of 3 min $^{-1}$, at 29°C, in $[Ca]_e$ of 2.5 mM. (From Weisfeldt et al., ref. 52, by permission of the American Physiological Society.)

be compared over a range of resting lengths, as the relative effec-tiveness of the perturbations is highly length dependent (Fig. 10C).

In the preceding discussion, DT and dT/dt and changes in these parameters after various perturbations have been used to make inferences regarding the activation process. Measurements of these parameters, however, are also influenced by viscoelastic properties of the muscle. It is conceivable that in myocardium from aged animals, alteration in viscoelastic properties may mod-ify the expression of the activation process as measured by the parameters of the twitch. In classical muscle mechanics, viscoelas-tic properties of muscle have been depicted in analog models as passive (inert) springs. Perturbations such as quick stretch or quick release were employed to deduce information about these inert (passive) properties and to distinguish these properties from

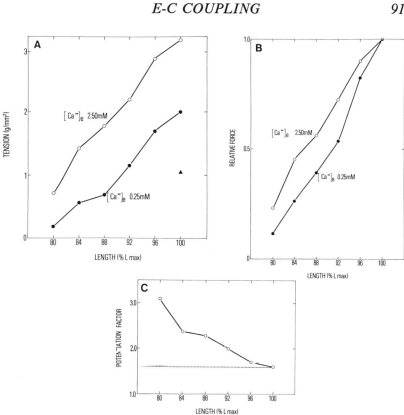

FIG. 10. A: Developed tension as a function of resting muscle length in a rat right ventricular papillary muscle, at 29°C, stimulated to contract at 24 min^{-1} (28). (○) [Ca]$_e$ 2.5 mM; (●) [Ca^{2+}]$_e$ 0.25 mM. Resting force at L$_{max}$ (▲) that length at which DT is optimal, is not altered by a change in [Ca^{2+}]$_e$. **B:** Data in **A** normalized to compare relative force at each [Ca]$^{2+}_e$ as a function of muscle length. **C:** Data in **A** expressed as the ratio $\dfrac{\text{DT in [Ca}^{2+}]_e \text{ 2.5mM}}{\text{DT in [Ca]}_e \text{ 0.25 mM}}$ at each muscle length. This ratio is designated as the potentiation factor. If the potentiation factor were equal at all lengths, the data would fall on the dotted line which is the response at L$_{max}$.

those of the contractile element (active properties). Interpretation of results utilizing these techniques is clouded by the fact that they both interfere with the activation process and the parameters which they measure do not appear to behave like purely passive materials (43).

Various other techniques including measurements of resting tension, stress relaxation, and dynamic stiffness have been employed to deduce information regarding age changes in viscoelastic properties of muscles. Muscles from senescent hearts exhibit less stress relaxation when compared to those from adult hearts (52), while resting tension is increased or unaltered as a function of age depending on the experiment (25,26,46,52). It is not certain, though, to what extent the information from these measurements in resting muscle can be extrapolated to the contraction phase. In addition, there is some evidence that suggests that resting tension and stress relaxation may also be intimately associated with crossbridge activation (5,42).

Dynamic stiffness (R), as defined as the change in stress to response to small sinusodial changes in length, has been measured in muscles both at rest and during contraction (31,46,49). During contraction and relaxation, R is increased in cardiac muscles from senescent compared to those from adult animals (46). R is a linear function of force ($R = AF + B$), where F is force and A and B are the stiffness coefficients. Table 1 indicates an age-related change in stiffness coefficient A. The recent evidence suggesting that a major portion of true stiffness of muscle resides

TABLE 1. *Active contraction and relaxation stiffness–force coefficients[a]*
($R = AF + B$) for male rats at L_{max}, 30 Hz

	Adult	Senescent	Age difference, *p*
Contraction			
n	6	9	
A	1.16 ± 0.03	1.77 ± 0.15	$p < 0.002$
B	5.99 ± 0.9	3.39 ± 0.7	NS
Relaxation			
n	6	9	
A	1.69 ± 0.06	2.2 ± 0.17	$p < 0.014$
B	3.85 ± 0.78	1.93 ± 0.97	NS

[a] The correlation coefficient (R) of active force versus active stiffness during contraction ranged from 0.97 to 0.99. Muscles were studied at 29°C in Krebs-Ringer bicarbonate solution, with $[Ca]_e$ of 2.5 mM.
Modified from Spurgeon et al. (46).

in the crossbridge itself (20,39,43) and the observation that R significantly increases during contraction may indicate an intimate association between this measurement and the activation process. The information realized from measurements of R during contraction, therefore, does not distinguish the purely passive properties of the muscle from those related to activation per se. Since purely passive properties during contraction cannot be measured separately from the activation process, it cannot be determined to what extent, if any, an age difference in purely passive properties modifies the expression of the activation process in measurements of DT and dT/dt. Simultaneous measurements of the twitch and extent of sarcomere shortening and velocity in muscles from adult and aged animals may provide information to clarify this issue. Age comparison of the parameters of an isometric twitch might also be made in purely isometric preparations, since excessive internal shortening, which is related to the damaged ends of the preparation, modify both the force and stiffness characteristics (24). However, in order to attribute age differences in the twitch to damaged ends of the preparation, an age difference in the extent of damage need pertain, and this possibility seems remote.

Relaxation

It has been demonstrated that contraction duration, both the time to peak tension and relaxation and/or half relaxation time ($RT_{1/2}$), is prolonged in cardiac muscle from aged rats, when compared to muscles from adult animals.[4] This has been demonstrated over a range of muscle lengths (2), $[Ca^{2+}]_e$, and frequencies stimulation (11,13,25,52) and is not dependent on an age differ-

---

[4] Prolongation of various phases of the isometric twitch has also been noted in aged rabbit (12) and dog (50) hearts. Age differences in time to peak tension and relaxation time have been demonstrated over a wide range of stimulation frequencies in the guinea pig papillary muscles (see footnote 2). Also indirect assessment of isometric relaxation in man demonstrates significant prolongation in normal healthy men (15).

ence in tissue catecholamine content (26). Interpreted in the context of the model in Fig. 1, contraction duration is related to the duration of activation. In order for force to dissipate, the A-M interaction must terminate. This requires that the sarcoplasmic [Ca^{2+}] be lowered by the relaxing apparatus (SR in Fig. 1). It is apparent that in those muscles in which it has been studied, the decline in myoplasmic free [Ca^{2+}] begins very early in the twitch, about the time of peak dT/dt (14,48). Thus, an alteration in the properties of Ca^{2+} sinks may alter both time to peak tension as well as $RT_{1/2}$.

The rate of Ca^{2+} accumulation in SR has been measured in microsomal preparations isolated from hearts of young adult and aged rats (Fig. 11). The data indicate that over a range of [Ca^{2+}] the velocity of Ca^{2+} accumulation is greater in SR from hearts

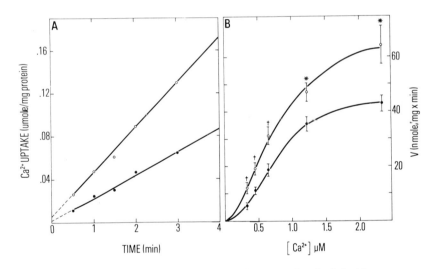

FIG. 11. Ca^{2+} accumulation in microsomal preparation isolated from young adult and aged rat hearts. **A:** Ca^{2+} uptake vs. time in microsomes from single hearts of a (○) 6-month and (●) 25-month-old rat. **B:** The velocity of Ca^{2+} accumulation over a range of Ca^{2+} concentrations was derived for each heart from a plot as in **A.** Each point is the mean ± SE of 11 preparations. *, $p < 0.02$; †, $p < 0.01$. (Redrawn from Froehlich et al., ref. 8.)

of adult animals compared to that from hearts of aged animals. One possible mechanism for the prolonged twitch in the aged muscle may relate to this age-associated decline in the velocity of Ca^{2+} accumulation. It should be noted, however, that the velocities of Ca^{2+} in Fig. 11 are steady state measurements and are several fold lower than the theoretical velocities required to effect relaxation of the twitch (23,53). An age difference in measurements of the rapid transient kinetics of Ca^{2+} accumulation would add additional support to the hypothesis that prolonged contraction in aged myocardium is related to an age alteration in Ca^{2+} accumulation by the SR. In addition, measurement of the dissociation rate of Ca^{2+}-troponin in adult and aged myocardium would be needed to solidify the hypothesis. Currently no such measurements in cardiac muscle are available.

In contracting muscles, age-related differences in SR function may become manifest under experimental conditions designed to stress SR function. A situation that provides a stress for the intracellular Ca^{2+} sinks occurs during recovery from exposure to hypoxia. During this time, depending on the conditions of the experiment, contraction duration is prolonged greatly in excess of control, and this is followed by a gradual return to control levels. As indicated in Fig. 12, this overshoot in the duration of contraction is significantly greater in and persists for a longer time in myocardium from aged compared to that from adult animals.

An additional method of stressing the capabilities of the SR is the experiment in Fig. 3. According to the model in Fig. 1, the mechanical response to a second stimulus delivered at short coupling intervals is dependent on Ca^{2+} transfer from the SR to the Store for subsequent release (Fig. 1, step 4). A delay in Ca^{2+} accumulation by the SR may alter the transfer of Ca^{2+} to the Store, and could be linked to the age related EMD *(vide supra)*.

Factors in addition to SR function may influence contraction duration. Excessive shortening during an isometric contraction may shorten contraction duration (22). If the extent of internal

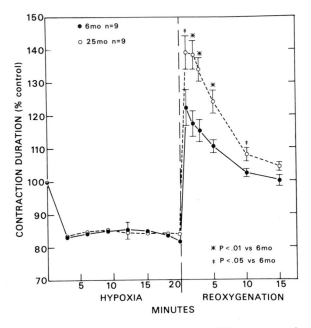

FIG. 12. Effect of age on contraction duration (CD) expressed as percent control hypoxia and reoxygenation. During reoxygenation, the CD overshoot above baseline is greater in the aged myocardium. Muscles were studied at L_{max} while stimulated at 24 mm^{-1} at 29°C in Krebs-Ringer bicarbonate solution $[Ca^{2+}]_e = 1.0$ mM. Mean control values for CD were 254.2 msec in the 6-month-old group and 282 msec in the 25-month-old group. Control DT and dT/dt were not age related. (From Lakatta et al., ref. 26, with permission of the *Journal of Clinical Investigation.*)

shortening during the twitch is less in aged compared to that in adult myocardium, contraction in the aged muscle may appear relatively prolonged. This can be tested by measurements of internal shortening during the twitch in both age groups. Contraction duration may also be affected by an alteration in purely passive elements in the muscle. However, complex models would be required to explain the age difference in contraction duration since simple alteration in series compliance have not altered the twitch in a manner to that found in aged muscle (36).

SUMMARY

It is evident that in some aspects of muscle contraction, hearts of senescent animals are similar to those of adults, while in others there is an age-associated alteration. I have attempted to interpret these similarities and differences in terms of a general model of the E-C coupling process. It should be recognized that neither the model nor the interpretations of the literature on aging in the context of such a model are definitive but rather serve to organize concepts and stimulate further research. In order for age differences in properties of the various components of such a model to be more fully characterized, additional and more precisely focused experiments must be implemented. Some of these are currently technically feasible, as I have indicated in the preceding discussion, while others have not as yet been performed in cardiac or any other muscle. Precise elucidation of the mechanisms responsible for age-associated changes which can consistently be demonstrated will undoubtedly be useful to our understanding of the E-C coupling process in muscle per se.

REFERENCES

1. Allen, D. G., Jewell, B. R., and Wood, E. H. (1976): Studies of the contractility of mammalian myocardium at low rates of stimulation. *J. Physiol.*, 254:1–17.
2. Alpert, N. R., Gale, H. H., and Taylor N. (1967): The effect of age on contractile protein ATPase activity and the velocity of shortening. In: *Factors Influencing Myocardial Contractility,* edited by R. D. Tanz, F. Kavaler, and J. Roberts, pp. 127–133. Academic Press, New York.
3. Bassingthwaighte, J. B., and Reuter, H. (1972): Calcium movements and excitation–contraction coupling in cardiac cells. In: *Electrical Phenomena in the Heart,* edited by W. C. DeMello, pp. 353–395. Academic Press, New York.
4. Brandt, P. W., and Hibberd, M. G. (1976): Effect of temperature on the pCa-tension relaxation of skinned ventricular muscle of the cat. *J. Physiol.,* 258:76P–77P.
5. Butler, T. M., Siegman, M. J., and Davis, R. E. (1976): Rigor and resistance

to stretch in vertebrate smooth muscle. *Am. J. Physiol.*, 231(5):1509–1514.

6. Cavoto, F. V., Kelliher, G. J., and Roberts, J. (1974): Electrophysiological changes in the rat atrium with age. *Am. J. Physiol.*, 226:1293–1297.

7. Dhalla, N. S., and Braxton, A. (1968): Influence of some inhibitors and ions on the positive inotropic action of epinephrine, tyramine and calcium. *J. Pharmacol. Exp. Ther.*, 161:238–246.

8. Fabiato, A., and Fabiato, F. (1973): Activation of skinned cardiac cells: subcellular effects of cardioactive drugs. *Eur. J. Cardiol.*, 1/2:143–155.

9. Fabiato, A., and Fabiato, F. (1975): Contraction induced by a calcium-triggered release of calcium from the sarcoplasmic reticulum of single skinned cardiac cells. *J. Physiol.*, 249:469–495.

10. Forester, G. V., and Mainwood G. W. (1974): Interval dependent inotropic effects in the rat myocardium and the effect of calcium. *Pfluegers Arch.*, 352:189–196.

11. Froehlich, J. P., Lakatta, E. G., Beard, E., Spurgeon, H. A., Weisfeldt, M. L., and Gerstenblith, G. (1978): Studies of sarcoplasmic reticulum function and contraction duration in young adult and aged rat myocardium. *J. Mol. Cell. Cardiol.*, 10:427–438.

12. Frolkis, V. V., Berzrukov, V. V., and Shevchuk, V. G. (1975): Hemodynamics and its regulation in old age. *Exp. Gerontol.*, 10:251–271.

13. Gerstenblith, G., Spurgeon, H. A., Froehlich, J. P., Weisfeldt, M. L., and Lakatta, E. G. (1979): Diminished inotropic responsiveness to ouabain in aged rat myocardium. *Circ. Res.*, 44:517–523.

14. Gordon, A. M., and Ridgeway, E. B. (1976): Length-dependent electromechanical coupling in single muscle fibers. *J. Gen. Physiol.*, 68:653–669.

15. Harrison, T. R., Dixon, K., Russell, R. O., Jr., Bidwai, P. S., and Coleman, H. N. (1964): The relation of age to the duration of contraction, ejection, and relaxation of the normal human heart. *Am. Heart J.*, 67:189–199.

16. Heller, L. J., and Whitehorn, W. V. (1972): Age-associated alterations in myocardial contractile properties. *Am. J. Physiol.*, 222:1613–1619.

17. Henderson, A. H., Brutsaert, D. L., Forman, R., and Sonnenblick, E. H. (1974): Influence of caffeine on force development and force-frequency relations in cat and rat heart muscle. *Cardiovasc. Res.*, 8:162–172.

18. Henry, P. D., Ahumada, G. G., Friedman, W. F., and Sobel, B. E. (1972): Simultaneously measured isometric tension and ATP hydrolysis in glycerinated fibers from normal and hypertrophied rabbit heart. *Circ. Res.*, 31:740–749.

19. Honorati, M. C., and Ermini, M. (1974): Myofibrillar and mitochondrial ATPase activity of red, white, diaphragmatic and cardiac muscle of young and old rats. *Experientia*, 30:215–216.

20. Housman, Ph. R., and Brutsaert, D. L. (1976): Three-step yielding of load-clamped mammalian cardiac muscle. *Nature*, 262:56–58.

21. Jewell, B. R. (1977): A reexamination of the influence of muscle length on myocardium performance. *Circ. Res.*, 40:221–230.

22. Jewell, B. R., and Wilkie, D. R. (1960): The mechanical properties of relaxing muscle. *J. Physiol.*, 152:30–47.

23. Katz, A. M., and Repke, D. I. (1967): Quantitative aspects of dog cardiac microsomal calcium binding and calcium uptake. *Circ. Res.*, 21:153–162.

24. Krueger, J. W., and Pollack, G. H. (1975): Myocardial sarcomere dynamics during isometric contractions. *J. Physiol.,* 251:627–643.

25. Lakatta, E. G., Gerstenblith, G., Angell, C. S., Shock, N. W., and Weisfeldt, M. L. (1975): Diminished inotropic response of aged myocardium to catecholamines. *Circ. Res.,* 36:262–269.

26. Lakatta, E. G., Gerstenblith, G., Angell, C. S., Shock, N. W., and Weisfeldt, M. L. (1975): Prolonged contraction duration in aged myocardium. *J. Clin. Invest.,* 55:61–68.

27. Lakatta, E. G., and Henderson, A. H. (1977): Starling's law reactivated. *J. Mol. Cell. Cardiol.,* 9:347–351.

28. Langer, G. A., and Brady, A. J., editors (1974): *The Mammalian Myocardium,* Wiley, New York.

29. Langer, G. A., Frank, J. S., and Brady, A. J. (1976): The myocardium. In: *International Review of Physiology, Vol. 9: Cardiovascular Physiology II,* edited by A. C. Guyton and A. W. Cowley, pp. 191–237. University Park Press, Baltimore.

30. Lee, S. E., Mainwood, G. W., and Korecky, B. (1970): The electrical and mechanical response of rat papillary muscle to paired pulse stimulation. *Can. J. Physiol. Pharmacol.,* 48:216–225.

31. Loeffler, L., III, and Sagawa, K. (1975): A one-dimensional viscoelastic model of cat heart muscle studied by small length perturbations during isometric contraction. *Circ. Res.,* 36:498–512.

32. Luchi, R. J., Kritcher, E. M., and Thyrum, P. T. (1969): Reduced cardiac myosin adenosinetriphosphatase activity in dogs with spontaneously occurring heart failure. *Circ. Res.,* 24:513–519.

33. Malhotra, A., Bhan, A., and Scheuer, J. (1977): Biochemical characteristics of human cardiac myosin. *J. Mol. Cell. Cardiol.,* 9:73–80.

34. Masuoka, D. T., and Saunders, P. R. (1950): Positive inotropic action of ouabain on rat ventricle strips. *Proc. Soc. Exp. Biol. Med.,* 74:879–882.

35. Meijler, F. L. (1962): Staircase, rest contractions, and potentiation in the isolated rat heart. *Am. J. Physiol.,* 202:636–640.

36. Parmley, W. W., Chuck, L., Clark, S., and Matthews, A. (1973): Effects of added compliance on force–velocity relation calculated from isometric tension records. *Am. J. Physiol.,* 225:1271–1275.

37. Reuter, H. (1974): Exchange of calcium ions in the mammalian myocardium. Mechanisms and physiological significance. *Circ. Res.,* 34:599–605.

38. Roberts, J., and Goldberg, P. B. (1975): Changes in cardiac membranes as a function of age with particular emphasis on reactivity to drugs. In: *Advances in Experimental Medicine and Biology, Vol. 61: Explorations in Aging,* edited by V. J. Cristofalo, J. Roberts, and R. C. Adelman, pp. 119–148. Plenum Press, New York.

39. Rüegg, J. C., Kuhn, H. J., Herzig, J. W., and Dickhaus, H. (1975): Effect of calcium ions on force generation and elastic properties of briefly glycerinated muscle fibres. In: *Calcium Transport in Contraction and Secretion,* edited by E. Carafoli, F. Clementi, W. Drabikowski, and A. Margareth, pp. 547–554. North-Holland, Amsterdam.

40. Rumberger, E., and Timmermann, J. (1976): Age-changes of the force-

frequency-relationship and the duration of action potential of isolated papillary muscles of guinea pig. *Eur. J. Appl. Physiol.,* 35:277–284.

41. Schlettwein-Gsell, D. (1970): Survival curves of an old age rat colony. *Gerontologia,* 16:111–115.

42. Siegman, M. J., Butler, T. M., Mooers, S. U., and Davies, R. E. (1976): Calcium-dependent resistance to stretch and stress relaxation in resting smooth muscles. *Am. J. Physiol.,* 231:1501–1508.

43. Simmons, R. M., and Jewell, B. R. (1973): Mechanics and models of muscular contraction. In: *Recent Advances in Physiology,* edited by R. J. Linden, pp. 87–147. Longman, New York.

44. Solaro, R. J., Wise, R. M., Shiner, J. S., and Briggs, F. N. (1974): Calcium requirements of cardiac myofibrillar activation. *Circ. Res.,* 34:525–530.

45. Speirs, R. L. (1959): Potentiation of contractions after rest in the isolated rat ventricle preparation. *Nature,* 184:66–67.

46. Spurgeon, H. A., Thorne, P. R., Yin, F. C. P., Shock, N. W., and Weisfeldt, M. L. (1977): Increased dynamic stiffness of trabeculae carneae from senescent rats. *Am. J. Physiol.,* 232(4):H373–H380.

47. Takauji, M., and Honig, C. R. (1972): Shortening and ATPase activities of single cardiac fibrils of normal sarcomere length. *Am. J. Physiol.,* 222:1–9.

48. Taylor, S. R., Rudel, R., and Blinks, J. R. (1975): Calcium transients in amphibian muscle. *Fed. Proc.,* 34:1379–1381.

49. Templeton, G., Adcock, R., Willerson, J. T., Nardizzi, L., Wildenthal, K., and Mitchell, J. H. (1976): Relationships between resting tension and mechanical properties of papillary muscle. *Am. J. Physiol.,* 231:1679–1685.

50. Templeton, G. H., Willerson, J. T., Platt, M. R., and Weisfeldt, M. (1978): Contraction duration and diastolic stiffness in the aged canine left ventricle. In: *Recent Advances in Studies on Cardiac Structure and Metabolism, Vol. 11: Heart Function and Metabolism,* edited by T. Kobayashi, T. Sano, and N. S. Dhalla, pp. 169–173. University Park Press, Baltimore.

51. Van Winkle, W. B., and Schwartz, A. (1976): Ions and inotropy. *Annu. Rev. Physiol.,* 38:247–272.

52. Weisfeldt, M. L., Loeven, W. A., and Shock, N. W. (1971): Resting and active mechanical properties of trabeculae carneae from aged male rats. *Am. J. Physiol.,* 220:1921–1927.

53. Will, H., Blanch, J., Smeltan, G., and Wollenberger, A. (1976): A quench-flow kinetic investigation of calcium ion accumulation by isolated cardiac sarcoplasmic reticulum. Dependence of initial velocity on free calcium ion concentration and influence of preincubation with protein kinase, MgATP, and cyclic AMP. *Biochim. Biophys. Acta,* 449:295–303.

54. Wood, E. H., Heppner, R. L., and Weidmann, S. (1969): Inotropic effects of electric currents. I. Positive and negative effects of constant electric currents or current pulses applied during cardiac action potential. II. Hypothesis; calcium movement, excitation-contraction coupling and inotropic effects. *Circ. Res.* 24:409–445.

The Aging Heart (Aging, Vol. 12),
edited by Myron L. Weisfeldt.
Raven Press, New York © 1980.

Chapter 5

Nervous Control of the Heart and Cardiovascular System

James A. Joseph and B. T. Engel

Gerontology Research Center, National Institute on Aging, Baltimore City Hospitals, Baltimore, Maryland 21224

In this chapter we will review and summarize the literature concerning the possible relationships between age-related changes in the cardiovascular (CV) system and the central nervous system (CNS). It will be seen from this review that investigations which attempt to examine these putative contingencies must take into account at least three considerations: First, one must distinguish between the necessary and sufficient effects of central neural activity—i.e., evidence that a particular region in the CNS can influence CV function does not mean that it must be involved in normal function. Peripheral effects may be mediated by more than one system and, in fact, as a result of the considerable redundancy within the CNS, may be mediated by different systems under different conditions. A second consideration is that the CNS is necessarily highly plastic in its function. One of its (CNS) major functions is to modify peripheral performance on the basis of prior experience under related conditions. This rule of plasticity applies as strongly to autonomically mediated responses as it does to somatically mediated responses. Thus, as a result of maturation and experience, there are likely to be wide individual differences in the way specific CV effects are mediated in different subjects. Third, both the CV and the CN systems age, but at different rates with respect to one another. Even within the CNS different structures age differently. As an example, dopamine-stimulated adenyl cyclase activity has been shown to be lowered in the striata but not in the retinas of aged rats (12). Moreover, each system may make adaptations to limitations of the others. Consider that as a person grows older his ability to respond motorically, his pulmonary functional capacity, and his muscle mass all show decrements with age. Additionally, his CV system changes and his neuroendocrine and neurotransmitter functions show alterations. It becomes increasingly apparent, then, that investigations in which age-related changes are examined must consider both the within- and the between-system homeostatic adjustments that are taking place.

There are several lines of evidence that indicate that cardiac function per se is age dependent. Physiological indices of cardiac function have been extensively studied in the aged rat (e.g., ref. 28) and in the human (e.g., ref. 15). In a review by Roberts and Goldberg (24) it was pointed out that, to some extent, the heart of the senescent rat exhibits: (a) an increased stiffness, (b) an increased sensitivity to lidocaine, (c) an increase in myocardial lipofuscin, and (d) a decrease in cardiac output. A later review (10) has shown that in the resting state the duration of cardiac contraction and relaxation appears to be prolonged, peripheral vascular resistance is increased, cardiac output is lowered, and impedance to left ventricular exertion is greater in the aged rat and human. Moreover, these changes become maximized during physical stress such as exercise, wherein maximal heart rate, stroke volume, and arteriovenous oxygen differences are all lowered in the senescent organism (10). These findings are discussed in more detail elsewhere in this volume. Of more relevance to this discussion is the contribution that the nervous system may make toward mediating these changes. The importance of the nervous system in influencing and modulating cardiac function is very well known, but that this interaction may be particularly important in aging stems from at least three lines of evidence. First, catecholamine content of the heart decreases with increasing age (23) (from 1.27 μg/g at 1 month of age to 0.46 μg/g at 28 months of age, whole heart), suggesting that there may be a presynaptic deficit in catecholamine metabolism of the cardiac sympathetic nerves.

Second, the heart rate response to various maneuvers declines with age. Rothbaum et al. (25) studied the reflex increase in heart rate in response to a standard blood pressure rise elicited by phenylephrine. It was seen that the baroreceptor reflex was more reactive in mature (12-month-old) than old (24-month-old) Wistar rats. Similar findings have been reported in man by Gribbin et al (13), who found that baroreceptor sensitivity, defined as the change in heart period/change in systolic blood pressure following phenylephrine infusion, was lower in older individuals. They studied a group of 61 men and 20 women ranging in age from 19 to 66 years. None of their subjects was receiving antihypertensive medication at the time of the study although some of them were patients who had been referred because of high blood pressure. They also found that baroreflex sensitivity was lower in patients with higher blood pressures. Despite this apparent reduction in baroreceptor sensitivity with age, several clinical investigators have reported that older patients show evidence of "carotid sinus hypersensitivity." This "hypersensitivity" is characterized by bradycardia, sometimes to the point of asystole, and in some patients by hypotension. Clinical signs include dizziness and syncope (20,22,26). Although it is likely that this "hypersensitivity" is associated with complications of peripheral vascular disease (13,21), one cannot rule out the possibility of cerebral ischemia (27) or neural hyperactivity. It would be valuable to develop an animal model in which this phenomenon could be studied more fully. More recent evidence (17) has shown that in older individuals (50 to 59 versus 20 to 29 years of age) there was a general tendency for heart rate accelerations to decrease in magnitude during various phases of the Valsalva maneuver whether the individuals were sitting, standing, or in a supine position. For example, when tests were done in a sitting position the mean heart rate change from the start of the Valsalva maneuver to its completion was 34 beats/min for the old subjects and 40 beats/min for the young subjects. Other studies (e.g., ref. 11) have reported that there is a decline in the magnitude of bradycardia seen in aged subjects during breath holding with face immersion. Gooden et al. (11) have shown that subjects ranging in age from 35 to 45 years showed a maximum deceleration in heart rate of 20 beats/min while subjects 48 to 65 years of age showed a maximum heart rate fall of 5 beats/min at 20 sec after the start of face immersion.

A third line of evidence linking age-related changes in the CNS to changes in the CV system comes from studies which have shown that covariations between changes in respiratory activity and changes in heart rate—i.e., respiratory sinus arrhythmia—decline with age. Hellman and Stacy (15) studied two age groups of volunteer men (21 to 39, young; 40 to 65, old). Respiratory airflow and electrocardiogram (EKG) were measured. The EKG was amplified and routed to an R-wave detector which differentiated the signal and produced a 3-msec, 5-V pulse triggered by the EKG. The leading edge of the pulse occurred very early in the rising phase of the R wave. Instantaneous heart rate was determined by measurement of the time between pulses. The subjects were asked to couple their respiratory rate to a rhythm produced by a light that remained on for 6 cardiac cycles, and off for 6 cardiac cycles. A ratio was calculated of the amplitude of the instantaneous heart rate to the average heart rate over the respiratory cycle. This value was called PB.

Results showed that the mean PB for the younger group was 13.6 ± 4.55 (mean $\pm$ SD) while that of the older group was 5.0 ± 3.20, indicating a significant decline for the older subjects. When the data were subjected to linear regression analysis, it was seen that there was a continuous linear decrease of PB with age over the age range studied ($r = -0.83$). This trend showed little correlation with amount of exercise that an individual regularly engaged in, but did show some correlation with general clinical health as obtained by questionnaire data. Similar findings have been reported by Davies (5), who characterized these changes in terms of possible diminished autonomic reactivity of the vagus or of physical changes in the sinoatrial (SA) node. This conclusion is supported by Lev's findings (19). He showed that as subjects age, the SA node contains an increasing amount of connective tissue and fat and that the nodal (pacemaker) cells decrease in number and their shape becomes more irregular. Further research is needed to delineate the mechanisms underlying this phenomenon, both at the end-organ and at the presynaptic portion of the system, so that the possible morphological and physiological changes that occur with senescence may be determined. At present the exact mechanisms of these age changes is unclear. It may be, for example, due to alterations in sensory receptors, afferent nerves, portions of the CNS, efferent nerves, or even the end-organ autonomic receptors.

Probably the most extensive series of studies carried out to further investigate these putative, age-related pre- and postsynaptic changes of the CV-CN systems are those of Frolkis and his colleagues. In recent reviews Frolkis et al. (9) and Frolkis (8) summarized many years of extensive work using a variety of animal models, especially rabbits and rats. They have reported a number of systematic age differences in CV function and in the CV response to electrical square wave or chemical stimulation of many regions of the brain (9) using the following stimulus parameters: a frequency of 100 pulses/sec, a 1-sec pulse duration, a 1-msec pulse width; a 15- to 20-sec stimulus duration; and a 5- to 10- or 300- to 500-mamp current intensity. Stimulation was monopolar. Chemical stimulation with acetylcholine, epinephrine, norepinephrine, and atropine was accomplished by injecting 1-ng doses of these substances intracerebrally. The subjects were adult rabbits 10 to 14 and 48 to 54 (old) and rats 8 to 10 and 24 to 26 months of age, respectively. Both males and females were used.

The electrical stimulation of the various CNS structures showed that the excitability of the "hemodynamic centers" (9) changed differentially in senescence. Old rabbits developed threshold blood pressure (BP) reactions at higher current intensities than adult rabbits in the sensorimotor cortex, medial amygdaloid nucleus, lateral hypothalamus, and caudal part of the fourth ventricular floor when compared with adult animals. However, the piriform cortex, central amygdaloid nucleus, and anterior and posterior hypothalamus all showed decreases in threshold stimulation for pressor responses in old animals. In stimulating the anterior hypothalamus, for example, the maximal increase in BP was 130% in the adult and 90% in the old animal. It was 110 and 80% in the lateral hypothalamus and 100 and 60% in the posterior hypothalamus for adult and old animals, respectively. Systemic vascular resistance also showed differential changes during electrical stimulation of the brain (ESB) in the anterior, posterior, and lateral hypothalamus respectively (anterior, 540% young, 330% old; posterior, 400% young; 300% old; lateral, 200% young, 170% old). The pressor elements of the hippocampus, reticular nuclei of the pons, and tegmentum responded similarly in both age groups to ESB. Interestingly, when epinephrine or acetylcholine (1 ng) were injected into different brain structures, more pronounced BP shifts occurred in old animals, suggesting that, at least at these low doses, old animals may be showing actual increases in sensitivity to the direct application of these biogenic amines. At larger doses of these drugs the differences between the groups became less distinct. Similar findings have recently been obtained in our laboratory (16), where it was shown that rotational behavioral strength following lesions of the substantia nigra was similar in young and old rats with peripherally administered high doses (5 mg/kg) of apomorphine (a dopamine receptor agonist).

Frolkis and his colleagues also showed that there may be qualitative as well as quantitative differences in the CV responses to ESB in old animals. They showed that although both young and old animals responded with pressor responses at low-intensity hypothalamic ESB and pressor responses at high-intensity ESB, the senescent animals seemed to use a different mechanism to accomplish these hemodynamic changes. As an example, when ESB was applied to the anterior hypothalamus of adult animals, all pressor reactions were induced by increasing systemic vascular resistance and decreasing cardiac output, whereas in old animals the pressor shifts were accomplished by increasing cardiac output and decreasing systemic vascular resistance. Depressor responses in old animals, induced by increasing hypothalamic ESB, were more frequently characterized by decreased cardiac output than in young animals. Thus, there seem to be changes in response patterns as well as response sensitivity of CNS structures with senescence. These changes include: (a) loss of presynaptic effectiveness contributing to an altered postsynaptic receptor sensitivity, (b) some loss of function differentially in various CNS structures, and (c) qualitative changes in hemodynamic homeostatic adjustment following limbic stimulation. On the basis of their findings Frolkis et al. (9) concluded that "the irregular threshold changes in influences of various CNS structures on circulation can account for the finding that in old age shifts in circulation recorded during various motor and behavioral acts may be different in both size and duration."

Strikingly similar changes to those reported centrally were obtained with peripheral electrical and chemical stimulation by Frolkis et al. (9)—i.e., raised thresholds to bradycardia in the old rat with electrical stimulation of the vagus (young, 0.35 ± 0.04 V; old, 0.53 ± 0.04 V) and increased sensitivity to low doses of intravenously administered norepinephrine (0.05 μg/kg). Norepinephrine at this dose level produced increases in blood pressure, cardiac output, and stroke volume in the old rabbit but not in the young. These findings are, however, at variance with those of other investigators (29) who found that the heart rate in both senescent dogs and rats is less responsive to isoproterenol stimulation. Clearly, more work is needed to resolve these differences, but the importance of these studies is that without them it is impossible to know whether alterations in target organ behavior, in neural activity, or both, are responsible for any observed effects; as we have suggested, both are involved.

On the basis of this research, Frolkis (8) has proposed that the changes that are taking place in the autonomic nervous system and in the CNS structures which mediate its function create decreases in the organism's adaptive capacities, in the reliability of the homeostatic regulatory mechanisms, and in the ability of the organism to withstand disruption of its regulatory mechanisms. In other words, older individuals are less able to respond, or may respond inappropriately rather than effectively and efficiently, to a variety of challenges which variations in environmental conditions demand of them. This decline in adaptability is particularly evident in experiments in which attempts are made to relate behavioral manipulations to cardiovascular responses.

Cohen and Shmavonian (4) noted that comparisons between young and old subjects in studies of classically conditioned vasomotor responses show that older subjects (average age, 69 years) produce smaller conditioned responses than do younger subjects (average age, 20 years). This study consisted of pairing a 512-Hz tone (conditional stimulus; CS) with an electric shock (unconditional stimulus; UCS) to the finger and measuring changes in urinary output of catecholamines, electrical skin conductance, vasomotor tone, and respiration. The subjects were given 10 reinforcement trials (CS + UCS) and 10 extinction trials. Old subjects tended to show smaller skin conductance changes than young ones during both conditioning and extinction. Similar results were seen with vasomotor reactivity measured by photoelectric plethysmography. There was only minimal conditioning seen with both these measures. There is some indication, however, that these differences may be secondary to peripheral changes since there was evidence that the vessels of the aged were either vasoconstricted or arteriosclerotic. Furthermore, there is evidence that the aged subjects may have been more aroused than the young subjects initially. Baseline cortical beta wave density in the aged subjects was almost three times that of the young subjects, and that level was maintained throughout conditioning. Norepinephrine and epinephrine levels also were elevated at the start of the experiment.

One interpretation of these data (6) is that the aged response pattern includes a state of cortical activation and that this state exerts influences on lower centers. A second hypothesis is that hypothalamic degenerative changes in the aged may alter control functioning. The hypothesis set forth by the authors was that there is an inability of the vessels to react to autonomic or neuroendocrine excitatory influences. This latter suggestion, as we have seen from the Frolkis et al. (9) data (at least insofar as neuroendocrine excitation is concerned) is probably not true.

Studies of cardiac function also have reported smaller conditioned responses in older subjects. Lang et al. (18) reported that older subjects emitted smaller operantly conditioned heart rate responses than did younger subjects. The subjects were instructed to speed or slow their heart rates and were given feedback from an oscilloscope on which the R–R interval was displayed as a horizontal line. The word "good" was flashed on the screen when a subject performed correctly. While there was some indication that older subjects had lower baseline rates than younger subjects, the differences were not statistically significant [however, see Jose and Collison (15), who showed convincingly that intrinic heart rate—following vagal and β-adrenergic blockade—falls with age]. Older individuals did show less labile heart rate than their younger counterparts. For both speeding and slowing conditions the young subjects showed larger changes overall in heart period than aged subjects (young: speed 0.07 sec, average interpulse interval, slow 0.075 sec; old: 0.04 sec, 0.06 sec, respectively). However, it was shown that at least for slowing, the older subjects tended to perform as well as the younger subjects, especially during the late trials. This finding would suggest that it might be possible to modify deficits in CV functioning with proper training.

Further evidence for the importance of training comes from the "try" condition discussed by Lang et al. (18) in which the subjects were instructed to alter their heart rates without feedback. College students were superior to aged subjects, especially in speeding. The deficit, thus, may depend on the nature and the amount of feedback that is given. It would appear, then, that some deficits in behavior of normal aged subjects in tasks which integrate CV and CNS functioning may be highly dependent upon the experimental conditions under which the measurements are made.

To further illustrate this suggestion, consider the following study by Birren et al. (2). These investigators reported that there were significant differences in reaction time (RT) among young adults, depending on the phase of the cardiac cycle in which the imperative stimulus (the cue to press a button) was presented. Subsequently, Birren (1) reported that the effect was absent in older subjects. This procedure offered a useful model for testing age-related differences in CNS/cardiac interactions. However, two later studies (3,7) failed to replicate this effect or to show age differences. In the first of these experiments Botwinick and Thompson (3) showed that Birren's findings were highly dependent on the foreperiod or preparatory interval (PI)—that is, the duration of time between the warning signal and a stimulus calling for a response. As pointed out by Botwinick and Thompson (3), "the reaction time varies with the duration of the PI and any variation in the PI, however slight, if systematically linked with the different phases of the cardiac cycle, may result in spuriously high relationships between RT and cardiac phase." Their PI was 1.15 sec which began after a 0.5-sec warning signal (a 400-Hz tone). The stimulus (a 1,000-Hz tone) following the PI was begun by the subject's R wave and terminated by a finger lift response. Reaction time and EKG were recorded from each individual. The findings were that time from the R wave in the cardiac cycle was not a determiner of reaction time. It was suggested that exact control of the PI is necessary in RT-physiological relationship determinations.

Similar findings were reported by Engel et al. (7), who tried to systematically analyze the effects of age, sex, mode of responding, cardiac cycle phase, and breathing cycle phase on reaction time. The stimulus was presented during each of three phases of the cardiac cycle: (a) the P-R interval, (b) the occurrence of the R wave, and (c) the occurrence of the T wave and during two phases of the breathing cycle (inspiration or expiration). Again, there was no evidence that individuals or groups emitted RTs which were in any way determined by the electrical events of the cardiac cycle. Thus, experimental situational determinants can affect age differences.

This brings the discussion to an important question. Is it possible through experimental manipulations to reduce the deficits seen in some areas of cardiac function in aged subjects? We have some evidence that this may be possible from the study of Lang et al. (18) cited earlier, wherein it was shown that in the later training trials aged subjects slowed their hearts as well as young subjects. Moreover, the older individuals have present, at least to some degree, the neural facilities necessary for the application of instrumental conditioning to the CNS-CV control systems (6). Thus, an important topic for future research should be to determine the extent to which older individuals can learn to improve their function. Successful application of these techniques will utilize the large plastic capabilities of the nervous system so that a deficit in this system need not be translated into a functional behavioral deficit.

Other important topics for future research include: (a) characterizing more clearly the neural–cardiovascular deficits with senescence, (b) determining whether these deficits are neuroendocrine, electrical, or both in nature, (c) determining the extent to which the deficiencies can be reduced pharmacologically by using agents which can amplify or reduce various aspects of neuronal transmission. We believe that such investigations should not only attempt to characterize the deficits which one is likely to see in the older subject, but also help to determine if these deficits can be overcome. To summarize, then, it appears that with senescence there may be (a) intrinsic changes in the cardiovascular system itself; (b) changes within the postsynaptic element, e.g., loss of receptor sensitivity; and (c) changes in the threshold firing rates of central neurons coupled with some loss of the integrative functions of these systems as evidenced by the various behavioral studies reviewed.

SUMMARY

This chapter reviewed and summarized the literature concerning the possible relationships between age-related changes in the cardiovascular system and those of the central nervous system. The studies reviewed indicated that there are neural, receptor, and end-organ changes in these systems with senescence. Specifically, there appears to be decreased baroreflex sensitivity, decreased responsiveness to intracerebral electrical stimulation, and perhaps altered responsivity to centrally and peripherally administered α- and β-agonists. From available data it is at times difficult to distinguish which of these factors is most important in contributing to the CV changes seen in senescence. However, these changes are believed to have contributed to the reduced response sensitivity and subsequent response deficits which were clearly revealed during conditioning procedures that examined operantly conditioned heart rate responses in older subjects. The senescent individuals emitted smaller responses than younger subjects. However, it was suggested that through the manipulation of such factors as trial length, amount of feedback given, and trial number, some of the response deficits seen in older subjects could be overcome.

REFERENCES

1. Birren, J. E. (1965): Age changes in speed of behavior: Its central nature and physiological correlates. In: *Behavior, Aging, and the Nervous System,* edited by A. T. Welford and J. E. Birren, pp. 191–216. Charles C Thomas, Springfield, Illinois.
2. Birren, J. E., Cardon, P. V., Jr., and Phillips, S. L. (1963): Reaction time as a function of the cardiac cycle in young adults. *Science,* 140:195–196.
3. Botwinick, J., and Thompson, L. W. (1971): Cardiac functioning and reaction time in relation to age. *J. Genet. Psychol.,* 119:127–132.
4. Cohen, S. I., and Shmavonian, B. M. (1967): Catecholamines, vasomotor conditioning and aging. In: *Endocrines and Aging,* edited by L. Gittman, pp. 102–141. Charles C Thomas, Springfield, Illinois.
5. Davies, H. E. F. (1975): Respiratory change in heart rate, sinus arrhythmia in the elderly. *Gerontol. Clin.,* 17:96–100.

6. Engel, B. T., and Bleecker, E. R. (1974): Application of operant conditioning techniques to the control of the cardiac arrhythmias. In: *Cardiovascular Psychophysiology,* edited by P. A. Obrist, A. H. Black, J. Brener, and L. V. DiCara, pp. 456–476. Aldine, Chicago.

7. Engel, B. T., Thorne, P. R., and Quilter, R. E. (1972): On the relationships among sex, age, response mode, cardiac cycle phase, breathing cycle phase, and simple reaction time. *J. Gerontol.,* 27:456–460.

8. Frolkis, V. V. (1977): Aging of the autonomic nervous system. In: *Handbook of the Psychology of Aging,* edited by J. E. Birren and K. W. Schaie, pp. 177–189. Van Nostrand, New York.

9. Frolkis, V. V., Bezrukov, V. V., and Shevchuk, V. G. (1975): Hemodynamics and its regulation in old age. *Exp. Gerontol.,* 10:251–271.

10. Gerstenblith, G., Lakatta, E. G., and Weisfeldt, M. L. (1976): Age changes in myocardial function and exercise response. *Prog. Cardiovasc. Dis.,* 19:1–21.

11. Gooden, B. A., Holdstock, G., and Hampton, J. R. (1978): The magnitude of the bradycardia induced in patients convalescing from myocardial infarction. *Cardiovasc. Res.,* 12:239–242.

12. Govani, S., Loddo, P., Spano, P. F., and Trabucchi, M. (1977): Dopamine receptor sensitivity in brain and retina of rats during aging. *Brain Res.,* 138:565–569.

13. Gribbin, B., Pickering, T. G., Sleight, P., and Peto, R. (1971): Effect of age and high blood pressure on baroreflex sensitivity in man. *Circ. Res.,* 29:424–431.

14. Hellman, J. B., and Stacy, R. W. (1976): Variation of respiratory sinus arrhythmia with age. *J. Appl. Physiol.,* 41:734–738.

15. Jose, A. D., and Collison, D. (1970): The normal range and determinants of the intrinsic heart rate in man. *Cardiovasc. Res.,* 4:160–167.

16. Joseph, J. A., Berger, R., Engel, B. T., and Roth, G. (1978): Age related changes in the nigrostriatum: A behavioral and biochemical analysis. *J. Gerontol.,* 33:643–649.

17. Kalfleisch, J. H., Stowe, D. F., and Smith, J. J. (1978): Evaluation of the heart rate response to the Valsalva maneuver. *Am. Heart J.,* 45:707–715.

18. Lang, P. J., Troyer, W. G., Jr., Twentyman, C. T., and Gatchel, R. J. (1975): Differential effects of heart rate modification training on college students, older males, and patients with ischemic heart disease. *Psychosom. Med.,* 37:429–446.

19. Lev, M. (1954): Aging changes in the human sino-atrial node. *J. Gerontol.,* 9:1–9.

20. Levy, M. N., and Zieske, H. (1969): Autonomic control of cardiac pacemaker activity and atrioventricular transmission. *J. Appl. Physiol.,* 27:465–470.

21. Manikar, G. D., and Clark, A. N. G. (1975): Cardiac effects of carotid sinus massage in old age. *Age Ageing,* 4:86–94.

22. Ritch, A. E. S. (1975): The significance of carotid sinus hypersensitivity in the elderly. *Gerontol. Clin.,* 17:146–153.

23. Roberts, J., and Goldberg, P. B. (1975): Changes in cardiac membranes as a function of age with particular emphasis on reactivity to drugs. In: *Explorations in Aging, Vol. 61: Advances in Experimental Medicine and Biology,* edited by V. J. Cristofalo, J. Roberts, and R. C. Adelman, pp. 119–148. Plenum Press, New York.

24. Roberts, J., and Goldberg, P. B. (1976): Changes in basic cardiovascular activities during the lifetime of the rat. *Exp. Aging Res.,* 2:487–512.

25. Rothbaum, D. A., Shaw, D. J., Angell, C. S., and Shock, N. W. (1974): Cardiac performance in the unanesthetized senescent male rat. *J. Gerontol.,* 28:287–292.

26. Smiddy, J., Lewis, H. D., and Dunn, M. (1973): The effect of carotid massage in older men. *J. Gerontol.,* 27:209–211.

27. Uesu, C. T., Eisenman, J. I., and Stemmer, E. A. (1976): The problem of dizziness and syncope in old age: Transient ischemic attacks versus hypersensitive carotid sinus reflex. *J. Am. Geriatr. Soc.,* 24:126–135.

28. Vizek, M., and Albrecht, I. (1973): Development of cardiac output in male rats. *Physiol. Bohemoslov.,* 22:573–580.

29. Yin, F. C. P., Spurgeon, H. A., Greene, H. L., Lakatta, E. G., and Weisfeldt, M. L. (1979): Age-associated decrease in heart rate response to isoproterenol in dogs. *Mech. Ageing Dev.,* 10:17–25.

The Aging Heart (Aging, Vol. 12),
edited by Myron L. Weisfeldt.
Raven Press, New York © 1980.

Chapter 6

Coronary Vasculature of the Aging Heart

Robert J. Tomanek

*Department of Anatomy, College of Medicine, University of Iowa,
Iowa City, Iowa 52242*

The coronary circuit assumes special significance since the myocardium is continuously active and incapable of sustaining an oxygen debt. Clinically, myocardial perfusion has received considerable attention, since an estimated 675,000 patients die each year from ischemic heart disease and its complications (4). Considerable advances during the last decade have contributed to our understanding of coronary blood flow and its regulation. The use of radioactive inert gases and microspheres, cytochemical and biochemical techniques, and α- and β-receptor blocking drugs are some of the technical approaches which have contributed to our knowledge.

In spite of these advances, the processes which may limit the ability of the coronary vasculature adequately to perfuse the myocardium under varied conditions throughout the lifespan remains ill defined. At the same time, it is generally recognized that aging is a significant factor in myocardial performance and disease and that coronary artery disease is common during old age. Studies of humans, based primarily on histological assessment at necropsy, indicate some of the trends which accompany aging. The lack of a controlled environment and experimental design are some obvious limitations of these studies. Animal models have provided some basic insights and demonstrated certain changes which occur with aging in the absence of pathology.

In considering the normal developmental sequence of changes which constitute aging of the coronary vasculature, it is imperative to recognize both the limitations of available data and the conditions under which they were obtained. Absence of anatomical change does not necessarily negate a functional alteration, nor does normality under basal conditions preclude a decrement under enhanced functional demand. Also, the uniqueness of the coronary vasculature should be kept in mind so as to avoid generalizations regarding the peripheral circulation which is discussed in Chapter 7.

STRUCTURAL CHANGES IN CORONARY VESSELS

Ischemic heart disease is invariably associated with segmental atherosclerotic plaques in the coronary arteries. A review of studies pertaining to fatal ischemic heart disease indicates that in nearly every case at least one of the three major coronary arteries was narrowed by more than 75% (23). Middle-aged individuals have a high incidence of ischemic heart disease preceded by a relatively early development (second and third decades of life) of coronary artery lesions (16). Coronary arteriosclerosis and atherosclerosis have long been considered associated with aging; they may appear as early as the second decade (34) with a peak incidence in the sixth decade of life (31). Certainly not all lesions of the coronary arteries are known to lead to clinical manifestations, a fact which does not mitigate the possibility that morphological and biochemical changes occur during the aging process. The problem of distinguishing between changes which constitute aging and those which are age related is particularly difficult in studies on man, which are complicated by variations in diet, geography, occupation, and stress. However, the data from man when compared to that from animal models in controlled environments become more meaningful in the quest for elucidating aging events in the coronary vasculature.

Studies on Man

Race and sex are factors which influence the extent of coronary lesions and the mortality rates of ischemic heart disease. Age, however, as shown by Strong and McGill (25), is a factor which influences these parameters for each race-sex group. In this study the incidence and severity of atherosclerosis of coronary arteries in individuals aged 1 to 69 years was determined at the time of necropsy. The incidence by race-sex of the lesions, at all ages below 40 years was greatest in white males, lowest in white females, and intermediate for male and female Negroes. The authors concluded that after the age of 20, atherosclerosis is present to some degree in virtually all white males. A strong correlation between coronary atherosclerosis and ischemic heart disease was established. When the death rates from coronary artery disease of a specific race-sex group in the 45- to 54-year-old group were compared to the incidence and severity of coronary artery lesions in the corresponding race-sex group studied at necropsy, the risk of dying from ischemic heart disease for each of the four race-sex groups could be established. Thus, consistent with the incidence and severity of coronary lesions, mortality rates related to ischemic heart disease were highest in white males, lowest in white females, and intermediate for Negro males and females. Since the incidence and severity of atherosclerotic lesions in individuals aged 20 to 29 years demonstrated the same race-sex association, this data could be used to predict the mortality rates in the corresponding 45- to 54-year-old group.

Strong and McGill's study (25) also considered the progression of atherosclerotic plaques to complicated plaques in evaluating the development of the disease.[1] For each group the incidence

---

[1] Fatty streaks, which may be reversible, are characterized by numerous cells containing lipid in a minimal intimal thickening. The fatty streaks progress to fibrous plaques as lipid is released from the cells and incites an inflammatory response followed by deposition of collagen and some small elastic fibers. Clinically manifest disease occurs as hemorrhage within the plaque and thrombosis over the plaque reduce the size of the lumen. At this stage calcification is common and the plaque is a complicated lesion.

of fatty streaks increased at an early age (10 to 20 years), while fibrous plaques were most severe after 30 years of age in the group most prone to atherosclerosis, white males. Calcification, characteristic of complicated plaques, became evident in about 10% of the white males aged 50 to 60 years, but was extremely rare in the other groups until the seventh decade of life. It has been established that the extent (amount of vessel area involved) increases with age and is directly related to the frequency of coronary artery stenosis (28). In summary, these data suggest that age is a factor in the development of coronary atherosclerosis and that the latter is directly related to ischemic heart disease and mortality. While race and sex modify the incidences of these factors, the relationship between coronary artery disease, age, and ischemic heart disease mortality rates is evident within each race-sex group.

As fatty streaks progress with age they are manifest as raised lesions, but have a lower incidence and demonstrate a less severe atherosclerosis in women than in men (7). The protective effect of female sex hormones may be suggested by the fact that women have less extensive raised lesions than men at all ages until the seventh decade, at which time the percentage of the intimal surface involved with these lesions becomes similar. The significance of local factors in the coronary artery is implied by data showing that women have more fatty streaks in the abdominal aorta than men. Accordingly, it is imperative that data regarding aging and pathogenesis be viewed with regard to specific vessels or regional circulation.

Consistent with the evidence demonstrating a relatively early onset of changes in the coronary arteries are data which show a drop in the percent of elastic tissue and an increase in nonelastic tissue of the tunica media after the third decade of life (1). This shift in relative composition of the media appears to be related to the incidence of arteriosclerosis. While both the right and the anterior interventricular (a branch of the left coronary) arteries show this trend, the incidence is higher for the latter and supports the observation that arteriosclerosis is more frequent in the left than in the right coronary artery.

While the large (epicardial) coronary arteries are preferentially affected by arterio- and atherosclerosis, the intramyocardial branches have been found to be affected by "cushion-like" lesions which protrude far into the lumen and consist of modified muscle cells, elastin, and structureless material (10). In persons under 40 years of age the cushions were not seen, while their frequency increased significantly in men over 40. The authors speculated that hemodynamic mechanisms are important in their pathogenesis. Presumably, the lesion develops over a long period of time and may represent either an aging response of the cells of the vessel or simply an adaptation to hemodynamic stress.

Animal Models

Swine have been employed as experimental animals for studies on spontaneous changes in the coronary arteries since the lesions in this species are similar to those found in man. French et al. (8) studied atherosclerosis with light and electron microscopy in pigs and described the progression of the disease in relation to age.

In the proximal segments of the coronary arteries of young pigs they found evidence of changes which may be indicative of atherogenesis. Muscle cells of the media protruded into the subendothelial region in areas where fragmentation of the internal elastic membrane occurred. Electron micrographs revealed what was interpreted as new elastin located adjacent to the protruding muscle cells. The marked progression of the disease was evident in old pigs, where the intimal thickenings became widespread in all coronary arteries. Intimal thickenings consisted almost entirely of smooth muscle surrounded by collagen and elastic fibers. The role of vascular smooth muscle in fibrilogenesis is clearly indicated by these observations and suggests that this cell is the first type involved in early alterations contributing to the development of atherosclerosis. As the lesions progressed they accumulated lipid and formed a hyperplastic layer, which contained more collagen than elastin. This more advanced change involved some cells which had ultrastructural characteristics different from smooth muscle and appeared to resemble fibrocytes. These observations demonstrate an early onset of cell and fiber changes which are involved in the development of atherosclerosis. Although more advanced lesions involving calcification were rare, the basic changes comprising atherosclerosis, intimal thickenings and a hyperplastic layer, were clearly related to aging and are consistent with the studies on man. It is not clear, however, whether these alterations are due to repeated endothelial injury which increases their severity and incidence over time or whether they reflect true senescent events.

Studies on the rat have also demonstrated an association between age and coronary artery disease. However, this species does not appear to be a good model for atherosclerosis owing to its apparent resistance to this lesion. An exception to most findings is Humphreys' paper (11), in which she reported that atheromatous plaques were found in 60% of the rats more than 500 days old. She described the plaques as marked fibrous thickenings of the intima consisting of collagenous tissue, hyaline material, swollen endothelial cells, and fat droplets. The incidence of atherosclerosis was not altered when the animals were fed high-fat diets. A lack of evidence from other strains of rats demonstrating athcrosclerosis has undoubtedly dampened interest in the use of this species as a model of spontaneous atherosclerosis.

The rat has, however, been widely used as a model of coronary artery aging and has provided a variety of data. In a systematic study on 487 rats it was concluded that, with the exception of infectious diseases, cardiovascular disease is first evident late in the second year (middle age) and reaches a maximum incidence during the third year (old age) (32). While the changes in the rat do not lead to marked occlusion, many are similar to those found in man. Arteriosclerosis of the coronary arteries and other vessels is a consistent finding in repeatedly bred male and female rats and is also common to old virgin females (30). Medial thickening and myocardial fibrosis were found to be the two most common age-related changes and appeared to be highly related (33). The involvement of the intramuscular arteries may contribute to the focal changes which occur with aging in this species, i.e., myocardial degeneration and fibrosis. The rat also appears to be a good model for studies on the aging of the coronary arteries since the changes are fairly constant (33). Sclerotic changes in the intramural coronary arteries, typical in aged rats, have also been reported in old dogs (6).

Indeed, the smooth muscle cell is implicated in age-related structural changes in coronary arteries and has been the subject of several experimental studies in the rat. A summary of the data from these studies is presented diagrammatically in Fig. 1. Oka and Angrist (19) studied adenosine monophosphatase (AMPase) and nicotinomide adenine dinucleotide-diaphorase (NADH-diaphorase or DPNH-diaphorase) histochemically in order to identify the role of aging on these enzymes and determine the relationship of changes in their activities to vascular sclerosis. While they found no reaction for AMPase in the media of rats up to 23 months of age, focal positive reactions typified the coronary arteries of animals older than 23 months. This enhanced focal activity of AMPase was accompanied by variation in NADH-diaphorase activity which stained as coarse clumps or disappeared. AMPase activity appears to be directly related to vascular aging but not atherosclerosis; this activity, determined biochemically in humans, increased with age but was similar in atherosclerotic and nonsclerotic vessels (15). NADH-diaphorase activity on the other hand, has been shown to be lower in the atherosclerotic aorta and the arteriosclerotic segments of the coronary arteries in man, but does not appear to be altered by age (14).

Oka and Angrist (19) cited evidence that the altered NADH-diaphorase activity may suggest mitochondrial damage, while increased AMPase activity may be significant because of its relationship to thrombus formation (AMP inhibits platelet aggregation). Considering this role of AMP, the enhanced AMPase activity during aging might represent an attempt to minimize thrombus formation which is a factor in the pathogenesis of atherosclerosis. Since lipids were not detectable in the muscle cells, the enzyme

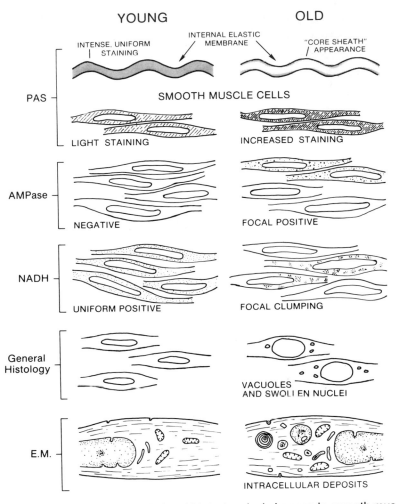

FIG. 1. A summary of structural and histochemical changes in smooth muscle cells and the internal elastic membrane of coronary arteries of aged rats. (Based on refs. 13, 19, and 20.)

changes observed preceded lipid accumulation and may represent early manifestations of a degenerative process. It is noteworthy that the enzymatic alterations were more common in the large coronary arteries and their branches (the vessels most frequently affected by lesions in man) than in the small segments. While these changes represent two cellular alterations which are associated with aging and pathogenesis, the relationship between NADH-diaphorase and AMPase activity changes is not clear. Several important questions arise from these findings: (a) Do these enzyme alterations contribute to functional changes in the vessels? (b) Do they underlie mechanisms which may trigger cellular aging or are they the byproduct of such mechanisms? and (c) Might increased AMPase activity simply constitute a protective activity related to an increased susceptibility to thrombus formation in the aged?

Phagocytosis of fragments from necrosis by the smooth muscle cell has been suggested by a study utilizing electron microscopy (13). Although no ages were indicated, in rats weighing between 65 to 535 g the intracellular accumulation of debris increased with the size of the animal. The presence of the intracellular deposits (small vesicles, myelin figures, small granules and structures which appeared to be remains of phagosomes) was considered to be evidence of inadequate digestive processes which may limit the life span of the arterial wall. These deposits are not identifiable by light microscopy and routine histological stains, which explains why they were not described in other studies. The early onset of the phagocytic activity (65-g rats are approximately 1 month old) supports the contention that the process may be a cellular aging phenomenon. The focal nature of the changes suggests that certain regions of the coronary arteries, i.e., those near the origin of a branch, are more susceptible to the accumulation of debris.

The consequences of certain cellular changes which are linked with aging may be evident only when the artery is exposed to potential insult. Patek and colleagues (20) considered several consistent histochemical and histological alterations evident in 25-month-old rats compared to 5-month-old animals. The authors noted three distinct changes: (a) a wide core, negative for periodic acid-Schiff reagent (PAS), characterizing the internal elastic lamina; (b) a dramatic increase in PAS positive material in the tunica media; and (c) an indistinct morphology and the presence of vacuoles in the cells of the media. PAS staining is dependent on the availability of aldehydes, and since both desmosine and isodesmosine, components of elastin, are composed of lysine residues, the authors postulated that an age-associated loss of PAS staining in the internal elastic membrane was because of an increase in cross-linkages with a decrease in the available lysine aldehydes. When colloidal carbon was injected intravenously, a lesion characterized by a slight thickening and occasional rupture of the internal elastic lamina with elastin proliferation developed; in the area of the rupture smooth muscle cells were disoriented. In the younger animals the lesion was not evident until 5 months following the injection, while in the older animals it appeared within 7 days. These findings are in concert with the supposition that aging phenomena enhance the susceptability of the coronary arteries to pathological changes.

In summary, there is evidence that coronary arteries undergo age-related changes which may be linked to pathological alterations. Some phenomenon indicative of early pathogenesis appears to be operational in young experimental animals. Both the smooth muscle cell and the internal elastic membrane are implicated in morphological changes which become evident in old animals. While these alterations may represent aging processes and appear to comprise or contribute to vascular pathogenesis, the relationship between aging and arterial lesions as well as the relationship between the various events themselves is not clear. The key to establishing aging phenomena in these vessels lies in elucidating sequential events. Such data are, at present, unavailable.

Myocardial Microvasculature

Oxygen extraction in the coronary circulation is unusually high, i.e., about 70%. Accordingly, any significant enhancement of myocardial work and O_2 demand is dependent on increased coronary blood flow, which in turn is dependent on an adequate number of capillaries.

The extent of the myocardial capillary bed has been quantified by counting the number of capillaries in cross-sectional fields. Since nearly all of the capillaries run parallel to the long axis of the myocardial cells, this approach provides a reasonable estimate of the capillary bed. Capillary density (the number of capillaries per unit area) remains fairly constant throughout growth. In the rat the capillary/myocardial cell ratio is approximately $1:4$ in the neonate and rises to $1:1$ during the second month of postnatal life (22). The similar capillary density for the two groups is accounted for by increase in cell size accompanied by capillary proliferation.

Studies on the rat indicate that aging is associated with a decrease in capillary density (22,26). These studies also demonstrated a drop in the capillary/myocardial cell ratio in old rats (26 to 27 and 22 months old, respectively). The decrement in the ratio may be owing to one or a combination of two events. First a loss of capillaries, as part of the degenerative process, may have occurred. Second, enhanced branching of the myocardial cell, as seen by electron microscopy (27) may have contributed to an increased number of cell profiles in cross-sectional fields. The decreased capillary density which is evident in the rat as early as 14 to 15 months (9), could be because of either of these factors along with a slight increase in cell diameter (26).

The ability of the heart of an old animal to enhance its capillary bed is supported by data demonstrating greater numbers of capillaries per square millimeter in exercised than in nonexercised rats (26). This increase presumably was due to capillary proliferation since capillary/cardiocyte ratio was also increased, and no evidence of cardiocyte necrosis in the exercised animals was evident.

Only recently has attention been focused on the microvascular bed of man. Ichikawa and Matsubara (12) stereoscopically examined the human myocardium after injecting silicone rubber and found spotty areas reflecting insufficient injection in the inner layer of the myocardium of the left ventricle of older persons. In middle aged persons this appearance was seen less often, and it was not observed in infants. Since only the inner third of the myocardium was affected, the deficit in perfusion is probably not owing to changes in the larger coronary arteries, but rather to subendocardial terminal branches. The patchy filling pattern suggests subendocardial ischemia and is consistent with the high incidence of infarction in this region.

The deficit in perfusion, as indicated by this study, may be owing to an increased arteriolar resistance. Quantitative data on the wall thickness of coronary arterioles indicates an age-related increase in both ventricles of men (2). The largest increase occurs in the left ventricle; when compared to men under 45 years of age, arteriolar wall thickness is increased by 37% in the 45- to 49-year-old-age group and by 69% in the 70 and above age group.

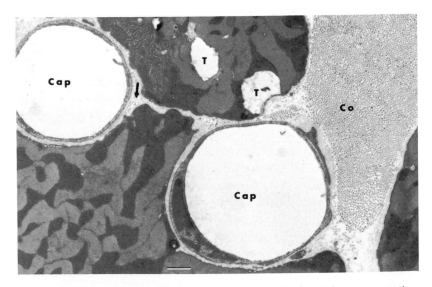

FIG. 2. Electron micrograph of two capillaries (Cap) cut in cross-section from a male rat aged 27 months. A marked accumulation of collagen (Co) is seen adjacent to one side of one capillary. Scattered profiles of collagen fibrils also occur *(arrow)*. Marked dilatations of transverse tubules (T) are seen in the cardiocyte in the upper portion of the micrograph. The dilatations are found in the region of the intercalated disc (seen to the left of the cell). The *bar* represents 1 μm.

Specific ultrastructural alterations in capillaries have not been described; however, enhancement of collagen around the capillaries of old rats has been demonstrated (27). Whether the presence of increased numbers of collagen fibrils (Fig. 2) represents a barrier to transcapillary exchange is not clear. Greatly enhanced collagen deposition is usually limited to one side of the capillary. Degenerative changes in capillaries appear to be limited to areas where myocardial cell degeneration is evident. In most capillaries the endothelial cell does not show structural changes which might reflect decrements in transport, i.e., cleft junctions appear normal, pinocytotic vesicles numerous, and the basal lamina intact. The possibility of more subtle changes cannot be excluded.

CORONARY FLOW AND OXYGEN EXTRACTION

While structural alterations in the coronary vasculature are associated with aging, the consequences of these alterations have received little attention. A decrement in myocardial performance in old rats is indicated by data which show a lower aortic flow in 24-month than in 12-month-old rats (24). This senescent change may be due to an increased ventricular volume in the absence of an increase in ventricular wall thickness. Thus the dilated heart of aged rats is at a disadvantage in that it must develop a greater wall tension for any given intraventricular pressure. This demand for increased wall tension requires increased oxygen utilization and thereby may contribute to the relatively poor performance of the heart during senescence. It is possible that, with constant or unchanged peripheral resistance, reduced aortic flow and pressure may be factors to be considered in aging where coronary blood flow may be compromised.

Weisfeldt et al. (29) studied the nonworking, nonblood-perfused Langendorff heart preparation from rats in order to determine whether blood flow and O_2 diffusion are altered during senescence. Heart preparations from 12- and 24- to 27-month-old rats were compared under a wide range of perfusate arterial Po_2. The percent of O_2 extracted by the hearts of the two groups was similar

TABLE 1. *Coronary flow and coronary flow per gram dry heart weight in hearts from 12- and 24- to 27-month-old male rats*

Age (months)	n	Dry heart wt (g)	Coronary flow at $Pao_2 = 250$ mm Hg		Maximal coronary flow[a]	
			ml/min	ml/min/g	ml/min	ml/min/g
12	11	0.2430 ± 0.0059	16.8 ± 0.4	68.9 ± 1.2	17.5 ± 0.4	72.0 ± 1.9
24–27	10	0.2615 ± 0.0098	16.2 ± 0.5	63.0 ± 1.8[b]	16.9 ± 0.4	65.9 ± 2.0[c]

[a] Maximal coronary flow = maximal flow at any arterial PO_2. Maximal flow occured at 200 to 250 mm Hg in all hearts. No increase in flow was noted between 200 and 150 mm Hg.
[b] $p < 0.01$ versus 12-month-old group.
[c] $p < 0.05$ versus 12-month-old group.
From Weisfeldt et al., ref. 29, with permission.

over a range of 650 to 200 mm Hg PO_2 and suggested that O_2 extraction is not impaired in the old rat. However, under severe hypoxia (arterial $PO_2 = 200$ to 250 mm Hg), O_2 consumption per gram dry weight was lower in the old group and was attributed to a decreased coronary flow (Table 1). These data have demonstrated that a decrement in myocardial O_2 consumption and maximal coronary flow both become evident in the heart of the senescent animal only on attainment of severe hypoxia.

The authors noted that the decrement in blood flow is consistent with a number of possible age-associated alterations: (a) an absolute decrease in the coronary vascular bed, (b) a decrease in vascular reactivity, or (c) a failure of the vascular bed to increase in proportion to heart weight. The latter increased by 7.6%, while coronary flow decreased by 8.5%. A fall in capillary density during aging (9,22,26) is well established and, as previously suggested, may be brought about in part by an absolute loss of capillaries. Thus, a relative reduction in the capillary bed may be the major factor limiting maximal coronary flow, although, pending data to the contrary, changes in vascular reactivity cannot be excluded. In addition, the supposition that the decrease in maximal coronary flow is owing to changes in the microvascular bed is supported by the observation that the coronary arteries of the old rats were free of occlusive lesions which might reduce blood flow (29).

DIRECTIONS FOR FUTURE RESEARCH

Whether or not aging of the cells and extracellular components of the coronary arteries predisposes these vessels to pathological changes is a question which requires considerable attention. Obviously, the elucidation of the factors which lead to a vulnerability of the coronary arteries to sclerotic changes requires the isolation of a process or processes from the overall complicated variables to which an organism is subject over time. In man this task is particularly difficult when one considers just a few of the variables which reputedly contribute to atherosclerosis—genetics, diet, hormones, neurogenic influences, metabolic defects, and exercise. Thus, the accumulation of many factors over a lifetime may be reflected in this age-associated disease. The coronary artery is a vessel highly susceptible to vascular disease; data from other arteries cannot be used convincingly to draw conslusions regarding phenomena in the coronary artery.

While the pathological changes common to coronary vessels in the aged may not constitute a senescent phenomenon, they may be a consequence of cellular aging. Bertelsen (3) pointed out that age changes in the media of arteries must be considered solely as fundamental factors in the development of atherosclerosis since in themselves they are insufficient to form fibrous plaques. He noted that mineralization of the media precedes intimal proliferation and plaque formation. This relationship between events which may reflect aging phenomena in the media and the development of atherosclerosis in the intima provides a potential major link between aging and atherosclerosis. Elucidating this potential link and the contributing factors requires that future studies focus attention on the life cycle of the major cells implicated in age-related diseases, i.e., endothelial, smooth muscle, and fibroblast.

Cell culture represents a promising approach with considerable potential for elucidating aging changes in the absence of hemodynamic and other influences. This method lends itself to the incorporation of a variety of biochemical and cytological techniques and represents a "pure" model for the study of the cell in a sequence of time. The demonstration of specific enzymatic or cytological changes in aging cells may provide the essential clues to the pathogenesis of coronary artery diseases such as atherosclerosis and arteriosclerosis.

As shown by histochemical and ultrastructural methods, vascular smooth muscle is clearly implicated in alterations which may represent cellular aging and deserves continued attention. In addition to its contractile role, the smooth muscle cell secretes components of the extracellular matrix and may become phagocytic. These noncontractile functions must be considered by using cytological techniques designed to define exocytosis and endocytosis in the vascular smooth muscle cell. Radioautography, cell fractionation, and cell culture represent a few important approaches to the problem of defining biochemical and localizing subcellular events which may constitute aging. If the vascular smooth muscle cell lacks intrinsic changes which define aging phenomena, it may be the victim of extrinsic factors which, over time, render it increasingly susceptible to vascular disease. In this regard vasoactive substances, hormones, and mechanical factors must be considered.

Exploration of senescent changes within the coronary arteries requires an active interest in collagen, elastin, and the matrix as research on numerous organs implicates these components in general aging phenomena. Arterial aging is characterized by a disproportional increase in heparin sulfate to total glycosaminoglycans and appears to be related to hyperproliferation of the intima as seen in Hurler's syndrome (17). Lipid and lipoprotein metabolism and repair of damaged cells are functions which can be restituted when chondroitin sulfates, which decrease during old age, are restored (18). Calcification of the tunica media may be facilitated by the age-associated increase in dermatin sulfate which tightly binds calcium (18). Such findings implicate cellular components involved in the synthesis and secretion of the extracellular matrix in aging phenomena. Considerable emphasis must be placed on the localization of subcellular defects which may alter the products of secretion. Certainly the collaborative efforts of the biochemist and cell biologist should be particularly useful as an approach to a critical problem and one which may play the most fundamental role in many age-associated changes.

A variety of cell processes may be advantageously studied in conditions stimulating collateral growth. This phenomenon involves lysis, phagocytosis, connective tissue reaction, cell division, and formation of new extracellular material. The inability of the myocardium to adapt to decrements in coronary circulation by collateral growth has not been demonstrated; such a limitation would indicate a loss of basic cellular response. Thus, knowledge of collateral growth or its limitations should prove useful in distinguishing aging changes in a variety of cells.

Our knowledge concerning the microvascular bed is limited. Although a decrement in capillary density occurs with aging, the consequences of this change may not be evident under basal conditions. As previously stated, decrements in myocardial O_2 consumption and maximal blood flow are demonstrable under hypoxic conditions in old rats and may be due to the decreased capillary density. If transcapillary exchange in the myocardium during senescence is altered is not known. Certainly age changes in the endothelial cell could limit transcapillary exchange even in the absence of arterial disease or decrements in blood flow. Definite priority to the studies of blood flow, transcapillary exchange, and endothelial cell cytology seems warranted if we are to understand the role of the vascular system in age-related changes in the myocardial cell. It is essential that future experiments explore these variables under varying hemodynamic and oxygen-utilizing conditions since limitations of the coronary circulation, as well as those of the myocardial cell, may be evident only under conditions which place demands on the coronary reserve.

Finally, it is essential to recognize the gradient of vulnerability of coronary vessels to disease processes. A metabolic heterogeneity within the coronary vasculature has been demonstrated particularly with regard to the larger coronary arteries and the arterioles (5). The latter deserve long overdue attention with regard to their role in the microcirculation. Smooth muscle metabolism in coronary arterioles has a high aerobic capacity. This provides a distinct contrast with its counterpart in large coronary arteries, which has a weak aerobic potential. Such metabolic variation requires that arterioles be considered separately from larger coronary vessels. Comparisons of these vessels may in fact prove useful in elucidating the rationale for the differences in their vulnerability to age and disease.

SUMMARY

Coronary arteries undergo age-associated pathological changes. Epidemiological studies on man have suggested that atherosclerosis may have its onset relatively early in life and, if sufficiently advanced, leads to ischemic heart disease during middle and old age. Since coronary atherosclerosis, although common, is not inevitable in middle and old age, it should be considered a senile rather than a senescent process. Cellular aging, however, cannot be excluded as a factor in susceptibility to the disease. The role of early accumulation of glycosaminoglycans and subsequent mineralization of the media have been linked to the development of plaques in the intima. Therefore, medial changes are more likely to reflect aging events, a contention that is supported by data on experimental animals.

Most of the experimental work on coronary vessels and aging is based on the rat. Associated with the thickening of the tunica media are a variety of specific morphological and histochemical changes, most of which concern the smooth muscle cell and the intercellular components. Basic aging patterns may include altered enzyme functions and intracellular accumulation of lipid and debris. They may explain the susceptibility to vascular injury in old animals. The hemodynamic and metabolic consequences of these alterations are not well established, since occlusion of the coronary arteries in the rat is rare. Although relatively little work has focused on myocardial circulation, the significance of the available data is evident. A decrement in capillary density is consistent with a decrease in maximal coronary flow in the senescent rat. If transcapillary exchange is limited in the aged is not known.

It is concluded that aging phenomena in the coronary vasculature of the rat involve both the coronary arteries (epicardial and intramural) and the microvascular bed. These alterations are of particular significance in that they are not complicated by the age-related atherosclerosis common to man. It is suggested that these events may (a) predispose the arteries to pathological changes and (b) limit the response of the coronary bed to enhanced functional demands.

Future research must consider a number of areas in order to provide data which will elucidate the specific effects of aging on coronary vessels. Some avenues for exploration include: (a) experimental designs which consider coronary artery disease in aging experimental animals, (b) biochemical and cytochemical studies aimed at defining the role of the extracellular matrix and its fibers in aging and their relationship to coronary artery disease, (c) *in vitro* (cell culture) and *in vivo* studies on the role of the smooth muscle cell in aging and pathogencsis, and (d) studies correlating regional blood flow, capillary permeability, and endothelial cell alterations under various physiological conditions.

ACKNOWLEDGMENTS

This work was supported in part by funds from the National Institutes of Health Grant No. HL-18629.

REFERENCES

1. Ahmed, M. M. (1970): Age and sex differences in the structure of tunica media of coronary arteries in Chinese subjects. *J. Anat.,* 106:202.
2. Auerbach, O., Hammond, E. C., Garfinkel, L., and Kirman, D. (1971): Thickness of walls of myocardial arterioles in relation to smoking and age. *Arch. Environ. Health,* 22:20–27.
3. Bertelsen, S. (1963): The role of ground substance, collagen, and elastic fibers in the genesis of atherosclerosis. In: *Atherosclerosis and its Origin,* edited by M. Sander and G. F. Bourne, pp. 119–165. Academic Press, New York.

4. Braunwald, E. (1976): Introductory remarks. In: *Protection of the Ischemic Myocardium,* edited by E. Braunwald, pp. 1–2. American Heart Association, Monograph 48.

5. Cook, B. H., Granger, H. J., and Taylor, A. E. (1977): Metabolism of coronary arteries and arterioles. A histochemical study. *Microvasc. Res.,* 14:145–159.

6. Detweiler, D. K., Patterson, D. F., Hubben, K., and Botts, R. P. (1961): The prevalence of spontaneously occurring cardiovascular disease in dogs. *Am. J. Public Health,* 51:228–241.

7. Eggen, D. A., and Solberg, L. A. (1968): Variation of atherosclerosis with age. *Lab. Invest.,* 18:571–579.

8. French, J. E., Jennings, M. A., and Florey, H. W. (1965): Morphological studies on atherosclerosis in swine. *Ann. N.Y. Acad. Sci.,* 127:780–799.

9. Gauthier, D., Martini, J., and Coraboeuf, E. (1964): Etude comparative de la densité capillaire coronaire chez le rat et le cobaye. *J. Physiol. (Paris),* 56:356–357.

10. Haerem, J. W. (1969): Cushion-like intimal lesions in intramyocardial arteries of man. Their relationship to age, sex, coronary atherosclerosis and certain diseases. *Acta Pathol. Microbiol. Scand.,* 77:598–608.

11. Humphreys, E. M. (1957): The occurrence of altheromatous lesions in the coronary arteries of rats. *Q. J. Exp. Physiol.,* 42:96–103.

12. Ichikawa, H., and Matsubara, O. (1977): Studies on the microvasculature of human myocardium. *Bull. Tokyo Med. Dent. Univ.,* 24:53–65.

13. Joris, I., and Majno, G. (1974): Cellular breakdown within the arterial wall. An ultrastructural study of the coronary artery in young and aging rats. *Virchows Arch. [Pathol. Anat.],* 364:111–127.

14. Kirk, J. E. (1962): The diaphorase and cytochrome with reductase activities of arterial tissue in individuals of various ages. *J. Gerontol.,* 17:276–280.

15. Kirk, J. E. (1963): Enzyme chemistry of the vascular wall. In: *Fundamentals of Vascular Grafting,* edited by S. A. Weschowski and C. Dennis, pp. 32–62. McGraw-Hill, New York.

16. McGill, H. C., Jr., Geer, J. C., and Strong, J. P. (1963): Natural history of human atherosclerotic lesions. In: *Atherosclerosis and Its Origin,* edited by M. Sandler and G. H. Bourne, pp. 39–65. Academic Press, New York.

17. Meyer, K. (1964): Mucopolysaccharide composition of the vessel wall. In: *Small Blood Vessel Involvement in Diabetes Mellitus,* edited by M. D. Siperstein, p. 193. American Institute of Biological Sciences, Washington, D.C.

18. Morrison, L. M., Schjeide, O. A., and Meyer, K. (1974): *Coronary Heart Disease and the Mucopolysaccharides (glycosaminoglycans),* pp. 93–108. Charles C Thomas, Springfield, Illinois.

19. Oka, M., and Angrist, A. (1967): Histoenzymatic studies of vascular changes in the aorta and coronary arteries in the aged rat. *J. Gerontol.,* 22:23–31.

20. Patek, P. R., deMignard, V. A., and Bernick, S. (1968): Changes in structure of coronary arteries: Susceptibility to arteriosclerosis in old rats. *Arch. Pathol.,* 85:388–396.

21. Rakusan, K., and Poupa, O. (1963): Changes in the diffusion distance in the rat heart muscle during development. *Physiol. Bohemoslov.,* 12:220–227.
22. Rakusan, K., and Poupa, O. (1964): Capillaries and muscle fibers in the heart of old rats. *Gerontologia,* 9:107–112.
23. Roberts, W. C. (1975): The coronary arteries in coronary heart disease: Morphologic observations. *Pathobiol. Annu.,* 5:249–282.
24. Shreiner, D. P., Weisfeldt, M. L., and Shock, N. W. (1969): Effects of age, sex, and breeding status on the rat heart, *Am. J. Physiol.,* 217:176–180.
25. Strong, J. P., and McGill, H. C., Jr. (1962): The natural history of atherosclerosis. *Am. J. Pathol.,* 40:37.
26. Tomanek, R. J. (1970): Effects of age and exercise on the extent of the myocardial capillary bed. *Anat. Rec.,* 167:55–62.
27. Tomanek, R. J., and Karlsson, U. L. (1973): Myocardial ultrastructure of young and senescent rats. *J. Ultrastruct. Res.,* 42:201–220.
28. Vikhert, A. M., and Zhdanov, V. S. Kaltsinoz koronarnykh arterii serdtsa. (1975): *Kardiologiia,* 15:102–108.
29. Weisfeldt, M. L., Wright, J. R., Shreiner, D. P., Lakatta, E., and Shock, N. W. (1971): Coronary flow and oxygen extraction in the perfused heart of senescent male rats. *J. Appl. Physiol.,* 30:44–49.
30. Wexler, B. C. (1964): Spontaneous arteriosclerosis in repeatedly bred male and female rats. *J. Atheroscler. Res.,* 4:57–80.

The Aging Heart (Aging, Vol. 12),
edited by Myron L. Weisfeldt.
Raven Press, New York © 1980.

Chapter 7

The Aging Vasculature and Its Effects on the Heart

Frank C. P. Yin

Cardiology Division, Department of Medicine, Johns Hopkins Medical Institutions, Baltimore, Maryland 21205

In evaluation of the influence of age on heart function *in toto,* it is important to consider not only the effects of age on the intrinsic performance of the heart, but also the effects of age on the properties of the vascular system. This is because the ventricle and the vascular system into which blood is ejected can be viewed in simplistic terms as a pump working against a load. The functioning of the ventricle is determined in part by its intrinsic contractile properties and in part by the properties of the vasculature. However, the vasculature is not a rigid system presenting a fixed resistance to the pump. Rather, it is an extensible system that acts as a buffer to convert the pulsatile flow from the heart into a more or less continuous flow that is more suitable for use by the peripheral beds. Because of the pulsatile flow and the extensible nature of arterial walls, the load presented by the vasculature to the ventricle has both static and dynamic components. In other words, the static and dynamic mechanical properties of the vascular system together determine the load faced by the ventricle and the efficiency with which the external work of the heart is converted into delivery of blood.

Besides its direct effect on the ventricle, the vascular system has an important role in hemodynamics. The properties of the vessel wall together with the arrangement of its various branches determine the amplitude and configuration of the pressure and flow waves and the transmission characteristics of the pressure and flow pulses in the system. Once the blood enters the vasculature, the properties of the system determine how the blood is distributed to the various peripheral beds. All of these factors can then act via metabolic or reflex pathways to influence the overall function of the entire organism. It is clear, then, that any age changes in the properties of the vascular system could have a profound influence on the functioning of the heart and other organ systems.

This chapter reviews what is currently known about the effects of age on both the structure and function of the pulmonic and systemic arterial trees. Since aging and not development is of major concern herein, the discussion will be limited to examination of the changes with age from maturation to senescence. Occasionally developmental aspects will be discussed for clarification or emphasis. Since the primary focus of this book concerns the aging heart, emphasis will be placed on delineating the age changes in these two vascular systems that affect the functioning of the heart. Space limitations preclude any extensive discussion of the aging effects of the venous system and microvasculature. Likewise, there is extensive literature concerning the intrinsic metabolic and biochemical changes with age in the systemic vascular tree which are not included except where pertinent to structure and function. Much of the non-English literature, especially the extensive German and Russian works, was not reviewed in detail.

For ease of presentation, this chapter is divided into sections. The first section reviews the changes with age, from both the macroscopic and microscopic viewpoints, in first the systemic then the pulmonic vascular systems. The second section reviews the influence of age on the mechanical properties of each vascular system. In the next section an attempt is made to relate the structural changes discussed in the prior section to the mechanical property changes. The next section reviews the aging aspects of the pharmacologic responsiveness of vascular smooth muscle. The fourth section discusses the implications of the age changes in each vascular system on the function of its associated ventricle as well as on the functioning of the cardiovascular system as a whole.

STRUCTURAL CHANGES WITH AGING

Systemic Vasculature

The systemic arterial tree consists of the aorta and its major branches, each of which sequentially branches until the arteriolar level is reached. It is the proximal portion of the tree that has the major influence on left ventricular function during ejection. Despite the marked changes in size as one progresses from the central to the peripheral vessels, the structure of the vessel wall retains basically three layers: the intima, media, and adventitia. Each layer contains elastin, collagen, smooth muscle as well as other cells, and ground substance. The amount of each component varies depending on the location in the vascular tree. Furthermore, within a given location the arrangement of each of these components depends on the degree of distention of the vessel wall. Thus, when speaking of the architecture of the vessel wall, it is necessary to specify where and under what conditions the structure is examined.

There has been a long and continued interest in the effects of age on the structure of the vascular system. The studies in this area have been of several types. One approach has been to delineate the changes per se in the histological features of aging vascular tissue. Another approach has been to attempt to correlate age changes in structure and function. Since arteriosclerosis is a process that becomes increasingly evident with advancing age, another area of continuing investigation and controversy is the ascertainment of whether or not this process is a precursor, is an adjunct, or is unrelated to the structural changes seen in aging tissue.

The aging process differentially affects each layer as well as each region of the vascular tree. There also appear to be rate and species differences in the aging process. Therefore, the problem of delineating the age changes in the structure of the arterial tree is complex and is responsible for some of the confusing interpretations in the literature. An extensive review (95) of this subject was published in 1965, and what follows is a summary of that review together with an update of more recent work. Before proceeding with a discussion of age changes, the normal histology of the blood vessel wall is reviewed.

The normal mature tunica intima (Fig. 1) consists of a layer of flattened endothelial cells packed in an orderly side-by-side fashion forming the luminal surface of the vessel. The cells are very uniform in size, only rarely binucleate, and are polarized with their long axes along the longitudinal axis of the vessel (34). The cells rest on a thin basement membrane composed of a mixture of collagen, elastin, reticulum, smooth muscle, histiocytes, fibroblasts, and ground substance. Beneath this subendothelial layer lies the internal elastic membrane, which is composed of closely packed concentric laminae of elastin.

The tunica media begins beneath the internal elastic membrane. In the undistended state it consists of concentric, corrugated lamellae of elastin interconnected by a network of fine elastin fibrils (Fig. 1). Collagen fibers and bundles, which are distributed randomly, appear to pass through fenestrations in the elastic lamellae without any apparent connections to the elastin. On the other hand, smooth muscle cells have frequent attachments to the elastin and accompany the fine elastic network as it interlaces among the elastin lamellae. With increasing vessel distention, the random orientation of the collagen and smooth muscle is lost and all the components become aligned into a low-pitched helical arrangement (95).

The collagen and elastin content of the media varies greatly depending on the site of the vascular tree examined. Human thoracic aorta has been shown by a number of studies to be comprised of about 50% elastin plus collagen (50,74,108). Simi-

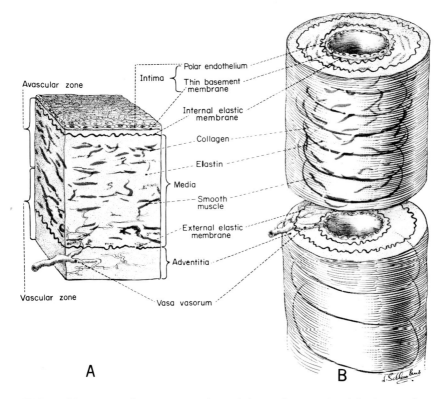

Polar endothelium
Intima {
Thin basement membrane

Avascular zone

Internal elastic membrane

Collagen

Elastin

Media

Smooth muscle

External elastic membrane

Adventitia

Vascular zone

Vasa vasorum

A

B

FIG. 1. Diagrammatic representation of the major structural features of a mature artery. **A:** Cross-sectional view of wall. **B:** Longitudinal view of vessel. (From Milch, ref. 95, with permission.)

larly, 50% of the dry weight of the dog thoracic aorta was comprised of collagen plus elastin (72). In the carotid artery and femoral artery, however, the percentage of collagen plus elastin was considerably higher (70% and 60% respectively). The proportion of collagen to elastin appeared to be clearly demarcated by anatomic boundaries, with the intrathoracic arteries being comprised of 50 to 60% elastin and the extrathoracic arteries being only 30% elastin.

Bounding the media is another layer of concentrated elastin lamellae, the external elastic membrane, which blends imperceptibly into the tunica adventitia. This outermost adventitial layer is a thin layer of tissue comprised of loosely meshed lipid, connective tissue, and amorphous ground substance (Fig. 1). The vasa vasorum runs in this layer. Because of its thinness and amorphous nature, many investigators prefer to remove the adventitia when studying vessel wall properties. Thus, the properties, composition, and function of the adventitia are not as well defined as the other two layers.

With aging, certain histological changes in the arterial vessel wall are manifested (Fig. 2). The changes in the intima appear to be similar in all the species that have been examined. Studies in man (34,68,104,106), rat (60), and monkey (93) demonstrated that with age the endothelial cells became more irregular in size and shape and increased numbers of giant multinucleated cells appeared. These changes were most prominent in the aorta and least prominent in the renal artery (34). The subendothelial layer became thickened with an increase in connective tissue content (95). This layer often became diffuse, and sublayers of elastic-hyperplastic and musculoelastic lamellae became evident. In the coronary arteries, as with other arteries, the changes first appeared in the proximal portion of the vessel and eventually involved the entire vessel with the distal portion having the most prominent changes (44). The changes became manifest at different times in different coronary arteries with the right and posterior descending arteries showing changes only after the fifth decade. The elastic laminae became less dense and were split into bands with individual fibers appearing thinned, frayed, and fragmented (Fig. 2). In the very late stages of aging, calcification and lipid deposition occurred in close proximity to the internal elastic membrane. A similar temporal sequence of aging changes was seen in the human lower extremity arteries. Pariera et al. (118) found that the subendothelial layer thickened with age and contained more elastic fibers and calcium. The popliteal and tibial arteries showed these changes earlier than the dorsalis pedis artery, and the digital arteries showed these changes later than all of the other vessels.

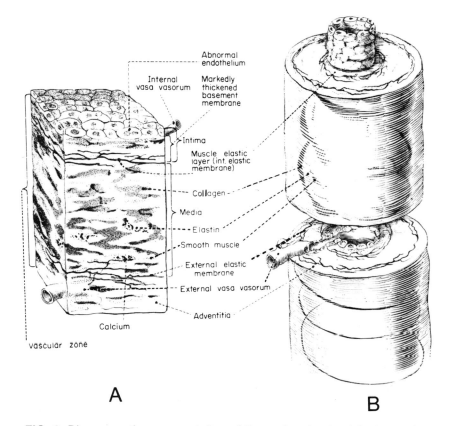

Abnormal endothelium

Internal vasa vasorum

Markedly thickened basement membrane

Intima

Muscle elastic layer (int. elastic membrane)

Collagen

Media

Elastin

Smooth muscle

External elastic membrane

External vasa vasorum

Adventitia

Calcium

vascular zone

A

B

FIG. 2. Diagrammatic representation of the major structural features of a senescent artery. **A:** Cross-sectional view of wall. **B:** Longitudinal view of vessel. Elastin fragmentation, calcification, and increased amount of collagen as compared to Fig. 1 are depicted. (From Milch, ref. 95, with permission.)

In the media, changes similar to those seen in the intima occur with advancing age. The most conspicuous changes are thickening of the media with elastin fragmentation and calcification. Auerbach et al. (7) found medial thickening in the walls of arteries and arterioles of numerous structures including the trachea, bronchi, stomach, and adrenals. Wellman and Edwards (158), in human autopsy specimens, noted that during the first five decades of life the aortic media increased in thickness from 1.21 to 1.67 mm. However, they did not study the histological changes responsible for this thickening. Wolinsky (165) demonstrated regional differences in the histology of the thickened human aorta. In the thoracic aorta thickening was due to an increase in the number of elastic laminae, whereas in the abdominal aorta it was due to thickening of each lamina with concomitant smooth muscle proliferation. Schlatman and Becker (135) found fragmentation of the elastic laminae in all aortas from persons older than 7 years of age. The fragmentation was more prominent in the ascending aorta and arch than in the descending aorta and was most pronounced in the inner layers of the media. A similar finding was noted in an earlier study by Guard and Bhende (68), who found that fragmentation was more pronounced in the inner two-thirds than in the outer one-third of the media. The latter study also demonstrated that the elastic laminae thickened only up to the second decade of life before the deterioration began. Besides the structural changes in the elastin, calcification was shown to be a widespread and progressive process in human aorta specimens (19,89). By the fourth decade, 98% of the aortas examined demonstrated significant medial calcification. The calcification occurred in association with an increase in decarboxylic acid containing amino acids in the elastin and it was postulated that the calcium was bound to these acids (89). Identical age changes as those reported for the aorta media have been demonstrated for the arteries of the lower extremity (118). However, as in the intima, the time course of the elastin fragmentation and calcification appears to be delayed in the smaller caliber vessels.

Other species besides humans demonstrate some of the same age changes in the aortic media. In rats the media thickened from 60 μm at 1 week of age to 120 μm at 3 years of age (30). This thickening was accompanied by an increase in collagen content, a decrease in number of cell nuclei, no change in the number of elastic lamellae, and an increase in randomization of orientation. Each elastic fibril increased in thickness in the first year of life and then became progressively more frayed, ruptured, and thinned. An increase in extracellular debris was also seen. Smith et al. (143) found that the aortic media of mice increased from 25 to 59 μm from birth to age 2 years. This increase was owing to an increase in the interlamellar distance and was caused by an increase in the number of interlamellar elastic fibers. The elastic lamellae themselves did not thicken with age. In monkeys the aging aortic media demonstrated a progressive increase in thickness, collagen content, and number of fibroblasts (93). However, some species differences do seem to be present, as one study found no age changes in collagen or elastin content or in the ratio of collagen to elastin in any portion of the aorta in groundhogs (23).

Age changes in the adventitia are less specific and less well studied than in the other two layers. A nonspecific increase in the number of lymphocytes and collagen fibers was found in monkeys (93). An increase in fatty tissue and decrease in quantity of collagen fibers was found in guinea pigs (147). However, one study demonstrated no age change in aging human aortic adventitia (68).

The smooth muscle cells of the media also appear to undergo age changes. For unclear reasons, the histological changes with age in this important component of the vessel wall have not been extensively studied. Young rat thoracic aorta muscle cells were found to be smooth and to have blunt cytoplasmic projections, a large nucleus, few mitochondria, and a well-developed rough endoplasmic reticulum (148). On the other hand, old muscle cells were found to have a rough outer surface with multiple projections into the nearby fibrous matrix. Most of the cytoplasm consisted of myofibrils together with large numbers of mitochondria and plasmalemmal vesicles. These changes appeared to increase the cell surface area in the old rat, as they were accompanied by increases in both phospholipid and sphingomyelin content (148). Similar findings were seen in the muscle cells of mice (143). The muscle cells of mice aorta were smooth with narrow spaces between them and the elastic lamellae. With increasing age the cells became more vacuolated and the spaces widened and became filled with fine fibers which apparently emanated from the muscle cells.

From the macroscopic standpoint, age changes in the larger arteries appear to support the microscopic findings described above. An increase in aortic mass or increase in lumen size and wall thickness with age has been shown in humans (9,13,75, 103,158,161), monkeys (93), rabbits (54), guinea pigs (147), and rats (40). The rate of change of lumen size and wall thickness varies with age and site, so that the ratio of thickness to radius may increase or decrease with age in different arteries. An increase in this ratio was found in human renal and carotid arteries, whereas a decrease was seen in the aorta and femoral arteries (11). A progressive increase in thickness-to-radius ratio towards the periphery was shown in old human aortas (90), whereas young aortas demonstrated no site dependence of this ratio. However, not all studies agree with the above results. One study demonstrated a decrease with age in lumen size in rabbits (132). Another study demonstrated first an increase then a decrease in lumen size with advancing age in human iliac arteries, with no overall change in wall thickness (128).

Pulmonary Vasculature

In considering the structural changes with age in the large pulmonary arteries, it is desirable first to examine the spectrum of changes from fetal life to senescence since the great majority of change occurs in the early postnatal period. In the fetus, the structures of both the pulmonary artery and aorta are similar but not identical. The media of both are of the same thickness, ranging from 300 to 400 μm (76). Unlike the aorta, however, the elastin fibrils in the pulmonary artery are fewer and less regular. They are also coarser, shorter, and often branched with occasional clublike expansions at the ends (76). This configuration persists until about 6 months of age, when the elastic fibrils appear divided transversely into many numerous, branched structures.

In the next 2 years, the pulmonary artery undergoes a transition into the mature form. The ratio of medial thickness of the pulmonary artery to aorta decreases from 1.0 at birth to about 0.4, and the elastin fibrils become quite sparse and irregular. By 2 years of age the pulmonary artery assumes its mature configuration with very sparse, fragmented elastic lamellae distributed at random. Fenestrations and clumping of amorphous material are common. However, at this age there is still a distinct internal elastic membrane composed of compressed elastic fibrils. At this stage of development there are also regional differences in the structure of the pulmonary tree. The elastin content is higher in the main pulmonary artery than in the right pulmonary artery (51). Smooth muscle becomes the predominant component in the periphery beginning in vessels of about 2,000 μm diameter (136). As one progresses towards the peripheral vessels, the muscle coat appears more tightly spiralled. In the very small arteries the wall is again composed primarily of collagen and elastin (136). There is evidence that for a vessel of given diameter the wall thickness is the same in either the upper or lower lobes and in either the right or left lungs (140).

As the human lung ages, other structural changes begin to appear. There is increasing medial fibrosis (76,136) and elastin degeneration with collagen replacing most of the elastin in the wall (140). One study (136) demonstrated no relationship between total wall thickness and age, whereas other studies (76,140) demonstrated that wall thickness increased with advancing age. Despite the variability of the wall thickness changes found with age, there is a consensus that the thickness-to-diameter ratio increases with age. A doubling of the thickness ratio from 2 to 3 to 4 to 6% was found in comparing groups of young and old human lungs (136,140). In both groups the thickness ratio varied in a predictable manner with the diameter of the vessel (140), with the old group exhibiting an increase in both relative and absolute thickness in vessels of all sizes. The transition from elastic-type to muscular-type arteries occurred more proximally in the old pulmonary artery, and intimal changes consisting of thickening with acellular material were found only in the nonmuscular proximal and very small arteries. Intimal hyperplasia has also been found in the pulmonary arteries of aging rabbits (156).

In summary, aging appears to affect both the systemic and pulmonic vasculature in a similar fashion. The difference is in the time course of the changes. Intimal hypertrophy is one of the earliest signs of the aging process. Elastic tissue disruption and fragmentation with migration of elastin fibrils into the intima and into the interlamellar spaces is another of the hallmarks of aging. Calcification in association with the elastin fibrils and gradual replacement of elastin by collagen are the late manifestations of aging and occur to varying degrees depending on the site.

MECHANICAL PROPERTY CHANGES WITH AGE

In the century since the publication of Roy's study (130) on the elastic properties of the arterial wall, there has been considerable interest in the changes with advancing age in the mechanical properties of the vascular system. Unfortunately, because of inexact nomenclature and because of species and regional differences, there is still some confusion regarding the relationship between age and vascular mechanical properties. Before proceeding with a review of the current status of knowledge in this area, it seems appropriate to review the principles of quantifying the mechanical properties of soft tissue, i.e., the relationship between the applied forces and the resulting deformations. This discussion will focus on the passive mechanical properties of blood vessels, that is, the properties in the absence of muscle contraction. The contribution of muscle contraction to the overall mechanical properties of the blood vessels is controversial (38,43,126). There are very few studies on the effects of age on the active mechanical properties (during muscle contraction) of vascular tissue, therefore, this aspect will not be discussed in detail. In principle, however, the concepts to be discussed for the passive properties are directly applicable to the active properties.

There are many different experimental and analytical methods used to quantify the mechanical properties of soft tissues such as blood vessels. However, not all of the methods are based on proper engineering principles and they only add confusion to an already complex field. From an engineering standpoint, the passive property of a material is completely described by its stress–strain–history relationship. Stress is a measure of the force acting over a unit area. Strain is a measure of the deformation of a portion of the material relative to a reference condition. History takes into account time-dependent phenomena. Use of unnormalized quantities such as pressure and radius or pressure and volume rather than stresses and strains not only limits one to a descriptive view of mechanics, but may also provide an inaccurate representation of the wall properties. This point will be amplified later. In order to compare different samples or to describe large changes in an individual sample, it is essential to use consistently normalized parameters.

Methods of Quantifying Mechanical Properties

Elasticity

For linearly elastic materials with infinitesimally small deformations, the general relationship between stress and strain can be expressed in tensor notation as

$$\sigma_{ij} = E_{ijkl}\epsilon_{kl} \qquad [1]$$

where σ_{ij} is the second order stress tensor, ϵ_{kl} is the second order strain tensor, and E_{ijkl} is a fourth order material property tensor. [A full discussion of tensor analysis is beyond the scope of this review. The interested reader is referred to the excellent book by Fung (55) for details.] Since a fourth order tensor has 81 components, this number of components would be needed to fully describe the relationship between stress and strain in the most general case. However, symmetry considerations can be invoked to reduce the number of independent constants to 21 (55). Further reduction in the number of independent constants can be achieved by assuming symmetry about certain planes in the material. For example, a material that is symmetric about one plane has 13 independent constants and one that is symmetric across three orthogonal planes has 9 independent constants. The simplest case of a material that has uniform properties in all directions (an isotropic material) has two independent constants. It is clear that considerable experimental difficulties would exist in attempting to quantify the material constants in any case other than the isotropic one. Hence, most authors restrict attention to this very special case. However, even in isotropic materials, the geometry of the structure leads to multiple components of stress and strain that need to be taken into account. For instance, a two-dimensional axisymmetric structure, such as the transverse section of a blood vessel, has six components of stress and strain. To measure these components experimentally is still a difficult task. Thus, for further simplicity, attention is usually restricted to the one-dimensional (uniaxial in most instances) case. For purposes of illustration, this simplest of all cases will be used to describe the procedures necessary to quantify the mechanical properties of tissue.

In this simplest of all cases, the relationship between stress and strain for isotropic, linearly elastic materials with small deformations reduces to the familiar form

$$\sigma = E\epsilon \qquad\qquad [2]$$

where σ is the force acting along the uniaxial direction divided by the area perpendicular to the axis, ϵ is the infinitesimal strain defined as the change in axial length due to the stress divided by a reference length (usually the unstressed length), and E is a material constant called the modulus of elasticity. For this very special case, since there are no shear forces involved, that is, all forces act along the direction of the long axis, E uniquely describes the property of the material and is the measure of the elasticity of the material. The terms "Young's modulus" and "stiffness" can be used synonymously with E. Frequently, however, when mention is made of "elasticity" of a material, what is meant is not E but $1/E$. This is an incorrect use of the term "elasticity," but unfortunately the usage has pervaded much of the literature. To prevent such confusing nomenclature, the parameter $1/E$ should be called "extensibility" or "compliance." These definitions of elasticity and extensibility will be adhered to in the remainder of this chapter.

Most biological materials, however, do not behave according to Eq. 2. The stresses and strains are (a) not linearly related, and (b) the material usually has a history- or time-dependent component. Furthermore, the deformations involved are not small. Thus, in the uniaxial case the appropriate relationship between the stresses and deformations must be described in a functional form such as

$$\sigma = f(\lambda, t) \tag{3}$$

where f is a nonlinear function, λ is the stretch ratio defined as the instantaneous length divided by the reference length and is the large deformation definition of strain,[1] and t represents time and accounts for the time-dependent behavior of the material.

While the functional notation of Eq. 3 suffices for a general description of the material properties, more specific forms must be used in order to quantify these properties. The time dependence and nonlinearity add immensely to the complexity of the problem. Consider first the problem of the nonlinear relationship between stress and strain as illustrated for vascular smooth muscle in Fig. 3. A graphical description of the relationship using terms such as "s-shaped," "sigmoid," "concave," etc. is commonly used. Use of these terms is purely descriptive. While providing some idea of the relationships involved, this approach is not precise and does not lend itself to quantification. Specific functions can be chosen to try to quantify the material properties under certain conditions, but each has limitations in that the entire curve cannot

---

[1] The question of the appropriate reference length to use for biologic materials is still unresolved. The unstressed length is difficult to determine accurately because most tissues curl or fold when completely unstressed. Therefore, most workers use the length under an arbitrary load as the reference (57).

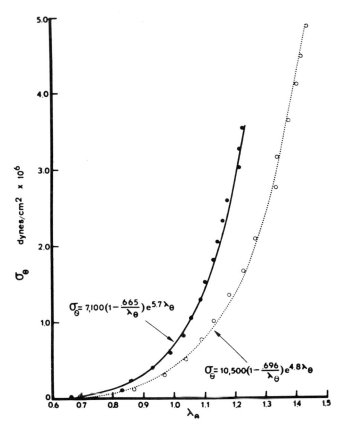

FIG. 3. Circumferential stress–strain relationship of a dog carotid artery based on large deformation theory. (●) During smooth muscle contraction induced by norepinephrine; (○) in the absence of smooth muscle contraction after poisoning with cyanide. (From Doyle et al., ref. 43, with permission.)

be described adequately with any one function. Another approach is to linearize the curve in a piecewise fashion and talk about the relationship between stress and strain over a small range of strain. For instance, incremental stiffness can be defined as the incremental stress divided by the incremental strain. For a non-linear stress–strain curve incremental stiffness has a different value at each point on the curve. A value for stiffness has meaning only if one specifies the exact point on the curve at which it is measured. Whatever route is chosen, it is clear that terms such as "stiffness," "elasticity," or "extensibility," which were precisely defined in the linear case, are no longer sufficient in the nonlinear case.

As an example of the functional approach, a particularly useful function is the exponential. Many biologic materials including heart muscle, striated muscle, ureters, tendons, elastin, and skin have been shown to have an exponential relationship between stress and strain over at least a certain range of strains (56,82, 124,127,144,149,170). One can express this relationship in the form

$$\sigma = (\sigma^* + A)\, e^{B(\lambda\,-\,\lambda^*)} - A \qquad [4]$$

where A and B are material constants and λ^* and σ^* are integration constants which uniquely describe the curve over the range that Eq. 4 applies. For this very special case the stiffness, defined as $d\sigma/d\lambda$, takes the simple and useful form

$$\frac{d\sigma}{d\lambda} = B\sigma + A \qquad [5]$$

In other words, for an exponential stress–strain relationship the stiffness is a linear function of the stress with slope defined by the constant B and intercept defined by the constant A (Fig. 4). It must be emphasized that Eqs. 4 and 5 apply only to a limited range of strains. A complete stress–strain curve may be composed of several exponentials each of which could then be described as in Eq. 5 over each strain range. An example of the multiexponential nature of the stress–strain relationship for ureteral smooth muscle is shown in Fig. 5.

There are numerous studies in which the relationship between pressure and either diameter or volume is used to describe the mechanical properties of the vessel wall (70). Examples are the pressure–diameter modulus $\left(\dfrac{R\,dP}{dR}\right)$ used by some authors (67,107) or the volume distensibility modulus $\left(\dfrac{dV}{V\,dP}\right)$ used by others (8). These indices do not take into account the geometry of the vessel and do not relate wall stresses to the strain components; therefore,

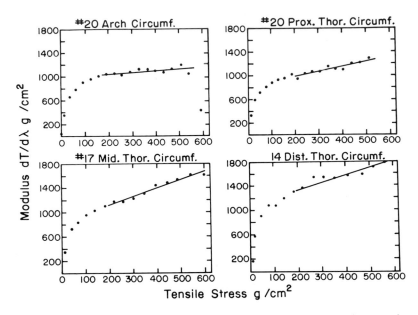

Fig. 4. Circumferential stiffness–stress relationships of various dog arteries during the loading process. The straight line portion of the curve represents Eq. 5 and is seen to be applicable only in the stress range 200–600 g/cm². (From Fung, ref. 57, with permission.)

they do not accurately reflect the properties of the vessel wall. There are methods of calculating the circumferential stress in a cylindrical tube subjected to a uniform transmural pressure. Once the stress is obtained the circumferential strain can be related to the stress to yield the circumferential stress–strain relationship. However, each method of calculating the stress is based on simplifying assumptions that may not be valid for blood vessels. For example, the Laplace relationship in the form

$$T = PR \qquad\qquad [6]$$

where P is pressure, T is wall tension and R is radius is not appropriate for blood vessels. Use of Eq. 6 assumes that the wall is infinitesimally thin so that the units of tension are dynes per centimeter rather than dynes per square centimeters. This approach is certainly not valid for blood vessels.

The modified Laplace relationship

$$\sigma = \frac{PR}{h} \qquad [7]$$

where σ is circumferential stress and h is wall thickness assumes a very thin wall with uniform stress distribution across the thickness. Again these assumptions are of doubtful validity when considering blood vessels.

Krafka (85) and Bergel (14) suggested the use of an incremental stiffness modulus based on a thick-walled cylindrical tube of internal radius R_i, outer radius R_o, and Poisson's ratio v in the form

$$E = 2\frac{\Delta P}{\Delta R_o}\frac{(1-v^2)R_i^2 R_o}{(R_o^2 - R_i^2)} \qquad [8]$$

Eq. 8, however, assumes that the deformations are small and linearly related to stress over the range of interest. In addition, the assumption is made that the material is isotropic. The isotropy and small deformation assumptions restrict the use of this relation considerably when blood vessels are being considered.

More recent works by Doyle and Dobrin (43), Simon et al. (139), Patel et al. (120), and Mirsky and Janz (102) have proposed alternative methods of quantifying the stress–strain characteristics of blood vessels by employing large deformation theory and allowing for tissue anisotropy. The last paper, using an approach suggested by Blatz et al. (18) pointed out clearly how the wall stiffness is comprised of many other factors besides VdP/dV. A detailed discussion of these more general approaches is beyond the scope of this review. In the discussion to follow, the method used by each author to quantify the stress–strain relationship of intact blood vessels will be pointed out.

Viscoelasticity

The discussion thus far has neglected the factor of the time dependence of the mechanical properties. The early studies of

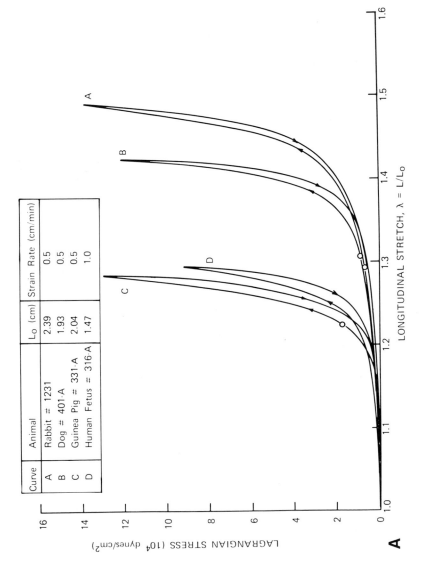

Curve	Animal	L_0 (cm)	Strain Rate (cm/min)
A	Rabbit # 1231	2.39	0.5
B	Dog # 401-A	1.93	0.5
C	Guinea Pig # 331-A	2.04	0.5
D	Human Fetus # 316-A	1.47	1.0

LONGITUDINAL STRETCH, $\lambda = L/L_0$

LAGRANGIAN STRESS (10^4 dynes/cm^2)

A

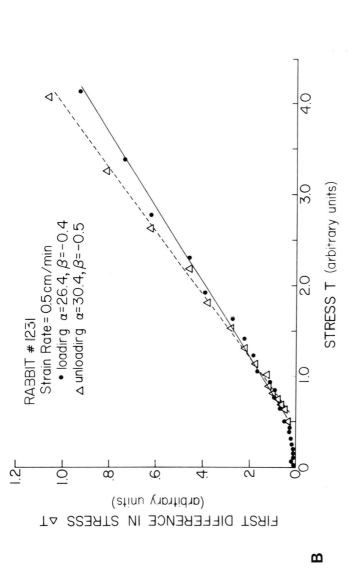

FIG. 5. A: Longitudinal stress–strain curves of various mammalian ureters during loading and unloading. **B:** Stiffness–stress relationship of the rabbit ureter (curve A), demonstrating that two straight line segments are needed to fit the data. Each line is applicable over the range of stress indicated. (From Yin and Fung, ref. 170, with permission.)

Remington (126), Peterson et al. (122), and Apter et al. (3) documented the time dependence of vascular properties.

Fung (57) has presented the most complete and unifying discussion of this aspect of mechanics for biologic tissues in general. For most materials, the stress depends not only on the amount of strain but also on the past history of the strain. For instance, if one stretches and then returns the material to its original length the stress-strain curve will describe a loop as shown in Fig. 6. At a given strain level the stress is no longer uniquely determined by the strain, but depends on whether one is on the loading or unloading portion of the curve. This behavior is termed hysteresis. For a linearly viscoelastic material, the size of the hysteresis loop depends on the speed with which the loading and unloading occurs. In order to quantify the hysteresis, one must apply the concepts previously discussed for both the loading and unloading portions of the curve for each rate of loading and unloading.

The time dependence of tissue properties can be demonstrated directly by certain maneuvers. If one rapidly stretches the tissue to a new length and then holds it at that length, the stress will gradually decrease to an asymptotic value with a time course vary-

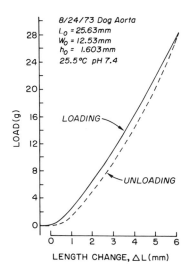

FIG. 6. Longitudinal load–extension curve of dog aorta loading *(solid line)* and unloading *(dashed line)* at a stretch rate of 0.02 lengths/sec. The difference between loading and unloading represents hysteresis. (From Tanaka and Fung, ref. 150, with permission.)

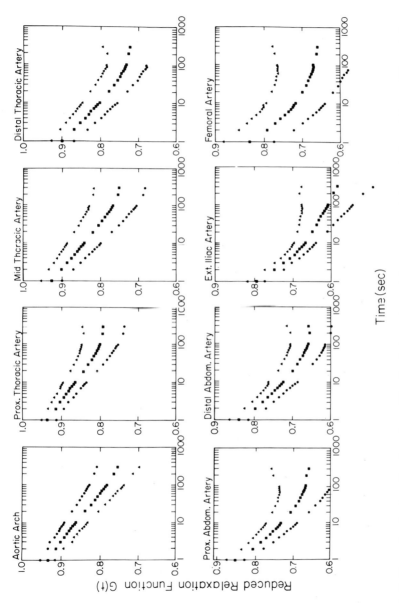
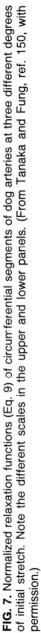

FIG. 7. Normalized relaxation functions (Eq. 9) of circumferential segments of dog arteries at three different degrees of initial stretch. Note the different scales in the upper and lower panels. (From Tanaka and Fung, ref. 150, with permission.)

ing from less than 1 sec to several hours, depending on the tissue, temperature, speed of initial stretch, amount of stretch, and other factors (Fig. 7). This behavior is called stress relaxation and is another manifestation of the time-dependent behavior of biologic tissues including blood vessels. Stress relaxation is easier to quantify than hysteresis and, thus, has been more widely studied (150). One promising method of quantifying stress relaxation has been proposed by Fung (57), who found that the stress–strain–history relationship could be expressed as

$$\sigma(\lambda, t) = G(t) * \sigma^{(e)}(\lambda) \qquad [9]$$

where G(t) is the so-called reduced relaxation function, $\sigma^{(e)}$ is the elastic response to an instantaneous change in length as described by Eq. 4, and the asterisk denotes convolution. The beauty of this formulation is that the time-dependent behavior has been separated from the stretch response, so that each can be obtained separately from suitable experiments.

If one subjects tissue to a constant stress, the tissue will gradually elongate over a prolonged period of time (Fig. 8). This behavior is called creep. It is the converse, both experimentally and

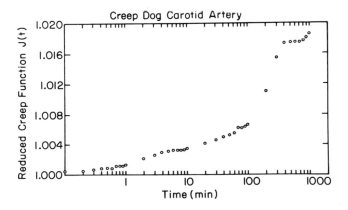

FIG. 8. Normalized creep function of a dog carotid artery. The *ordinate* represents the change in strain due to a step change in loading. (From Tanaka and Fung, ref. 150, with permission.)

mathematically, of stress relaxation and should be amenable to a similar type of analysis as in Eq. 9. Often a tissue will not return to its original length on removal of a load. This increase in unstressed length is one manifestation of creep and is owing to what is termed the irrecoverable portion of creep.

Another method of assessing time-dependent behavior of materials is to subject it to an oscillatory loading and unloading at varying frequencies. If the oscillatory (usually a sinusoid) load is made very small, the material can be assumed to behave linearly over the range of oscillations so that the complications of non-linearity are avoided. One can then measure the dynamic stiffness modulus, which is the ratio of the oscillatory stress to strain, and also the phase difference between the stress and strain as a function of frequency as shown in Fig. 9. The modulus and phase enable one to fully describe the time-dependent behavior.

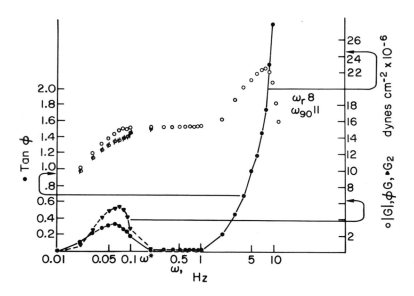

FIG. 9. The dynamic response of dog aortic elastin to a sinusoidal forcing function. *Open symbols* represent the dynamic stiffness modulus (stress/strain), and *closed symbols* represent the phase difference (stress phase − strain phase). (From Apter and Marquez, ref. 4, with permission.)

Hysteresis, stress relaxation, creep, and the oscillatory response are all manifestations of tissue viscosity and can be lumped under the general term viscoelasticity. Since they all derive from the same tissue property, any one type of test should be sufficient to describe fully the viscoelasticity of tissue. Theoretically, if the material were linearly viscoelastic, one could perform one type of test and be able to predict the results of the others. However, Remington (126) and Cox (42) in vascular tissue and Pinto and Fung (124) in heart muscle have shown that the hysteresis loop size is relatively independent of strain rates. Similarly, the dynamic stiffness is not strongly frequency dependent, and the phase lag does not have a sharp peak (3,124). These results imply that the time-dependent behavior of biologic tissue is not strictly linearly viscoelastic. Thus another complication is introduced into the picture. A unifying theoretical formulation has not yet been achieved, partly because of the nonlinearity and large deformations involved in this type of tissue. Until that goal is achieved, one is left with describing viscoelastic behavior in terms of one or more specific tests without being able to verify that the results of one corroborate the other. Fung (57) is working toward this end, and the reader is referred to his work for details.

Indirect Methods

An indirect means of measuring the viscoelastic properties of blood vessels is to measure the propagation velocity of either pressure or flow waves between two points. This method has its basis in the Moens-Korteweg equation which was formulated in 1878 and, in reality, was restricted to elastic tubes. This equation predicts the pulse wave velocity to obey the relationship

$$C = \sqrt{\frac{Eh}{2\rho R}} \qquad\qquad [10]$$

where C is the wave velocity, E the elastic modulus, h the thickness of the wall, ρ the density of the fluid, and R the radius of the tube. Obviously, this equation has limited application in the

actual vasculature because h and R are assumed to be constant at the two points of measurement and the tube is assumed to be linearly elastic. As the previous discussion indicated, none of these assumptions is correct.

Bramwell and Hill (21) modified Eq. 10 into a more useful form by using the equation for a thick-wall cylinder and arriving at the form

$$C = \sqrt{\frac{V}{P\,dV/dP}} \qquad [11]$$

where V is the volume and P is transmural pressure. In this form of the equation the pulse wave velocity is related to the volume distensibility of the vessel.

Experimentally, many earlier workers measured the pulse wave velocity by measuring the propagation time of a selected point on the pressure pulse, usually the foot of the pressure wave. From that measurement inferences were made regarding the "elasticity" or "distensibility" of blood vessels with increasing age (22,70,88,133,134,141). Because of the viscoelastic properties of the wall and because of reflections from the periphery, recent workers have pointed out deficiencies in the previous experimental methods used to measure wave velocity (36,111). These properties of the vessel wall produce wave distortions along the vasculature so that one cannot simply measure the propagation speed of a selected point in either the pressure or flow waves. Cox (36) and Nichols and McDonald (111) have proposed alternative methods of measuring the so-called true propagation coefficients, and the reader is referred to their works for details. Suffice it to say that the older literature regarding the changes in the pulse wave velocity with age should be interpreted qualitatively and not quantitatively.

What emerges from this brief discussion is a picture of the complexity of the relationship between stress and strain in living tissue. It is of little wonder that the many different experimental approaches and definitions used over the years have made the study of the relationship between age and vascular tissue proper-

ties a complicated and confusing area. What follows is an attempt to highlight the major age-dependent changes that have been found.

Directly Measured Mechanical Properties

Descriptive Studies

One of the earliest published reports concerned with mechanical property changes with age in the arterial system is that by Roy (130). He performed a variety of experiments including thermoelastic studies, force–elongation and pressure–volume studies of intact segments, and force–elongation studies of strips of aortic tissue from both humans and rabbits. Without attempting to quantify the data, he concluded that with advancing age, the distensibility (compliance) of arterial segments decreased. Mature arteries tended to be more compliant than very young aortas. He also found that the pressure–volume curves of different parts of the aorta had very similar shapes, as did those from femoral and carotid arteries.

Following Roy's publication have been numerous studies that have evaluated the mechanical properties of aging arteries in a descriptive manner without rigorous attempts to quantitate the results in an engineering framework. Yater and Birkeland (169) studied human aortic strips obtained at autopsy subjected to uniaxial loading and demonstrated that extensibility decreased with age. They found that the extensibility increased up to 27 years of age then decreased progressively. They found no dependence on sex or blood pressure in this decrease. Wilens (161) found both a site and a directional dependence of extensibility. Strips from the transverse lower abdominal and longitudinal thoracic aorta seemed to become less extensible earlier than other portions of the aorta. Winson and Heath (164), however, found that in the carotid sinus, there was no difference in extensibility between longitudinal and circumferential strips. Hass (74) studied isolated elastic tissue and ring segments taken from human thoracic aortas.

He showed that the extensibility of the isolated elastin was greater than that of the ring, whereas creep was greater in the ring specimens. There appeared to be no age dependence to the creep phenomena, but in both rings and isolated elastin the extensibility increased up to the fourth decade of life then decreased with further aging. He concluded that isolated tissue behavior did not predict the behavior of an intact ring. Ben-Ishai et al. (13) determined the amount of retraction resulting when two transverse cuts were made in human aortas and found that the retraction decreased with increasing age and was greater in males than females.

Quantitative Studies

A number of other investigators (8,26,54,67,107,109) have studied the mechanical properties of aging arteries by measuring the pressure–volume or pressure–diameter behavior of intact segments of vessels. Hallock and Benson (71) demonstrated that the percentage increase in volume because of a pressure increment (volume distensibility) progressively decreased with increasing age. By age 75 the distensibility was 25% of that in a young specimen. Butcher and Newton (26) studied volume distensibility as well as circumferential and longitudinal distensibility in thoracic and abdominal segments of human aortas. They found that the distensibility decreased in both the longitudinal and circumferential directions with age, with the maximum distensibility occurring at age 8. They also found regional differences, with the thoracic having greater volume distensibility than the abdominal aorta. The longitudinal distensibility was greater in the iliac than in the abdominal aorta, while the converse was true for the circumferential distensibility.

Bader (8) found that older aortas had larger volumes at zero pressure than young aortas and the percentage volume increase owing to a 100-mm Hg pressure step decreased linearly with age. Nakashima and Tanikawa (109) found the volume distensibility of human aortas that had been stored for 2 to 5 days to decrease progressively with increasing age. This decrease in distensibility was apparently not related to the degree of atherosclerosis.

Mozersky et al. (107) used a transcutaneous echo probe to measure femoral artery diameters and brachial artery sphygmomanometer pressures to estimate blood pressures in living human subjects. They found a decrease with age in percent volume distensibility and an increase with age in the normalized pressure–diameter modulus $\frac{R dP}{dR}$. Gozna et al. (67) measured the aortic pressures and diameters at the time of cardiac catheterization in man and, using the same modulus as Mozersky et al., found a linear increase with age.

Fronek and Fung (54) measured volume distensibility in various segments of 6- and 30-month-old rabbit aortas. They found that the old had larger volumes than the young with greater distensibilities as well. There were also regional differences, with the carotid artery having the greatest, the abdominal aorta an intermediate amount, and the iliac artery the least distensibility. The distensibility was 25% greater in the old iliac artery and 50% greater in the old abdominal aorta at 100 mm Hg luminal pressure. Thus, most of these studies show that in intact segments of aortas and large arteries, distensibility decreases with increasing age. There are some regional differences in this age dependence. The study by Fronek and Fung (54) demonstrates that rabbits may differ from humans in this age dependence.

There are several animal and human studies that have quantified the changes in the mechanical properties of blood vessels in accordance with the engineering principles outlined at the beginning of this section. Many studies have shown the nonlinear nature of the stress–strain relationship in rats (16,40,80), dogs (37,39,90,150), rabbits (132), and humans (128). The exponential nature of the relationship was demonstrated in dogs (150) and humans (90). Regional differences in the dynamic stiffness property changes with age have also been shown in human aortas (90).

The age dependence of these mechanical properties appear to depend on the species examined. Hume (80) subjected ring segments of rat aortas of 90, 180, and 600 days of age to various loads. He calculated the elastic modulus using the large deformation strain. There was a progressive decrease with advancing age in the modulus at each of the loads studied. With aging there was also a progressive decrease in the load necessary to cause fracture. Cox (40) studied intact segments of rat aortas and converted the pressure–diameter data to stress–strain data by assuming a uniform cylindrical geometry. There was an increase in the value of the modulus with increasing age. Viscoelasticity was demonstrated, with the amount of hysteresis in the stress–strain curve being highest in the middle age group. Berry et al. (16) found no age difference in the incremental modulus in rats. However, they did not convert their pressure data into stresses and this latter fact may account for the discrepancy between their data and those of the previous two studies.

Saxton (132) subjected rings of rabbit aortas to increments of load and calculated the passive elastic modulus at loads of 20, 60, 100, and 160 g after allowing 5 min for creep to equilibrate. He demonstrated that at every load there was a progressive decrease with age in the value of the modulus with 5-month- and 5-year-old rabbits differing by about 30%. The older aortas had less creep recovery (retraction) on release of each load. In each age group regional differences were noted with a decrease in the modulus in the distal compared to the proximal aorta.

Cox (37,39) studied canine arterial vessels using a modified incremental modulus based on Eq. 8 as proposed by Bergel (14). He found that in iliac, renal, mesenteric, and carotid arteries, as well as the aorta, the circumferential and radial moduli increased with age. In the carotid artery the longitudinal modulus decreased during maturation and then increased with aging.

More recently Cox (41,42) demonstrated regional differences in both the passive and viscous properties in both the circumferential and longitudinal directions in dogs. The intercept of the stiffness–stress line (Eq. 5) decreased in the periphery in circumferen-

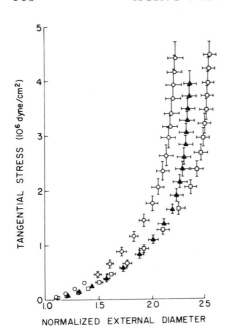

FIG. 10. Effect of age on the tangential stress–strain relationship of rat carotid arteries based on an incremental theory: (□) 2-month; (▲) 12-month; (○) 24-month. With increasing age the curves shift to the left, indicating increasing stiffness. *Bars* denote mean ± SEM. (From Cox, ref, 40, with permission.)

tial strips, whereas it increased in longitudinal strips. The slope, however, increased in the periphery in circumferential strips and decreased in longitudinal strips (Fig. 10). The viscoelastic behavior was not entirely consistent, since the amount of hysteresis and the slope of the stiffness–stress line were independent of strain rate but stress relaxation occurred. The rate and extent of this stress relaxation was greater in the peripheral vessels. The findings in this last study are compatible with the findings of Pinto and Fung (124) in heart muscle and Remington (126) in blood vessels, which suggest that tissue possesses nonlinear viscoelasticity.

Burton and co-workers (25,128) used the simplified Laplace law (Eq. 6) to convert pressure–volume data to stress and strain. They demonstrated that human iliac and brain vessels had an increased elastic modulus with increasing age. Mirsky and Janz (102) developed a more complete large deformation, anisotropic theory for soft tissues and applied it to the human pressure–volume data of Bader (8). They found that both the diameter

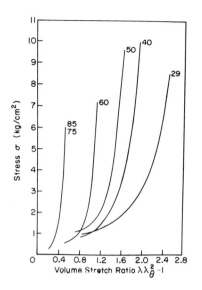

FIG. 11. Effect of age on the stiffness–stress relationship of human aortas based on a large deformation anisotropic theory. The arterial stiffness increases with age up to age 75. (From Mirsky and Janz, ref. 102, with permission.)

and the elastic stiffness increased with increasing age (Fig. 11). The larger diameter and the nonlinear nature of the stress–strain relationship, however, allowed the older aorta to operate at a level where the wall stiffness remained nearly the same as that in the younger aortas.

Two studies on the age dependence of dynamic stiffness have been conducted. Band et al. (10) demonstrated no age difference in the dynamic stiffness of aortas of rats in the frequency range of 1 to 5 Hz. Learoyd and Taylor (90), in a more complete study of human aortas, demonstrated that there was both an age and site dependence of dynamic stiffness. In the frequency range of 1 to 10 Hz the old thoracic aorta was stiffer than the young thoracic aorta. In the carotid and abdominal aorta there was no age difference. These findings are shown in Fig. 12. In the iliac and femoral arteries the young had a higher dynamic stiffness than the old.

In summary, these studies demonstrate that in humans there are definite mechanical property changes in the large vessels with advancing age. The consensus of the quantitative and qualitative data is that there is an increase in the elastic modulus or decrease

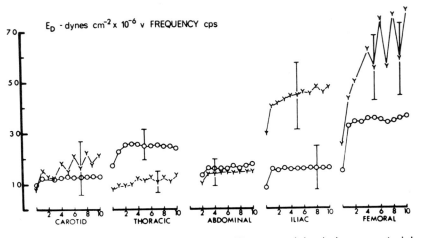

FIG. 12. Effects of age on the dynamic stiffness modulus in human arterial walls from various sites. All data obtained at 100 mm Hg intraluminal pressure. Only in the thoracic aorta do the old arteries have a higher modulus than the young. (From Learoyd and Taylor, ref. 90, with permission.)

in distensibility, respectively, in human vessels in old age. There are some regional differences and in a given region there is a directional dependence to this age change. The dynamic elastic properties in humans also appear to change with age but the change is complex and is quite site dependent. The aging dog appears to have changes similar to those of man. However, the age changes shown in the two rabbit studies cited are opposite to those seen in man. The data in rats is inconclusive, with one study showing no change, one an increase, and one a decrease in elastic modulus with age. Whether these are actual species differences or whether alterations in vessel properties are dependent on absolute rather than relative age is difficult to ascertain and needs clarification.

Indirectly Measured Mechanical Properties

As discussed previously, measurements of pulse wave velocity that do not account for reflections and viscoelastic properties of the vessel wall are quantitatively in error. Qualitatively, however, they indicate certain trends with advancing age. The pioneering work of Bramwell et al. (21,22) postulated the feasibility of using the pulse wave velocity as an indirect method of measuring the mechanical properties of large vessels in man. They demonstrated an increase with age in the pulse wave velocity from 5.8 m/sec at 15 years to 8.0 m/sec at 60 years of age. The calculated mean volume distensibility based on those figures decreased from 0.36 to 0.20 (mm Hg^{-1}). Since that time, there have been numerous studies on the change in pulse wave velocity with age in man (22,70,134,141). The conclusion from these human studies is that in every vessel studied thus far, the pulse wave velocity increases with advancing age. These data are supportive of the directly measured change in the mechanical properties discussed above.

Pulmonary Vasculature Mechanical Property Changes

The changes with age in the mechanical properties of the pulmonary circulation have not been studied as extensively as the systemic circulation. Roy (130) noted the curvilinear nature of the force–elongation curve in pulmonary arteries and also noted that they were more extensible than aortas. Harris et al. (73) measured the length–tension relationship of circumferential strips of the human pulmonary trunk with the adventitia removed. They also demonstrated that the extensibility was greater than that in the aorta. At stresses of 2,400 and 10,000 dynes/mm^2 there was a decrease in extensibility with increasing age (from 34.5 and 73.6%, respectively, in the second decade to 22 and 35%, respectively, in the eighth decade). They found that percentage extensibility could be expressed as an exponential function of age. Gozna et al. (67) used a pressure–strain modulus, with the strain measured from maximum to minimum diameter, as well as the pulse wave velocity to quantitate the age change in human pulmonary arteries. They found a linear increase in both the modulus and pulse wave velocity with increasing age.

Indirect studies have also demonstrated an increase in pulmonary circulation elasticity with age. Emirgil et al. (48) performed right heart catheterization in humans and measured the pulmonary vascular resistance index as a function of both age and exercise. They found a linear relationship between pressure and flow for both young and old subjects. The old (60 years and older) subjects had almost twice as high a value of pulmonary vascular resistance index as the young subjects. Robinson and Gillespie (129) measured diffusing capacity and pulmonary capillary volume in beagles between 1 and 10 years of age and found that there was a decrease in both parameters with increasing age. They found no change in pulmonary artery pressures and attributed the decrease in the latter to a loss of exchange area due to encroachment by alveolar ducts.

In summary, the few studies on pulmonary vascular mechanics indicate that the pulmonary artery is more extensible than the aorta but that, like the aorta, there is an age-associated decrease in this extensibility with age.

RELATION OF STRUCTURAL AND MECHANICAL AGE CHANGES

Background

The mechanical properties of the vessel wall reflect both its structural composition and its architecture. The latter is, in turn, strongly dependent on the degree of distention of the vessel. As discussed above, aging is accompanied by changes in the composition and intrinsic architecture of the vessel wall as well as by increases in vessel diameters. All of these factors contribute to the age change in the mechanical properties of the blood vessels. Some aspects of the relationship between structure and function of blood vessels will be reviewed before considering the effects of age on this relationship.

Because of the thinness of the endothelial lining, both Remington (126) and Burton (24) considered it extremely unlikely that the endothelium contributed significantly to the overall mechanical properties of the blood vessel. A similar although tacit assumption has been made by most workers regarding the role of the adventitia. Indeed, many studies on vessel properties have been conducted on vessels stripped of adventitia. Thus, the major contribution to vessel properties is assumed to arise from the inner intima and the media, which consist mainly of smooth muscle, elastin, and collagen. The effects of each of these components, individually and collectively, determine the mechanical properties of the vessel wall. The following discussion is a brief overview of some aspects of this complex interaction between structure and function.

Wilens (161) observed that passive smooth muscle exhibited mainly plastic rather than elastic behavior under normal stress levels. That is, once the muscle was loaded, it failed to retract to its original length when the load was removed. Since this behavior was very dissimilar to that of the vessel wall, he considered it unlikely that the muscle contributed significantly to the passive wall properties. Berry et al. (16) directly measured the incremental modulus of rat aorta before and after stimulating muscle contraction with norepinephrine. They found that muscle contraction had no effect on the modulus. However, Doyle and Dobrin (43), using finite deformation theory, demonstrated that muscle contraction due to norepinephrine increased the passive stiffness of dog carotid arteries. Wilens (161) also felt that collagen was not a major contributor to wall properties since it underwent only a 6% elongation compared to the 30 to 50% overall wall elongation at normal stresses. He thus felt that elastin must be the major contributor to the mechanical properties of the wall.

Burton (24) extended and quantified the findings of Wilens. Burton estimated that the Young's modulus for noncontracting smooth muscle was a very low 6×10^4 dynes/cm^2, making it far more extensible than the vessel wall. However, during rapid loading the modulus for muscle increased and could exceed that of the vessel wall. Using Hass' data (74) demonstrating a linear relationship between force and elongation for isolated elastic tissue, Burton estimated its Young's modulus to be 3×10^6 dynes/ cm^2. This value is still quite low, being 5 to 10 times lower than that of natural rubber. Burton felt that this large extensibility did not represent the intrinsic property of the elastin fibers but was owing to their helical configuration, and that what was being measured was the elasticity of the helix. Finally, using unpublished data on collagenous tissue, Burton estimated its Young's modulus to be about 10^9 dynes/cm^2.

To account for the overall vessel properties, Burton proposed a functional model with the elastin in parallel with the collagen. The collagen was assumed to be slack and under no stress at normal distending pressures. The muscle was interspersed between the elastin and collagen, with some transverse attachments to the collagen. With small elongations or low distending pressures, the property of the vessel reflected that of the elastin alone. With higher loading rates, the viscoelastic properties reflected those of the smooth muscle. With more elongation or distention the collagen became taut, and only then did the vessel elasticity begin to reflect that of the collagen fibers. During muscle contraction the transversely attached muscle removes some of the slack from the collagen causing the vessel to become less distensible. This transverse arrangement of some muscle was needed to explain the decreased vessel distensibility during muscle contraction since the diameter decreases with contraction and should, theoretically, cause more slack in the collagen. It should be pointed out that Burton's schema with linear elastin and collagen stress–strain relationships cannot account for the curvilinearity in the vessel stress–strain curve. However, if the coiled elastin fibers behaved like a mesh, or a nonlinear spring, or if the elastin fiber itself were subjected to some tension and had a nonlinear stress–strain curve, this difficulty with the conceptual model would be removed.

There is some evidence for the above. Wolinsky and Glagov (166) demonstrated that at physiological distending pressures the elastin lamellae actually straighten out completely and both the interlamellar distance and lamellae thickness decrease. In addition, the thin interconnecting fibrils became more circumferentially oriented and began to restrain more lamellae. This change in geometry and evidence of actual stretching of elastin lamellae could produce the curvilinearity in the force–elongation curve. Carton et al. (27) demonstrated that the relation between stress and strain of single elastin fibers was exponential. Elastin was highly extensible at lower strain levels. Their findings do not answer the question of whether the elastin fibers themselves are supporting the stress or whether the curvilinear portion of the force–elongation curve is owing to a nonlinear springlike behavior of the elastin. Regardless of the mechanism, the nonlinearity of the elastin stress–strain curves helps resolve the difficulty with Burton's original schema.

Remington (126) envisioned the vessel to be composed of a loose jacket of collagen which was essentially inextensible. This jacket was thought to be attached in parallel to a network of elastic fibers which had a nonlinear stress–strain behavior. The overall stress–strain curve of the vessel at low strains was thought to be due to the elastic components and to the constraining collagen coat once the strain reached a given level. Remington thought that both the nonlinearity and viscoelasticity of the elastic fibers could be ascribed to a geometric arrangement akin to that of a mesh in a stocking. The changing tightness of the weave with larger strains produced the nonlinearity in stress. Varying amounts of lubricant between the fibers accounted for viscosity. In addition, the arrangement of the weave could be altered by muscle activity or previous stretches to account for altered mechanical properties due to these factors. However, Remington did not dismiss the possibility that elastin per se possessed a nonlinear stress–strain curve, since he demonstrated such behavior in ligamentum nuchae which is composed primarily of elastin. The idea of a constraining jacket of collagen was supported by the findings of Smith et al. (143) of circumferential hoops of collagenous fibers attached to the outer surfaces of the elastic membranes of rat aortic media.

Before addressing the question of the role of aging in modifying the relationship between structure and function, it is useful to consider the question of whether or not arteriosclerosis is a precursor, is a resultant, or is unrelated to the mechanical property changes seen with aging. Wilens (161) found that with age the increasing weight of the aortic intima correlated with the decrease in extensibility. However, in strips of aortic media denuded of intima and in pulmonary artery strips in which there were no intimal changes with age, there was still a progressive decline in extensibility with age. Furthermore, in aortas in which there was no intimal sclerosis the decrease in extensibility with age persisted. These findings led Wilens to conclude that the decline in extensibility with age was primarily influenced by age rather than the presence of intimal sclerosis. Subsequently, there have been many studies which support the viewpoint that age per se is the causative factor in the change in mechanical properties. For instance, Butcher and Newton (26) found that the decrease in volume distensibility with age in human arteries was no different in those vessels with or without advanced intimal disease or medial calcification.

Similarly, Nakashima and Tanikawa (109), in a study of Japanese and American aorta autopsy specimens, found that age rather than the severity of the atherosclerosis was the major factor accounting for the decrease in distensibility with advancing age. Thus, arteriosclerosis may actually be the result of alterations in mechanical properties producing localized regions of excessive trauma which then lead to the pathological state. There are differences of opinion on this matter, with many workers still favoring the view that intimal changes caused by blood-borne factors or caused by lipid migration through the vessel wall are the etiologic factors in plaque formation and that these intimal changes lead to the mechanical property changes. A detailed discussion is beyond the scope of this review; the reader is referred to the discussion by Milch (95).

Effect of Aging on Structure and Function

With the preceding discussion as a background, one can now examine the relationship between the age changes in the structural and mechanical properties of the larger blood vessels. Since the endothelium, the adventitia, and smooth muscle do not appear to contribute significantly to the passive mechanical properties, it is unlikely that the alteration in function in aged vessels is owing to the age changes in these components described earlier. Rather, it is more likely that the mechanical changes with age are related to the age changes in the intima and media. These changes could arise from age changes in the intrinsic properties of elastin and collagen, an alteration in the relative content of these two components, a change in the physical relationship (architecture) between the two, or a combination of all of these changes. A brief discussion of evidence for each of these possibilities follows.

Support for a change in architecture as the principal cause of the age change in properties comes from the study of Wilens (161), who found that aging was accompanied by a loss of undulation of the elastic fibers. When vessels were formalin fixed at pressures greatly exceeding those achieved during life, the elastin fibers were still found to be slightly wavy. Only at extreme loadings of 1,500 g or greater did the fibers appear to become straight. Thus, he postulated that the loss of extensibility of the vessel wall with age was due primarily to the change in architecture (increased stretch) of the elastic fibers rather than a change in the intrinsic material properties of the elastin. It should be pointed out that Wilens' findings suggest that the elastin helix behaves like a nonlinear spring with age determining at which portion of the force–elongation curve the vessel operates. Krafka (85) found no correlation between the wall thickness and decreased extensibility with age. He felt that the change in properties was owing more to an architectural change than to an increase in number of collagen fibers with age.

Butcher and Newton (26) postulated that the decreased distensibility seen in the abdominal compared to the thoracic aorta was because of a change in the helical arrangement such that longitudinal distensibility decreased whereas circumferential distensibility was not altered. Futhermore, they found that the aging changes were more prominent in the lower pressure ranges, where the collagen tended to be less stretched. They postulated that aging somehow caused a change in the unstretched collagen length such that the collagen effect became more prominent at shorter lengths. Finally, since they found no different age effect on distensibility in vessels with marked arteriosclerosis or medial elastin calcification, they felt that elastin fragmentation was not an etiologic factor in the mechanical property changes with age.

Roach and Burton (128) also found that the increased elasticity with age was not related to a change in medial thickness. Their finding of an increased modulus at zero stretch in aged vessels was interpreted as reflecting a larger population of collagen with shorter unstretched lengths since there was no change in elastin content. They postulated that this population arose because of increased cross-linking of collagen fibers with advancing age.

Many studies have demonstrated directly or indirectly an alteration in the elastin and collagen composition with aging in both the intima and media (9,23,30,40). Bader and Kapal (9) ascribed the disappearance of the inflection point of the pressure–volume curve in advanced age to almost complete loss of elastic tissue. In addition, the calculated elastic modulus at age 85 approached that of pure collagen. Roach and Burton (128) also ascribed some of the age changes they found to an increase in number of collagen fibers. Cox (40) measured the collagen/elastin ratio as well as the absolute collagen content in rat carotid arteries of different ages and found a close relationship between the age increase in the ratio and the age increase in incremental modulus. In an earlier study, Cox et al. (42) demonstrated a similar result in maturing dog aortas.

Hass (75) demonstrated the multifactorial nature of the age relationship between structure and function. He found that isolated elastic tissue extensibility decreased with increasing age. In addition, collagen content increased with age. This increase occurred in the form of diffuse interlamellar deposits as well as increased number of splints on the surface of each lamella. He postulated that collagen disruption of the elastin owing to the splints caused the elastin to remain under tensile stress. Thus, the decrease in vessel extensibility with age was because of age changes in the intrinsic property of the elastin, an increase in total collagen content, and an architectural change with collagen disrupting the elastin.

Similarly, Cox (38,40) noted that in the low-strain region, there was essentially no age effect on the incremental modulus despite a marked decrease in elastin content and no change in collagen content. He therefore felt that there were elements other than elastin and collagen that contributed to the stress–strain behavior in this low-strain region. He suggested smooth muscle activation, intrinsic change in elastin properties, extracellular water, and complicated architectural effects as some possibilities to explain this effect.

Smith et al. (143) demonstrated increased interlamellar fiber density in old mouse aorta. They also demonstrated increased ground substance staining between the elastic lamella and increased number of circumferential collagenous hoops attached to the lamella. They postulated that all three of these age changes contributed to the decreased "efficiency" of elastin in the old mouse.

The few studies (10,90) on the age changes in viscoelastic behavior of the vascular system do not clearly elucidate the component(s) responsible for the viscous effect and do not elucidate which component(s) is (are) responsible for the aging effect. The studies of Apter et al. (3,4) show that it is likely that smooth muscle plays a major role in the dynamic vessel properties, but contributions from elastin and collagen, especially with respect to aging effects, are also possible and have not been evaluated.

The pulmonary vascular system is even less well studied than the arterial tree. There are no direct studies that attempt to relate age changes in structure to function. However, one can presume that the principles that govern the relationship between structure and function in the arterial system will also be extant in the pulmonary tree with quantitative but not qualitative differences. This presumption awaits further study.

From this brief overview, it is clear that the subject of the relation between structural changes and mechanical changes is extremely complicated because of its multifactorial nature. When the role of age is introduced, another complicating factor is added. With advancing age there are clearly definable alterations in the intrinsic structure of elastin, collagen, and smooth muscle as well as in the physical arrangement among these three major wall components. These alterations consist of (a) a decrease in inherent extensibility of elastin, (b) shorter unstressed lengths of both elastin and collagen, (c) increased stretch of elastin fibers, (d) increasing disruption of elastin by collagen and other fibrous tissues, and (e) increasing amount and content of collagen. The bulk of evidence favors the view that the mechanical property changes with advancing age cannot be ascribed solely to the changes in structure in any one component, but rather are owing to a multifactorial combination of intrinsic changes together with alterations in the physical arrangement between the components.

PHARMACOLOGIC CHANGES WITH AGING

Background

Aside from the earlier, brief discussion of pulse wave velocity changes with aging, the discussion thus far has considered the structural and mechanical changes with aging in isolated, noncontracting blood vessels. Before considering how aging of the vascular system affects cardiac function, it is useful to examine some pharmacologic changes with age, i.e., the response of the aged, intact vascular system to stimuli that are present in the body. In this setting, the role of smooth muscle, which was of secondary importance in the previous discussions, assumes primary importance because muscle tone is the one factor that can be altered on a moment-to-moment basis *in situ*. Alterations in smooth muscle tone, acting on the other structural components in the vessel wall, determine the functional mechanical state of the vascular system. The earlier discussion pointed out that the direct contribution of smooth muscle activation to the stress–strain properties of the vessel is still controversial. However, smooth muscle activation alters the intraluminal pressure and decreases the diameter of blood vessels and via this mechanism indirectly alters the mechanical properties of the vessel wall.

The muscle tone in the vascular system is determined by many factors, including the release of catecholamines by adrenergic nervous system activity, as well as by circulating levels of other vasoactive hormones. It is beyond the scope of this review to consider the age effects of the nervous system on vascular responsiveness. Rather, this discussion will focus on the age response of vascular tissue at the muscle level to catecholamines and other hormones. In general, stimulation of β-adrenergic receptors by pharmacologic or neurogenic means induces vasodilatation whereas α-adrenergic stimulation induces vasoconstriction. Stimulation by histamine, acetylcholine, 5-hydroxytryptamine (5-HT), or angiotensin causes vasoconstriction. The actual means whereby constriction or relaxation is attained by vasoactive drugs has not been clarified (20). One assumption is that the β-adrenergic response, as in other tissues, is triggered via receptors located on the surface of the muscle cell. Stimulation of the receptor by the pharmacologic agonist activates the enzyme adenylcyclase to make adenosine-3',5'-monophosphate (cyclic AMP), which acts as a messenger in the cell. Cyclic AMP formation causes a movement of divalent cations, primarily calcium, near the contractile apparatus, to produce the end result of muscle relaxation. The entire sequence of events from receptor stimulation to muscle relaxation is termed the β-adrenergic cascade. There is presumably another population of receptors on the cell surface which responds to α-adrenergic stimulation and causes vasoconstriction. The exact way in which α and β stimulation interact is also not known. It is clear that stimulation of one population of receptors modulates the tonic effect of the other set so that a constant balance between vasoconstriction and vasodilatation is maintained.

Age Changes

Hruza and Zweifach (79) infused epinephrine and norepinephrine to rats 3 and 14 months of age under pentobarbital anesthesia. They found no age difference in baseline blood pressures, but found a greater rise in pressure and a greater increase in blood flow in the old rats as compared to the young rats. When the catecholamines were applied directly to the mesentery, however, the old rats had a lesser response than the young. These results are difficult to explain, but Hruza and Zweifach ascribed this dichotomy of response to a regional age difference in responsiveness of vascular tissue to the catecholamines.

Fleisch et al. (53) studied the relaxation response of aortas of guinea pigs, rats, rabbits, and cats of various ages. Strips of aortas were first contracted with histamine or 5-HT and given an α-adrenergic blocking agent. The relaxation response to the β-adrenergic agonist isoproterenol was then tested. They found species and regional differences in the relaxation response. The thoracic aortas of guinea pigs, rabbits, and rats relaxed but that of the cat did not. The abdominal aortas did not relax with β-adrenergic stimulus, but did relax to sodium nitrate. The response of rabbit was greater than either rat or guinea pig. With increasing age the response to β-adrenergic stimulus decreased, but the relaxation response to nitrates was unchanged (Fig. 13). In a later (52) study involving rabbits and rats and a similar protocol, Fleisch and co-workers verified that the relaxation response to isoproterenol decreased with advancing age. Rabbits but not rats exhibited with age a decreased relaxation response to nitrates. In this later paper Fleisch et al. found that the agonist used to produce the initial contraction affected the amount of relaxation obtained. Less relaxation was obtained when histamine rather than potassium chloride was used initally to contract the muscle. They concluded that the relaxation deficit with increasing age was somewhere along the β-adrenergic cascade, but that the relaxation mechanism itself was intact since there was no age difference in response to the nonspecific relaxation caused by nitrates.

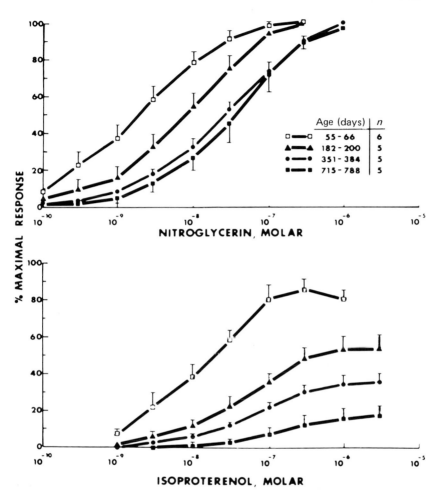

FIG. 13. Effect of age on the relaxation response of male rabbit thoracic aortas to both isoproterenol and nitroglycerin. There is a decreased response in the aged aortas to isoproterenol, but not to nitroglycerin. (From Fleisch and Hooker, ref. 52, with permission.)

Gulati et al. (69) compared isoproterenol-induced relaxation of aortas in rabbits of 2 to 3 months versus 6 months of age. They found that the young animals had a 15 to 25 times greater relaxation response to isoproterenol than the old ones. The fact that propranolol, a β-adrenergic blocker, did not block the relaxation response to isoproterenol in the old suggested to them that old aortas had an altered β-receptor population. In other words, old vessels appeared to have an α-adrenergic response to the isoproterenol that was not seen in the young rabbits.

Cohen and Berkowitz (31) studied the effects of various contracting and relaxing agents in old and young rat aortas. They found that the old aortas had a greater contractile response to 5-HT, potassium chloride, and norepinephrine than did the young ones. This age difference was thought not to be due to an α-adrenergic effect since it was present with the nonadrenergic drugs. Relaxation response was tested by administering cyclic AMP to aortic strips previously contracted with 5-HT. They found that the young relaxed to 50 to 60% of their maximum contraction, whereas the old only relaxed to 10%. Dibutyryl cyclic AMP, which is rapidly permeable across cell membranes, caused a similar age decline in relaxation as did administration of a phosphodiesterase inhibitor. However, there was no age difference in relaxation to nitroglycerin. These findings led them to conclude that the age-associated decrease in relaxation response was owing to a specific decrease in the vascular response to cyclic nucleotides rather than to age differences in cell permeability.

Ericsson and Lundholm (49) studied the isoproterenol-induced relaxation of 5-HT contracted thoracic aortic strips of rats aged 1, 3, and 6 months. With increasing age there was a diminution in isoproterenol-induced relaxation which was accompanied by a decrease in isoproterenol-stimulated cyclic AMP levels, an increase in basal and sodium fluoride-stimulated adenyl cyclase levels, and a decrease in phosphodiesterase levels. They concluded that the diminished ability of isoproterenol to increase cyclic AMP was not owing to a reduced ability to synthesize cyclic AMP nor to an increased rate of hydrolysis, but was because of the inability of isoproterenol to stimulate adenyl cyclase. This would place the age deficit at the level of the β-adrenergic receptors. They did not rule out the possibility that there was a reduced potency of cyclic AMP directly to induce relaxation since addition of cyclic AMP did not restore the relaxing ability of older aortas.

Tuttle (154) measured the response of rat aortas to norepinephrine and found an increase in the threshold and decreased maximum response in 2-year-old as compared to 1-year-old rats. Cox (40) also demonstrated a decreased maximum wall stress in 24-month-old as compared to 2- or 12-month-old rat aortas perfused with norepinephrine. However, there was no age decrement in the ability of muscle contraction to reduce the diameter of the blood vessel. These findings of a decreased contractile response in the old are opposite to the findings of Cohen and Berkowitz (31).

Fleisch and Hooker (52) found that the relaxation response to isoproterenol was decreased 50% in old compared to young pulmonary arteries. Like the aorta, there was no age difference in relaxation to the nonadrenergically mediated relaxant nitroglycerin. The above studies implicate changes in the β-adrenergic cascade for the decreased ability of aged vascular muscle to relax. The exact site or sites of the age defect have not been unequivocally determined. Age differences in the α-adrenergic contraction mechanism may also be present. Aside from these age changes, there are other sites in the link from central nervous system to muscle which could possess age changes. For example, Shibata et al. (138) employed catecholamine fluorescence to study adrenergic innervation in old and young rabbits. They found that the young had specific fluorescence in the muscle of the media. The old, however, had specific fluorescence only in the adventitia and adventitia–media junction. The young also had levels of tissue catecholamines twice as high as those of the old rabbits. They attributed their findings to degeneration with age in the adrenergic innervation of the media. A decreased innervation would explain a decreased *in vivo* response to adrenergic neural stimulation, but still would not explain the decreased pharmacologic responsiveness described earlier.

The degree of smooth muscle activation is a primary determinant of the size of the blood vessels, which, in turn, is a determinant of the mechanical properties in the intact vascular system.

As is discussed in the next section, these three interrelated factors (muscle tone, size, and mechanical properties) together dictate the functional state of the vascular system and its interaction with the heart. There are many other areas that require study in this complex field. The studies discussed above are just a beginning, but they indicate that definite age changes occur in the pharmacologic responsiveness of the vascular system. If one is eventually to delineate how the aging vascular system affects the function of the heart, these age responses must be clarified.

AGING AND THE VENTRICULAR–VASCULAR INTERACTION

Background

It is well known that the vascular system has a profound influence on the performance of the ventricle to which it is connected (81,153,155,162). For the purposes of this discussion, the general term "ventricular–vascular interaction" will be used to describe this physical interrelationship between the two systems. Probably the best-known example of the prolonged effect of an abnormal ventricular–vascular interaction is the development of right or left ventricular hypertrophy in response to pulmonary or systemic hypertension. Similarly, experimental hypertrophy has been produced by acutely altering the ventricular–vascular interaction by banding the pulmonary artery or aorta (17,92,113,145,163). Clinically, the principles of ventricular–vascular interaction have been applied empirically to improve left ventricular performance in acute left ventricular failure due to myocardial infarction (5,28,29) and in chronic failure due to other causes (32,33,96,105). Furthermore, the principles of mechanical cardiac assist devices such as aortic balloon counterpulsation (83,84,105) and aortic synchronized pulsation (87) are based on influencing the ventricular–vascular interaction in a direction favorable to the ventricle.

With regard to aging, changes that affect the vascular system might be expected to affect ventricular function independently of any intrinsic age alterations in ventricular function. As the previous sections have demonstrated, aging is associated with certain structural changes in both the systemic and the pulmonic vasculatures, including increase in vessel diameters, increase in collagen content, and loss of integrity of elastin. These structural changes are reflected in a change in the mechanical properties of the vessels of both systems such that the vessels become less extensible and their viscoelastic behavior is altered. Aging also alters the responsiveness of the smooth muscle of the vessels to vasoactive stimuli. This section will briefly discuss how these vascular changes can be integrated together to provide a picture of an age-associated change in the ventricular–vascular interaction. Since data in this area are scanty, there will, of necessity, be some speculative ideas that will need verification with future studies.

Vascular Impedance

In order for a concept as complex as the ventricular–vascular interaction to be useful, one must be able to measure and quantify some aspect of it. In the late 1950s Womersley (167,168) published a series of articles that paved the way for modern hemodynamics and established the foundations for using vascular impedance as a method of quantification of one aspect of the ventricular–vascular interaction.

Basically, the ventricle is considered to be a pulsatile pump ejecting blood into a series of elastic tubes which contain a Newtonian fluid. The fluid and the tubes represent a frequency-dependent resistance to the pump. Borrowing terminology from electrical engineering, this frequency-dependent resistance is called impedance. It has both real and imaginary parts and can be expressed as

$$Z = R + i\omega L \qquad [12]$$

where Z is the impedance, R is the steady state resistance, ω is frequency, and L is the inductance.

Following the work of Womersley, a number of other studies, both theoretical and experimental (1,6,15,47,58,60,97,99,100, 110,112,116,159), established that vascular impedance was a useful method of quantifying the load presented by the vascular system to the ventricle. Specifically, the efficiency with which the external work of the ventricle is transformed into forward blood flow can be calculated from measurements of vascular impedance. The impedance is determined by the physical characteristics of the vasculature (assumed to act as an elastic tube), including its elastic properties and size, as well as by the viscosity and density of the fluid contained within. A detailed discussion of vascular impedance is beyond the scope of this review. Excellent reviews of this subject can be found in refs. 94 and 98. The following section briefly covers some of the major quantitative aspects of vascular impedance.

Quantification of Impedance

Using the electric network analogy, Womersley (167) derived the vascular equivalents of R and L. The complete mathematical formulation of impedance is complicated and will not be presented here. However, examination of a limiting case is instructive, for it reveals the factors which comprise vascular impedance. If one considers an idealized system in which there are no wave reflections, one can calculate a characteristic impedance Z_0, the formula of which is

$$Z_0 = \frac{\rho V}{\pi R^2 \sqrt{1 - v^2} \sqrt{M}} e^{-i\phi/2} \qquad [13]$$

where V is the wave velocity given by Eq. 10, v is the Poisson's ratio of the tube, ρ is the fluid density, R is the radius of the tube, M is the modulus, and ϕ is the phase of the complex function

$$1 - \frac{2J_1(\alpha i^{3/2})}{\alpha i^{3/2} J_0(\alpha i^{3/2})} \qquad [14]$$

In this expression J_0 and J_1 are the Bessel functions of the first kind of order 0 and 1, i represents the imaginary number $\sqrt{-1}$, and α is a dimensionless number characterizing pulsatile flow. Womersley (167) defined α as

$$\alpha = R \frac{\sqrt{\omega}}{\nu} \qquad [15]$$

where ω is the frequency of oscillation and ν is the kinematic viscosity of the fluid. The specific dependence of impedance on the physical characteristics of the tube is delineated in this formula. This derivation assumes that the tube is elastic. More complex derivations that account for viscoelasticity of the wall have been proposed (35).

Experimentally, the impedance spectrum of the vascular tree is obtained by relating in terms of modulus and phase the corresponding frequency components of the pressure and flow waves at the entrance to the system. One way of doing this is by decomposing the pressure and flow waves into their Fourier components. The impedance modulus for a given harmonic is the ratio of the pressure to flow modulus at that harmonic, and the phase is the difference between the pressure and flow phase angles. This formulation can be expressed as follows. The flow wave can be expressed as

$$Q(t) = Q_0 + \sum_{n=1}^{N} Q_n \sin(n\omega t + \Phi_{Q_n}) \qquad [16]$$

where Q_0 is the mean flow, n is the harmonic number, Q_n is the amplitude of the nth harmonic, ϕ_{Q_n} is the phase of the nth harmonic, and ω is the frequency of pulsations. The pressure wave can be expressed in an analogous form. The impedance modulus on the nth harmonic is

$$Z_n = \frac{P_n}{Q_n} \qquad [17]$$

and the impedance phase is

$$\Phi_n = \Phi_{P_n} - \Phi_{Q_n} \qquad [18]$$

Examples of the aortic impedance modulus and phase using this formulation for the rat (Yin et al., *unpublished data*), dog (119),

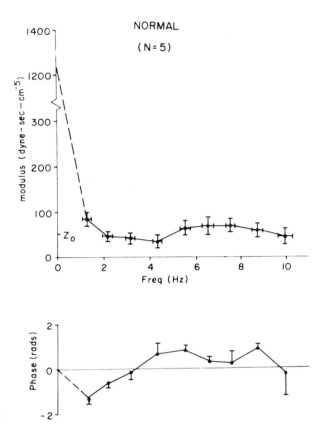

FIG. 14. (See pp. 190–192.) **A:** Aortic input impedance modulus and phase for man. (From Nicholas et al., ref. 110, with permission.)

and man (97) are shown in Fig. 14. The zero frequency term represents the mean peripheral resistance, i.e., mean pressure divided by the mean flow. The characteristic impedance is approximated by averaging the higher frequency components.

There are alternative methods to Fourier analysis for formulating the impedance. One such method, employing spectral analysis with randomly generated pressure and flow waves, has been proposed by Taylor (151).

From the modulus and phase data one can calculate the hydrau-

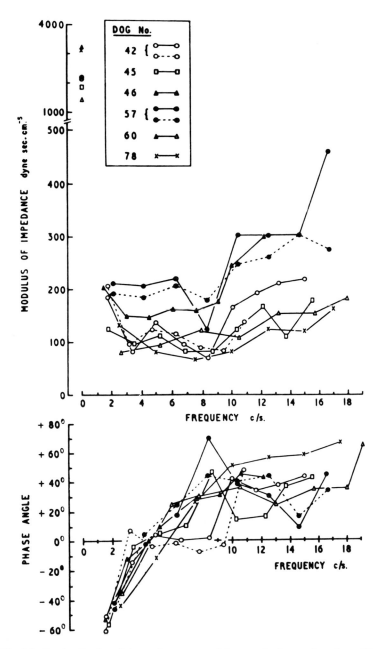

FIG. 14. B: Aortic input impedance modulus and phase for dog. (From Noble et al., ref. 112, with permission.)

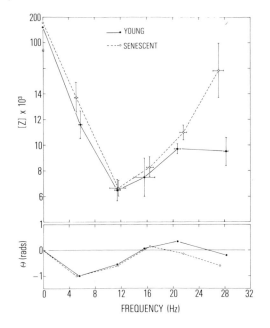

FIG. 14. C: Aortic input impedance modulus and phase for rat.

lic energy associated with the pulsatile waves. The energy per cardiac cycle is the average power. The hydraulic power consists of a steady and a pulsatile component. If one neglects the kinetic energy portion, which has been shown to be a small portion of the total energy (99), the total power can be expressed as

$$W = W_s + W_o \qquad [19]$$

where W_s is the steady component

$$W_s = P_0 Q_0 \qquad [20]$$

and W_o is the oscillatory component

$$W_o = \tfrac{1}{2} \sum_{n=1}^{N} (Q_n)^2 \, Z_n \cos(\Phi_n) \qquad [21]$$

where the terms on the right side of Eq. 21 are as defined in Eqs. 16 to 18.

The hydraulic power represents the power transferred from the left ventricle to the systemic vasculature. The mean power is that portion which is expended in moving blood and the oscillatory power is that portion which is lost in maintaining the pulsatile flow. Thus, the ratio of the pulsatile to the total power is an indication of the mechanical efficiency with which blood is pumped. The higher the ratio, the more energy is lost in the pulsatile components and the lower the efficiency of delivering blood to the periphery. For the aorta, several studies have demonstrated that the pulsatile fraction of total power is 10 to 15%, so that the efficiency of the left ventricle–systemic vasculature system is quite high (60,114,159).

A teleologic explanation for the similarity of the shape of the impedance spectrum across species was advanced by O'Rourke (115) and Mills et al. (97). They postulated that the anatomic configuration of most mammals can be visualized as an asymmetric T-tube with the upper extremities representing the short arm of the T. This configuration would theoretically cause the reflections from upper and lower extremities to cancel one another at the lower frequencies. Together with the attenuation of waves owing to the properties of the vascular wall, this results in the rather large drop from the mean term to the terms at the higher frequencies. This arrangement effectively uncouples the ventricle from the high impedances that occur in the peripheral arteries and is the physiologic means by which the vascular input impedance is matched to the ventricular output impedance. The efficiency of a mechanical system is optimized when input and output impedances are matched (1). Impedance matching thus allows the ventricle to deliver blood as efficiently as possible while also allowing the vascular system to buffer the pulsatile flow and convert it to a more continuous form. Viewed in this light, it is not surprising that mammals with such diverse sizes as the rat and the human have evolved with aortic impedances that are quite similar.

Many factors can alter the shape of the impedance spectrum and hence the ratio of pulsatile to total power. Factors that increase the ratio (i.e., decrease the efficiency of blood delivery) include decreasing the distensibility of the wall, vasodilatation and/ or a lowering of blood pressure, increasing cardiac output, slowing the heart rate, and moving the reflection sites more proximally (47,114,159). Vasoconstriction does not appear to have a significant effect on the pulsatile fraction of power (61,112,114). Increasing blood pressure per se, aside from its effects on extensibility, appears to decrease the pulsatile fraction (114). Thus, while the vasodilatory drugs that are being used for treatment of left ventricular failure may lower the total power output of the left ventricle by decreasing the mean term, they may actually decrease the efficiency of pumping by increasing the pulsatile fraction of total power. Whether or not this is beneficial to the heart in the long run and whether this is an optimum method of improving left ventricular function remains to be evaluated. In fact there are no direct studies on the effect of these vasodilatory drugs on aortic impedance.

The impedance of the pulmonary system differs considerably from that of the aorta. The impedance spectra of the pulmonary system for dogs (15) and man (100) are shown in Fig. 15. Calculations based on these data demonstrate a higher pulsatile power component (30 to 50% of the total) than in the aorta (99). Bergel and Milnor (15) also demonstrated that, unlike the aorta, the pulsatile power component was unchanged in the pulmonic system at heart rates up to 180 beats/min. Furthermore, some studies have shown that vasoconstriction in the pulmonary system increases the ratio of pulsatile to total power (123). This apparently does not occur in the aorta. However, the last point is still controversial, as one study showed no change in pulmonary impedance with vasoconstriction (117). The recent study by Piene and Hauge (123) demonstrated that at physiological pressures the pulsatile power component of the pulmonary artery was minimal. With either vasoconstriction or vasodilatation to pressures outside the normal range, the pulsatile component increased. While more data on the pulmonary impedance are needed before one can completely characterize its properties, it is evident that the pul-

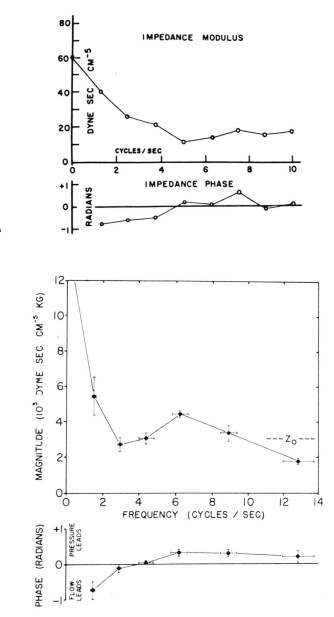

FIG. 15. Pulmonary vascular input impedance modulus and phase for **(A)** dog and **(B)** man. Compared to Fig. 14, it is seen that the higher frequency terms are more prominent. [From **(A)** Bergel and Milnor, ref. 15, and **(B)** Milnor et al., ref. 100, with permission.]

monic and systemic impedances differ both in the baseline state
and in response to vasoactive drugs. The higher fraction of pulsatile energy may be the most important difference between pulmonic and aortic impedances. The higher pulsatile component
in the pulmonic system presents the possibility that this term
actually becomes the dominant factor. Under certain conditions
the increase in the pulsatile energy term may outweigh the decrease in the steady energy term. This would certainly be detrimental to right ventricular function. This point will be emphasized in the later discussion.

Effects of Age on Impedance

Following this brief review of the concept of vascular impedance, one can now examine the effects of age. There are only
a few studies that have alluded to the question of age changes
in impedance in the systemic or pulmonic vascular trees, and
there are no studies that have directly measured age changes in
impedance. However, based on the knowledge of the age changes
in the vascular system and using the principles outlined above,
one can postulate how age might affect impedance. Learoyd and
Taylor (90) found an increase in dynamic stiffness and size in
old human thoracic aortas as compared to young ones. Since
the former would increase and the latter would decrease the impedance, the net result of age on aortic impedance would depend
on the relative influence of these counterbalancing factors.

It has been demonstrated that the left ventricle hypertrophies
mildly with advancing age (59,62,91,171). In rats it is also clear
that this hypertrophy is not owing to an elevation in mean arterial
pressure, as it occurs in the absence of an age-associated increase
in blood pressure (171). Since hypertrophy is caused by an increased loading on the heart, one possible explanation for this
age-associated hypertrophy is that the aged vascular system has
a slightly higher input impedance than the young one has. This
would place a greater load on the ventricle and result in the
mild hypertrophy. However, some preliminary measurements by

Yin et al. *(unpublished data)* suggest that under anesthesia there is no age difference in rat aorta input impedances. This finding would imply that at rest the old vascular system changes in such a way so as to enable the ventricle to continue to function at near optimum efficiency. Similarly, Cox (40) calculated the characteristic impedance in rat carotid arteries and found that Z_0 varied with transmural pressure and had a minimum at about 85 mm Hg. At all pressures Z_0 was actually higher in 2-month-old as compared to 24-month-old rats. Since aging of the rat systemic vasculature was shown previously to possess no clear age change in mechanical properties, these findings are not surprising. Nevertheless, if these findings are borne out by further studies in other species, one would have to postulate another mechanism besides increase in impedance to account for the ventricular hypertrophy with aging. On the other hand, Nichols et al. (110) found that Z_0 of patients with coronary disease was higher than that of normal controls. Since those with disease were older than the controls, they could not rule out age as one factor in the higher impedance in that group. Thus, the effect of age on vascular impedance in the normal state is not clear. Complicating factors of age differences in response to anesthesia, or age differences in vasomotor tone, etc., need to be examined.

All of the above studies were conducted without consideration of the effects of muscle contraction. As discussed earlier, the state of vasomotor tone may significantly alter both the aortic and, especially, the pulmonic impedances. The changes might be in disparate directions. Since the aged as compared to the young vascular smooth muscle has been shown to have an altered responsiveness to some vasoactive drugs, the combined effect of age and drugs on aortic and pulmonic impedances is complex and difficult to predict. The energy losses in the vasculature depend partially on its reflection characteristics. Vasodilatation changes these reflective properties. Aging, by virtue of producing changes in size and wall properties, also changes the reflective properties. Thus, the combination of age and vasodilatation might be synergistic such that large energy losses might be present.

Therefore, an aged individual could conceivably obtain fewer direct beneficial effects on left ventricular unloading from the use of vasodilatory drugs in the treatment of heart failure. In the pulmonary tree the pulsatile fraction of total power is large to begin with in the young and may be higher in the aged. If the finding of Piene and Hauge (123) discussed earlier is correct, than an intervention, such as vasodilatation, that increases this fraction might result in a net increase in total power as well as a decrease in efficiency and might actually increase the load on the right ventricle. Thus, the use of vasodilatory drugs for decreasing the load on the left ventricle might, in the aged, have a paradoxically deleterious effect on the right ventricle. The result of this on left ventricular function is discussed below.

Similarly, during exercise there is vasodilatation in many vascular beds, including the pulmonary bed, and vasoconstriction in other beds. The net effect of the vasomotor changes with exercise on aortic input impedance appears to be an increase in impedance (64,121). The effect of exercise on the pulmonary impedance is similar (45). Since the aortic impedance increases during exercise, the load on the left ventricle also increases. This increase in load may, in part, be the limiting factor for exercise capacity. If the impedance in either the pulmonary or aortic system increased more during exercise in the aged this might explain the decreasing exercise capacity (63) with increasing age. Thus, the effect of age on vascular impedance under stress conditions and during interventions that are actually meant to alter impedances are not known. This is clearly an area of study that would have important clinical implications.

Ventricular Interdependence

Up to this point the right ventricle–pulmonic vasculature and the left ventricle–systemic vasculature have been considered as separate entities. Alterations in ventricular function have been ascribed to changes in the vascular system into which it ejects. In reality, of course, the situation is quite different. The two ventricles are connected in series by the pulmonary vasculature. In addition, the two ventricles share a common wall, the interventricular septum, and are enclosed in a rather inextensible chamber, the pericardium. The pericardium is much less extensible than either ventricle (78,125) and effectively acts to maintain a constant total volume within its chamber. The physical arrangment is one in which alterations in the pressure or volume in one ventricle should affect the pressures and volumes in the other, i.e., ventricular interdependence exists.[2] There have been several studies that have demonstrated such ventricular interdependence. Laks et al. (86) and Taylor et al. (152) demonstrated that increasing right ventricular pressure and volume shifted and steepened the left ventricular pressure–volume relationship. Elzinga et al. (46) also demonstrated that increased filling on one side of the heart decreased the output from the opposite ventricle. This effect was more pronounced with an intact pericardium. Santamore et al. (131) and Bemis et al. (12) also demonstrated essentially similar findings. The significant role of the pericardium in the interdependence has been postulated and discussed by several authors (2, 65,66,146).

Thus, the pulmonary vasculature by virtue of its physical location, affects right ventricular function directly via its input impedance and indirectly affects left ventricular function via the interdependence mechanism. Clinically, this influence of the pulmonary vasculature has been known for years and is the postulated mechanism for the normal decrease in arterial pressure during deep inspiration (pulsus paradoxus). In this situation inspiration causes a sudden decrease in intrathoracic pressure which increases venous return to the right side of the heart (137). The increased right ventricular output is initially buffered by the ca-

---

[2] Note that, for purposes of this discussion, the pumping function of the heart is assumed to depend more on its chamber properties (pressure and volume) than on its wall properties (stress and strain). Mirsky (101) has demonstrated the complex relationship between chamber properties and wall properties and has shown that changes in chamber properties do not necessarily reflect changes in the properties of the wall.

pacitance effect of the pulmonic bed. The increased right ventricular volume and pressure transiently decrease left ventricular diastolic volume and hence cardiac output so that systemic arterial pressure decreases. This effect is exaggerated in conditions in which the ventricular volumes are constrained more than normally by the pericardium as in tamponade or constrictive pericarditis (137). Recently Weyman et al. (160) and Weiss et al. (157) have demonstrated clearly that the interventricular septum shifts towards the left ventricle during conditions that cause an overload on the right ventricle. Whether or not this septal shift influences left ventricular function is not yet clear.

The influence of the pulmonic vasculature in unloading the right ventricle has been postulated to be part of the beneficial effect obtained on left ventricular function when vasodilatory drugs are given for left ventricle failure (66). Sivak et al. (142) demonstrated that during nitroprusside infusion in dogs an increase in left ventricular cardiac output was obtained in conjunction with an increase in pulmonary blood volume and decrease in pulmonary vascular resistance. This effect was obtained prior to any change in mean arterial pressure. Presumably, nitroprusside dilated the pulmonary bed and thereby decreased the load presented to the right ventricle. Via the interdependence mechanism, this unloading of the right side allowed the left ventricular end-diastolic volume, and hence output, to increase even before a direct effect of the drug on aortic resistance or impedance was achieved. This study was only inferential, however, and no measurements of impedances were made. As discussed earlier, the impedance spectrum of the pulmonary bed together with its perhaps paradoxic response to vasoactive drugs preclude one from ascertaining without direct measurement the effect of a specific intervention. In fact, vasodilatation may actually cause a loading of the right ventricle, in which case the interdependence postulate for the beneficial effect of vasodilators would be incorrect.

The role of aging in ventricular interdependence has not been studied. From what has already been discussed, one could postulate several situations in which aging may play a significant role. During exercise, the pulmonary vascular bed of the aged might not be able to decrease its total power as much as in the young (perhaps owing to less efficient oxygenation or diminished pulmonary vascular response to catecholamines) (77). This would cause a relatively higher load on the right ventricle in the old and thus might impair left ventricular function, leading to the diminished exercise capacity.

Consider the use of vasodilatation for treatment of left ventricular failure. If the aged pulmonic vasculature had an altered response to the drugs such that input impedance were increased relative to that of the young, the old right ventricle would be less unloaded and the beneficial effect on the left ventricle might be diminished. On the other hand, as discussed earlier, if pulmonary vasodilatation actually caused a deleterious effect on right ventricular function and this effect were accentuated with age, this therapetuic modality would not be useful in the aged group.

As a final example of ventricular–vascular interaction, consider the effect of the left ventricle on the peripheral pulmonary system. It is known that ischemia causes both an increase in stiffness of myocardial tissue and a decrease in distensibility of the ventricular chamber. How age affects the response to ischemia is not known, but, as was discussed earlier, age causes similar changes in mechanical properties in the normal state. Thus, during ischemia (due to coronary artery disease, for example) the aged left ventricle (and atrium) might become much less distensible than a comparably diseased young left ventricle. This would be reflected in an elevated end-diastolic pressure and pulmonary capillary pressure, making the aged person more prone to developing pulmonary edema. Thus, the aged group might be more likely to present with pulmonary edema in addition to (or instead of) angina pectoris during ischemia. It is known that this feature of so-called "angina equivalence" exists. Its relationship to age has not been examined. Similarly, any other factor that causes an overload of the left ventricle would be more prone to manifest itself clinically with pulmonary symptoms in the aged because of the decreased distensibility of the ventricle (and presumably atrium) with increasing age.

From these brief comments, it is evident that the aging vascular system, particularly the pulmonic system, may play a key role in regulating the ability of the aged cardiovascular system to respond to stress. The pivotal role arises from its direct effects on the ventricular–vascular interaction with the right ventricle via its impedance spectrum and with the left ventricle via the interdependence mechanism. Further studies are needed to substantiate or repudiate the many speculations made in this section.

CONCLUDING REMARKS

This brief review has attempted to provide an overview of how the vascular system, particularly the larger arteries, changes with advancing age. First the structural and then the mechanical property changes with age in the systemic and pulmonic vasculature were examined. Next an attempt was made to relate the structural to the mechanical property changes. The next section examined the response to various vasoactive drugs in aging smooth muscle. Finally, an integrated view of how age changes in the vasculature affect ventricular performance, both directly via changes in input impedance and indirectly via ventricular interdependence, was examined. The major conclusions arising from this review are as follows:

1. There are definite histologic changes with aging in both the systemic and pulmonic vasculatures. These consist mainly of loss of endothelial uniformity, fragmentation, and degeneration of elastin with replacement by and proliferation of collagen.

2. With advancing age, most vessels increase in both diameter and wall thickness. This is especially true of the aorta. The age change in the ratio of radius to wall thickness depends on location in the vascular tree.

3. In general, the vessel wall becomes less extensible with ad-

vancing age. There are, however, species differences, with rabbit and rat showing either an increase or no change rather than a decrease in extensibility with age. There are also variations with age that are site dependent. The dynamic mechanical properties have not been well studied, but available data also indicate species and site differences in age changes.

4. The smooth muscle of the vessel wall appears to be less responsive to β-adrenergic stimulation with advancing age. The exact mechanism of this age deficit has not been established. The muscle also appears to have an altered response to other vasoactive hormones, but there is no alteration in response to nitrates.

It is clear that future investigation in many areas of this field is desirable. Many more studies on the effect of aging on the viscoelastic properties of the vasculature are needed before the species- and site-dependence question can be satisfactorily resolved. Studies on the changes with age in impedance, both systemic and pulmonic, would be of great benefit in helping to delineate the effect of the vasculature on ventricular function. Correlation of impedance changes in both pulmonic and systemic vasculatures during exercise and with vasoactive drugs would be of potential clinical use. Direct studies of the effect of age on ventricular interdependence would add to our basic understanding of this phenomenon. The role of the smooth muscle in affecting mechanical properties and its α- and β-adrenergic responsiveness must be studied in much more detail in order for the role of this important structural component to be better understood.

REFERENCES

1. Abel, F. L. (1971): Fourier analysis of left ventricular performance, evaluation of impedance matching. *Circ. Res.,* 28:119–135.
2. Alderman, E. L., and Glantz, S. A. (1976): Acute hemodynamic intervention shifts the diastolic pressure–volume curve in man. *Circulation,* 54:662–671.
3. Apter, J. T., Rabinowitz, M., and Cummings, D. H. (1966): Correlation

of viscoelastic properties of large arteries with microscopic structure II: collagen, elastin, and muscle determined chemically, histologically and physiologically. *Circ. Res.,* 19:104–121.

4.   Apter, J. T., and Marquez, E. (1968): A relation between hysteresis and other viscoelastic properties of some biomaterials. *Biorheology,* 5:285–301.

5.   Armstrong, P. W., Walker, D. C., Burton, J. R., and Parker, J. O. (1975): Vasodilator therapy in acute myocardial infarction. *Circulation,* 52:1118–1122.

6.   Attinger, E. O., Sugawara, H., Navarro, A., Ricetto, A., and Martin, R. (1966): Pressure–flow relations in dog arteries. *Circ. Res.,* 19:230–246.

7.   Auerbach, O., Hammond, E. C., and Garfinkel, L. (1968): Thickening of walls of arterioles and small arteries in relation to age and smoking habits. *N. Engl. J. Med.,* 278:980–984.

8.   Bader, H. (1967): Dependence of wall stress in human thoracic aorta on age and pressure. *Circ. Res.,* 20:354–361.

9.   Bader, H., and Kapal, E. (1957): Relationship between radius and wall thickness of human thoracic aorta at different ages and different pressures. *Physiologist,* 2:4.

10. Band, W., Goedhard, W. J. A., and Knoop, A. A. (1972): Effects of aging on dynamic viscoelastic properties of the rat's thoracic aorta. *Pfluegers Arch.,* 331:357–364.

11. Bazett, H. C., Cotton, F. S., Laplace, L. B., and Scott, J. C. (1936): The calculation of cardiac output and effective peripheral resistance from blood pressure measurements with an appendix on the size of the aorta in man. *Am. J. Physiol.,* 113:312–334.

12. Bemis, C. E., Serur, J. R., Borkenhagen, D., Sonnenblick, E. H., and Urschel, C. E. (1974): Influence of right ventricular filling pressure on left ventricular pressure and dimension. *Circ. Res.,* 34:498–504.

13. Ben-Ishai, Z., Abramowitz, A., Unger, H., and Laufer, A. (1961): The aging process of the aorta in relationship to atherosclerosis. *Bull. Res. Counc. Israel,* 9:176–177.

14. Bergel, D. (1961): The static elastic properties of the arterial wall. *J. Physiol.,* 156:445–457.

15. Bergel, D., and Milnor, W. R. (1965): Pulmonary vascular impedance in the dog. *Circ. Res.,* 16:401–415.

16. Berry, C. L., Greenwald, S. E., and Rivett, J. F. (1975): Static mechanical properties of the developing and mature rat aorta. *Cardiovasc. Res.,* 9:669–678.

17. Beznak, M. (1956): Changes in heart weight and blood pressure following aortic constriction in rats. *Can. J. Biochem. Physiol.,* 33:995–1002.

18. Blatz, P., Chu, B. M., and Wayland, H. (1969): On the mechanical behavior of elastic animal tissue. *Trans. Soc. Rheology,* 13:83–102.

19. Blumenthal, H. T., Lansing, A. I., and Wheeler, P. A. (1944): Calcification of the media of the human aorta and its relation to intimal arteriosclerosis, ageing, and disease. *Am. J. Pathol.,* 20:665–687.

20. Bohr, D. (1973): Vascular smooth muscle updated. *Circ. Res.,* 32:665–672.
21. Bramwell, J. C., and Hill, A. V. (1922): The velocity of the pulse wave in man. *Proc. R. Soc. Lond. [Biol.],* 93:298–306.
22. Bramwell, J. C., Hill, A. V., and McSwiney, B. A. (1923): The velocity of the pulse wave in man in relation to age as studied by the hot-wire sphygmograph. *Heart,* 10:233–249.
23. Brown, R. G., Walker, R. E., Aeschbacher, H. U., Boer, A. H., and Smith, M. C. (1974): Age-related changes in the composition of the aorta of the groundhog, *Marmota monax. Growth,* 38:295–300.
24. Burton, A. C. (1954): Relation of structure to function of the tissues of the wall of blood vessels. *Physiol. Rev.,* 34:619–642.
25. Busby, D. E., and Burton, A. C. (1965): The effect of age on the elasticity of the major brain arteries. *Can. J. Physiol. Pharmacol.,* 13:185–202.
26. Butcher, H. B., and Newton, W. T. (1958): The influence of age, arteriosclerosis, and homotransplantation upon the elastic properties of major human arteries. *Ann. Surg.,* 148:1–20.
27. Carton, R. W., Dainauskas, J., and Clark, J. W. (1962): Elastic properties of single elastic fibers. *J. Appl. Physiol.,* 17:547–551.
28. Chatterjee, J., Parmley, W. W., Ganz, W., Forrester, J., Walinsky, P., Crexells, C., and Swan, H. J. C. (1973): Hemodynamic and metabolic responses to vasodilator therapy in acute myocardial infarction. *Circulation,* 48:1183–1193.
29. Chiarello, M., Gold, H., Leinbach, R. C., Davis, M. A., and Maroko, P. (1976): Comparison between the effects of nitroprusside and nitroglycerin on ischemic injury during acute myocardial infarction. *Circulation,* 54:766–773.
30. Cliff, W. J. (1970): The aortic tunica media in aging rats. *Exp. Mol. Pathol.,* 13:172–189.
31. Cohen, M. L., and Berkowitz, B. A. (1974): Age-related changes in vascular responsiveness to cyclic nucleotides and contractile agonists. *J. Pharmacol. Exp. Ther.,* 191:147–155.
32. Cohn, J., and Franciosa, J. A. (1977): Vasodilator therapy of cardiac failure. *N. Engl. J. Med.,* 297:27–31; 254–258.
33. Cohn, J., Mathew, K. J., Franciosa, J. A., and Snow, J. A. (1974): Chronic vasodilator therapy in the management of cardiogenic shock and intractible left ventricular failure. *Ann. Intern. Med.,* 81:777–780.
34. Cotton, R., and Wartman, W. B. (1961): Endothelial patterns in human arteries, their relationship to age, vessel site, and atherosclerosis. *Arch. Pathol.,* 2:15–24.
35. Cox, R. H. (1970): Wave propagation through a Newtonian fluid contained within a thick-walled viscoelastic tube: the influence of wall compressibility. *J. Biomech.,* 3:317–335.
36. Cox, R. H. (1971): Determination of the true phase velocity of arterial pressure waves in vivo. *Circ. Res.,* 24:407–418.
37. Cox, R. H. (1974): Three-dimensional mechanics of arterial segments in vitro methods. *J. Appl. Physiol.,* 36:381–384.

38. Cox, R. H. (1975): Arterial wall mechanics and composition and the effect of smooth muscle activation. *Am. J. Physiol.,* 229:807–812.

39. Cox, R. H. (1976): Effects of norepinephrine on mechanics of arteries in vitro. *Am. J. Physiol.,* 231:420–425.

40. Cox, R. H. (1977): Effects of age on the mechanical properties of rat carotid artery. *Am. J. Physiol.,* 233:H256–H263.

41. Cox, R. H., Jones, A. W., and Fischerm, G. M. (1974): Carotid artery mechanics, connective tissue, and electrolyte changes in puppies. *Am. J. Physiol.,* 227:563–568.

42. Cox, R. H., Jones, A. W., and Swain, M. L. (1976): Mechanics and electrolyte composition of arterial smooth muscle in developing dogs. *Am. J. Physiol.,* 231:77–83.

43. Doyle, J. M., and Dobrin, P. B. (1971): Finite deformation analysis of the relaxed and contracted dog carotid artery. *Microvasc. Res.,* 3:400–415.

44. Ehrich, W., de la Chapelle, C., and Cohn, A. E. (1931): Anatomical ontogeny (B) Man. I. A study of the coronary arteries. *Am. J. Anat.,* 49:241–282.

45. Elkins, R. C., and Milnor, W. R. (1971): Pulmonary vascular response to exercise in the dog. *Circ. Res.,* 29:591–599.

46. Elzinga, G., von Grodelle, R., Westerhof, N., and van den Bos, G. C. (1974): Ventricular interference. *Am. J. Physiol.,* 226:941–947.

47. Elzinga, G., and Westerhof, N. (1973): Pressure and flow generated by the left ventricle against different impedances. *Circ. Res.,* 32:178–186.

48. Emirgil, C., Sobel, B. J., Campodonica, S., Herbert, W. H., and Mechkati, R. (1967): Pulmonary circulation in the aged. *J. Appl. Physiol.,* 23:631–640.

49. Ericcson, E., and Lundholm, L. (1975): Adrenergic beta-receptor activity and cyclic AMP metabolism in vascular smooth muscle: variations with age. *Mech. Ageing Dev.,* 4:1–6.

50. Faber, M., and Moller-Hou, G. (1952): The human aorta. V. Collagen and elastin in the normal and hypertensive aorta. *Acta Pathol. Microbiol. Scand.,* 31:377–382.

51. Farrar, J. F., Blomfield, Jr., and Reye, R. D. K. (1965): The structure and composition of the maturing pulmonary circulation. *J. Pathol. Bacteriol.,* 90:83–96.

52. Fleisch, J. H., and Hooker, C. S. (1976): The relationship between age and relaxation of vascular smooth muscle in the rabbit and rat. *Circ. Res.,* 38:243–250.

53. Fleisch, J. H., Maling, H. M., and Brodie, B. B. (1970): Beta-receptor activity in aorta, variations with age and species. *Circ. Res.,* 26:151–162.

54. Fronek, K., and Fung, Y. C. B. (1976): Age and distensibility of rabbit arteries. *Fed. Proc.,* 35:2367.

55. Fung, Y. C. B. (1965): *Foundations of Solid Mechanics.* Prentice-Hall, Englewood Cliffs, New Jersey.

56. Fung, Y. C. B. (1967): Elasticity of soft tissues in simple elongation. *Am. J. Physiol.,* 213:1532–1544.
57. Fung, Y. C. B. (1972): Stress–strain–history relations of soft tissues in simple elongation. In: *Biomechanics: Its Foundations and Objectives.* Prentice-Hall, Englewood Cliffs, New Jersey.
58. Gabe, J. T., Karnell, J., Porje, I. G., and Rudewald, B. (1964): The measurement of input impedance and apparent phase velocity in the human aorta. *Acta Physiol. Scand.,* 61:73–84.
59. Gardin, J. M., Henry, W. L., Savage, D. D., and Epstein, S. E. (1977): Echocardiographic evaluation of an older population without clinically apparent heart disease. *Am. J. Cardiol.,* 39:277.
60. Gerrity, R. G., and Cliff, W. J. (1972): The aortic tunica intima in young and aging rats. *Exp. Mol. Pathol.,* 16:382–402.
61. Gersh, B. J., Prys-Roberts, C., Reuben, F. R., and Schultz, D. L. (1972): The effects of halothane on the interaction between myocardial contractility, aortic impedance, and left ventricular performance. *Br. J. Anaesth.,* 44:767–774.
62. Gerstenblith, G., Fredericksen, J., Yin, F. C. P., Fortuin, N.J., Lakatta, E. G., and Weisfeldt, M. L. (1977): Echocardiographic assessment of a normal adult aging population. *Circulation,* 56:273–278.
63. Gerstenblith, G., Lakatta, E. G., and Weisfeldt, M. L. (1976): Age changes in myocardial function and exercise response. *Prog. Cardiovasc. Dis.,* 19:1–21.
64. Giolma, J., Murgo, J., and Altobelli, S. (1977). Aortic input impedance in man during rest and exercise. *Circulation,* 56:III–234.
65. Glantz, S. A., Misbach, G., Moores, W., Mathey, D., Lekven, J., Stowe, D., Parmley, W., and Tyberg, J. (1978): The pericardium substantially affects the diastolic pressure–volume relations in the canine left ventricle. *Circ. Res.,* 42:433–441.
66. Glantz, S. A., and Parmley, W. W. (1978): Factors which affect the diastolic pressure–volume curve. *Circ. Res.,* 42:171–180.
67. Gozna, E. R., Marble, A. E., Shaw, A., and Holland, J. G. (1974): Age-related changes in the mechanics of the aorta and pulmonary artery of man. *J. Appl. Physiol.,* 36:407–411.
68. Guard, H. R., and Bhende, Y. M. (1953): Changes due to aging in the abdominal aorta. *Indian J. Med. Res.,* 41:267–276.
69. Gulati, O. D., Methow, B. P., Parikh, H. M., and Krishnamurty, V. S. R. (1973): Beta-adrenergic receptor of rabbit thoracic aorta in relation to age. *Jpn. J. Pharmacol.,* 23:259–268.
70. Hallock, P. (1934): Arterial elasticity in man in relation to age as evaluated by the pulse wave velocity method. *Arch. Intern. Med.,* 54:770–798.
71. Hallock, P., and Benson, I.C. (1937): Studies on the elastic properties of human isolated aorta. *J. Clin. Invest.,* 16:595–602.
72. Harkness, M. L. R., Harkness, R. D., and McDonald, D. A. (1957): The collagen and elastin content of the arterial wall in the dog. *Proc. R. Soc. Lond. [Biol.],* 146:541–551.

73. Harris, P., Heath, D., and Apostolopoulos, A. (1965): Extensibility of the human pulmonary trunk. *Br. Heart J.,* 27:651–659.
74. IIass, G. M. (1942): Elastic tissue. II. A study of the elasticity and tensile strength of elastic tissue isolated from the human aorta. *Arch. Pathol.,* 34:971–981.
75. Hass, G. M. (1943): Elastic tissue. III. Relation between the structure of the aging aorta and the properties of the isolated elastic tissue. *Arch. Pathol.,* 35:29–45.
76. Heath, D., Wood, E. H., Dushane, J. W., and Edwards, J. E. (1959): The structure of the pulmonary trunk at different ages and in cases of pulmonary hypertension and pulmonary stenosis. *J. Pathol. Bacteriol.,* 77:443–456.
77. Hefner, L. L., Coghlan, H. C., Jones, W. B., and Reeves, T. J. (1961): Distensibility of the dog left ventricle. *Am. J. Physiol.,* 201:97–101.
78. Holt, J. P. (1970): The normal pericardium. *Am. J. Cardiol.,* 26:455–465.
79. Hruza, Z., and Zweifach, B. (1967): Effect of age on vascular reactivity to catecholamines in rats. *J. Gerontol.,* 22:469–473.
80. Hume, J. F. (1939): The tensility of the rat's aorta as influenced by age, environmental temperature, and certain toxic substances. *Am. J. Hyg. Sci.,* 29:11–23.
81. Imperial, E. S., Levy, M. N., and Zieske, H. (1961): Outflow resistance as an independent determinant of cardiac performance. *Circ. Res.,* 9:1148–1155.
82. Jewell, B. R., and Wilkie, D. R. (1958): An analysis of the mechanical components in frog's striated muscle. *J. Physiol. (Lond.),* 143:515–540.
83. Kantrowitz, A., Tjonneland, S., Krakauer, J. S., Phillips, S. J., Freed, P. S., and Butner, A. N. (1968): Mechanical intra-aortic cardiac assistance in cardiogenic shock. *Arch. Surg.,* 97:1000–1004.
84. Kantrowitz, A., Tjonneland, S., Freed, P. S., Phillips, S. J., Butner, A. N., and Sherman, J. L., Jr. (1968): Initial clinical experience with intra-aortic balloon pumping in cardiogenic shock. JAMA, 203:135–140.
85. Krafka, J. (1940): Changes in the elasticity of the aorta with age. *Arch. Pathol.,* 29:303–309.
86. Laks, M. M., Morady, F., Garner, D., and Swan, H. J. C. (1967): Volumes and compliances measured simultaneously in the right and left ventricles of the dog. *Circ. Res.,* 20:565–569.
87. Lang, T. W., Meerbaum, S., Lozano, J., Corrasco, H., and Corday, E. (1971): Ascending aorta synchronized pulsation (AASP): A new temporary circulatory assist technique for the treatment of cardiogenic shock. *Arch. Intern. Med.,* 128:258–264.
88. Landowne, M., (1958): The relation between intra-arterial pressure and impact pulse wave velocity with regard to age and arteriosclerosis. *J. Gerontol.,* 13:153–162.
89. Lansing, A. I., Alex, M., and Rosenthal, T. B. (1950): Calcium and elastin in human arteriosclerosis. *J. Gerontol.,* 5:112–119.

90. Learoyd, B. M., and Taylor, M. G. (1966): Alterations with age in the viscoelastic properties of human arterial walls. *Circ. Res.,* 18:278–292.
91. Linzbach, A. J., and Boateng, E. A. (1976): The ageing human heart. Presented at *European Congress of Cardiology,* Amsterdam, p. 171 (abstr.).
92. Malik, A. B., Shapiro, J. M., Yanics, J., Rojales, A., and Geha, A. S. (1974): A simplified method for producing rapid ventricular hypertrophy in rats. *Cardiovasc. Res.,* 8:801–805.
93. Maruffo, C. A., and Malinow, M. R. (1966): Postnatal changes in the aorta of howler monkeys *(Aluoatta caraya). J. Gerontol.,* 21:119–123.
94. McDonald, D. A. (1974): *Blood Flow in Arteries,* 2nd ed., Edward Arnold, London.
95. Milch, R. A. (1965): Matrix properties of the aging arterial wall. *Monogr. Surg. Sci.,* 2:261–341.
96. Miller, R. R., Awan, N. A., Maxwell, K. S., and Mason, D. T. (1977): Sustained reduction of cardiac impedance and preload in congestive heart failure with the antihypertensive vasodilator prazosin. *N. Engl. J. Med.,* 297:303–307.
97. Mills, C. J., Gabe, I. T., Gault, J. H., Mason, D. T., Ross, J., Jr., Braunwald, E., and Shillingford, J. P. (1970): Pressure–flow relationships and vascular impedance in man. *Cardiovasc. Res.,* 4:405–417.
98. Milnor, W. R. (1975): Arterial impedance as ventricular afterload. *Circ. Res.,* 36:565–570.
99. Milnor, W. R., Bergel, D. H., and Bargainer, J. D. (1966): Hydraulic power associated with pulmonary blood flow and its relation to heart rate. *Circ. Res.,* 19:467–480.
100. Milnor, W. R., Conti, C. R., Lewis, K. B., and O'Rourke, M. F. (1969): Pulmonary arterial pulse wave velocity and impedance in man. *Circ. Res.,* 25:637–649.
101. Mirsky, I. (1976): Assessment of passive elastic stiffness of cardiac muscle: Mathematical concepts, physiologic and clinical considerations, directions of future research. *Prog. Cardiovasc. Dis.,* 18:277–308.
102. Mirsky, I., and Janz, R. F. (1976): The effect of age on the wall stiffness of the human thoracic aorta: A large deformation anisotropic elastic analysis. *J. Theor. Biol.,* 59:467–484.
103. Moinian-Bagheri, M., and Meyer, M. M. (1967): Vergleichende untersuchung der Gewichte der Beckenarterien, der Aorta, und der Femoraliarterien und ihrer Beziehung zum Alter. *Frankfurt. Z. Pathol.,* 76:143–148.
104. Moon, H. D., and Rinehart, J. F. (1952): Histogenesis of coronary arteriosclerosis. *Circulation,* 6:481–488.
105. Moulopoulos, S. D., Topaz, S., and Kolff, W. J. (1962): Diastolic balloon pumping (with carbon dioxide) in the aorta: A mechanical assistance to the failing circulation. *Am. Heart J.,* 63:669–673.
106. Movat, H. Z., More, R. H., and Haust, M. D. (1958): The diffuse intimal thickening of the human aorta with aging. *Am. J. Pathol.,* 34:1023–1030.
107. Mozersky, D. J., Sumner, D. S., Hokanson, D. E., and Standness,

D. E., (1973): Transcutaneous measurement of arterial wall properties as a potential method of estimating age. *J. Am. Geriatr. Soc.,* 21:18–20.

108. Myers, V. C., and Lang, W. W. (1946): Some chemical changes in the human thoracic aorta accompanying the aging process. *J. Gerontol.,* 1:441–444.

109. Nakashima, T., and Tanikawa, J. (1971): A study of human aortic distensibility with relation to atherosclerosis and aging. *Angiology,* 22:477–490.

110. Nichols, W. W., Conti, C. R., Walker, W. W., and Milnor, W. R. (1977): Input impedance of the systemic circulation in man. *Circ. Res.,* 40:451–458.

111. Nichols, W. W., and McDonald, D. A. (1972): Wave velocity in the proximal aorta. *Med. Biol. Eng.,* 10:327–335.

112. Noble, M. I. M., Gabe, I. T., Trenchard, D., and Guz., A. (1967): Blood pressure and flow in the ascending aorta of conscious dogs. *Cardiovasc. Res.,* 1:9–20.

113. O'Kane, H. O., Geha, A. S., Kleiger, R. E., Abe, T., Salaymeh, M. T., and Malik, A. B. (1973): Stable left ventricular hypertrophy in the dog. *J. Thorac. Cardiovasc. Surg.,* 65:264–271.

114. O'Rourke, M. F. (1967): Steady and pulsatile energy losses in the systemic circulation under normal conditions and in simulated arterial disease. *Cardiovasc. Res.,* 1:313–326.

115. O'Rourke, M. F. (1967): Pressure and flow waves in systemic arteries and the anatomical design of the arterial system. *J. Appl. Physiol.,* 23:139–149.

116. O'Rourke, M. F., and Taylor, M. G. (1967): Input impedance of the systemic circulation. *Circ. Res.,* 20:365–380.

117. Pace, J. S. (1971): Sympathetic control of pulmonary vascular impedance in anesthetized dog. *Circ. Res.,* 29:555–568.

118. Pariera, M. D., Handler, F. P., and Blumenthal, H. T. (1953): Aging process in the arterial and venous systems of the lower extremities. *Circulation,* 8:36–43.

119. Patel, D. J., Defrietas, F. M., and Fry, D. L. (1963): Hydraulic input impedance to aorta and pulmonary artery in dogs. *J. Appl. Physiol.,* 18:134–140.

120. Patel, D. J., Janicki, J. S., and Carew, T. E. (1969): Static anisotropic elastic properties of the aorta in living dogs. *Circ. Res.,* 25:765–779.

121. Pepine, C. J., Nichols, W. W., Christie, L. G., and Conti, C. R. (1976): Divergence of left ventricular afterload components during exercise in man. *Fed. Proc.,* 35:73.

122. Peterson, L. H., Jenson, R. E., and Parnell, J. (1960): Mechanical properties of arteries in vivo. *Circ. Res.,* 8:622–639.

123. Piene, G., and Hauge, A. (1976): Reduction of pulsatile hydraulic power in the pulmonary circulation caused by moderate vasoconstriction. *Cardiovasc. Res.,* 10:503–513.

124. Pinto, J. G., and Fung, Y. C. (1973): Mechanical properties of the heart muscle in the passive state. *J. Biomech.,* 6:597–616.

125. Rabkin, S. W., and Hsu, P. H. (1975): Mathematical and mechanical modeling of stress-strain relationship of pericardium. *Am. J. Physiol.,* 229:896–900.

126. Remington, J. W. (1963): The physiology of the aorta and major arteries. In: *Handbook of Physiology, Sect. 2, Circulation,* Vol. 2, American Physiological Society, Washington, D. C.

127. Ridge, M. D., and Wright, V. (1964): The description of skin stiffness. *Biorheology,* 2:67–74.

128. Roach, M., and Burton, A. C. (1959): The effect of age on the elasticity of the human iliac arteries. *Can. J. Biochem. Physiol.,* 37:557–570.

129. Robinson, N. E., and Gillespie, J. R. (1975): Pulmonary diffusing capacity and capillary blood volume in aging dogs. *J. Appl. Physiol.,* 38:647–650.

130. Roy, C. S. (1880): The elastic properties of the arterial wall. *J. Physiol.,* 3:125–159.

131. Santamore, W. P., Lynch, P. R., Meier, G., Heckman, J., and Bove, A. A. (1976): Myocardial interaction between the ventricles. *J. Appl. Physiol.,* 41:362–368.

132. Saxton, J. A. (1942): Elastic properties of the rabbit aorta in relation to age. *Arch. Pathol.,* 34:262–274.

133. Schimmler, W. (1966): Correlation between the pulse wave velocity in the aortic iliac vessel and age, sex, and blood pressure. *Angiology,* 17:314–322.

134. Schimmler, W. (1974): Longitudinale Verlaufsstudie uber der Altersanstieg der Pulswellengeschwindigkeit in der Aorta iliaca bei Normo- und Hypertonikern. *Z. Kardiol.,* 63:887–895.

135. Schlatman, T. J. M., and Becker, A. E. (1977): Histologic changes in the normal aging aorta: Implications for dissecting aortic aneurysm. *Am. J. Cardiol.,* 39:13–20.

136. Semmens, M. (1970): The pulmonary artery in the normal aged lung. *Br. J. Dis. Chest,* 64:65–72.

137. Shabetai, R., Fowler, N. O., and Guntheroth, W. G. (1970): The hemodynamics of cardiac tamponade and constrictive pericarditis. *Am. J. Cardiol.,* 26:480–489.

138. Shibata, S., Hattori, K., Sakuvai, I., Mori, J., and Fujiware, M. (1971): Adrenergic innervation and cocaine-induced potentiation of adrenergic responses of aortic strips from young and old rabbits. *J. Pharmacol. Exp. Ther.,* 177:621–632.

139. Simon, B. R., Kobayashi, A. S., Strandness, D. E., and Wiederhielm, C. A. (1972): Reevaluation of arterial constitutive relations. *Circ. Res.,* 30:491–500.

140. Simons, P., and Reid, L. (1969): Muscularity of the pulmonary artery branches in the upper and lower lobes of the normal and aged lung. *Br. J. Dis. Chest,* 63:38–44.

141. Simonson, E., and Nakagawa, K. (1960): Effect of age on pulse wave velocity and aortic ejection time in healthy men and in men with coronary artery disease. *Circulation,* 22:126–129.

142. Sivak, E. D., Gray, B. A., McCurdy, H. T., and Phillips, A. K. (1977): Pulmonary vascular response to nitroprusside. *Circulation,* 55:III–163.

143. Smith, C., Seitner, M. M., and Wang, H. P. (1951): Aging changes in the tunica media of the aorta. *Anat. Rec.,* 109:13–39.

144. Sonnenblick, E. H. (1964): Series elastic and contractile elements in heart muscle: Change in muscle length. *Am. J. Physiol.,* 207:1330–1338.

145. Spann, J. F., Buccino, R. A., Sonnenblick, E. H., and Braunwald, E. (1976): Contractile state of cardiac muscle obtained from cats with experimentally produced ventricular hypertrophy and heart failure. *Circ. Res.,* 21:341–354.

146. Spotnitz, H. M., and Kaiser, G. A. (1971): The effect of the pericardium on pressure volume relations in the canine left ventricle. *J. Surg. Res.,* 11:375–380.

147. Stadeli, H. (1966): Der Einfluss des Lebenalters Auf die Wandstrucktur der isolierten ungedehnten Aorta thoracalis des Meerschweinchens. *Angiologica,* 3:213–225.

148. Stein, O., Eisenberg, S., and Stein, Y. (1969): Aging of aortic smooth muscle cells in rats and rabbits. *Lab. Invest.,* 21:386–387.

149. Stromberg, D. D., and Wiederhielm, C. A. (1969): Viscoelastic description of a collagenous tissue in simple elongation. *J. Appl. Physiol.,* 26:857–862.

150. Tanaka, T., and Fung, Y. C. (1974): Elastic and inelastic properties of the canine aorta and their variation along the aortic tree. *J. Biomech.,* 7:357–370.

151. Taylor, M. G. (1966): Use of random excitation and spectral analysis in the study of frequency-dependent parameters of the cardiovascular system. *Circulation,* 18:585–595.

152. Taylor, R. R., Covell, J. W., Sonnenblick, E. H., and Ross, J., Jr. (1967): Dependence of ventricular distensibility on filling of the opposite ventricle. *Am. J. Physiol.,* 213:711–718.

153. Tsontchev, J. (1975): Age-dependent changes in the complex of impedance plethysmographic and hemodynamic indices of the lung and aorta. *Bibl. Cardiol.,* 33:206–209.

154. Tuttle, R. S. (1966): Age-related changes in the sensitivity of rat aortic strips to norepinephrine and associated chemical and structural alterations. *J. Gerontol.,* 21:510–516.

155. Urschel, C. W., Covell, J. W., Sonnenblick, E. H., Ross, J., Jr., and Braunwald, E. (1968): Effects of decreased aortic compliance on performance of the left ventricle. *Am. J. Physiol.,* 214:298–304.

156. Vales, A. G. O. (1966): Estudio de la intima de las arterias pulmonares en conejos normales. *Rev. Soc. Argent. Biol.,* 42:50–55.

157. Weiss, J. L., Brinker, J. A., Lappe, D. A., Rabson, J. L., Summer, W. L., Permutt, S., and Weisfeldt, M. L. (1978): Leftward septal displacement during right ventricular loading in man: Demonstration by two-dimensional echo. *Am. J. Cardiol.,* 41:362.

158. Wellman, N. E., and Edwards, J. E. (1950): Thickness of the media of the thoracic aorta in relation to age. *Arch. Pathol.,* 50:183–188.

159. Westerhof, N., Elzinga, G., and Van den Bos, G. C. (1973): Influence of central and peripheral changes on the hydraulic input impedance of the systemic arterial tree. *Med. Biol. Eng.,* 2:710–722.
160. Weyman, A. E., Heeger, J. J., Kronik, G., Wann, L. S., Dillon, J. C., and Feigenbaum, H. (1977): Mechanism of paradoxical early diastolic septal motion in patients with mitral stenosis: A cross-sectional echocardiographic study. *Am. J. Cardiol.,* 40:691–699.
161. Wilens, S. L. (1937): The postmortem elasticity of the adult human aorta. Its relation to age and to the distribution of intimal atheroma. *Am. J. Pathol.,* 13:811–833.
162. Wilken, D. E. L., Charlier, A. A., Hoffman, J. I. E., and Guz, A. (1964): Effects of alterations in aortic impedance on the performance of the ventricles. *Circ. Res.,* 14:283–293.
163. Williams, J. F., Jr., and Potter, R. D. (1974): Normal contractile state of hypertrophied myocardium after pulmonary artery constriction in the cat. *J. Clin. Invest.,* 54:1266–1272.
164. Winson, M., and Heath, D. (1974): Extensibility of the human carotid sinus. *Cardiovasc. Res.,* 8:58–64.
165. Wolinsky, H. (1972): Long-term effects of hypertension on the rat aortic wall and their relation to concurrent aging changes. *Circ. Res.,* 30:301–309.
166. Wolinsky, H., and Glagov, S. (1964): Structural basis for the static mechanical properties of the aortic media. *Circ. Res.,* 400–413.
167. Womersley, J. R. (1957): An elastic tube theory of pulse transmission and oscillatory flow in mammalian arteries. WADC Tech. Rep. TR 56–614. Wright-Patterson Air Force Base, Dayton, Ohio.
168. Womersley, J. R. (1957): Oscillatory flow in arteries: The constrained elastic tube as a model of arterial flow and pulse transmission. *Phys. Med. Biol.* 2:178–187.
169. Yater, W. M., and Birkeland, I. W. (1929): Elasticity (extensibility) of the aorta of human beings. *Am. Heart J.,* 5:781–786.
170. Yin, F. C. P., and Fung, Y. C. (1967): Mechanical properties of isolated mammalian ureteral segments. *Am. J. Physiol.,* 221:1484–1493.
171. Yin, F. C. P., Spurgeon, H. A., Lakatta, E. G., Guarnieri, T., Weisfeldt, M. L., and Shock, N. W. (1977): Cardiac hypertrophy indexed by tibial length: Application in the aging rat. *Gerontologist,* 17:135.

The Aging Heart (Aging, Vol. 12),
edited by Myron L. Weisfeldt.
Raven Press, New York © 1980.

Chapter 8

Pharmacology

Paula B. Goldberg and Jay Roberts

*Department of Pharmacology, Medical College of Pennsylvania,
Philadelphia, Pennsylvania 19129*

It has been shown (e.g., refs. 52,81,82,86,93) that cardiac function changes with increasing age of an organism in such a way as to render the heart of an "old" individual functionally less efficient than the heart of a younger individual. The preceding chapters of this volume have reviewed structural, metabolic, functional, and pathological changes undergone by the heart as an animal ages. It seems quite reasonable to anticipate that responsiveness of the heart to various pharmacological substances could be altered by the aging process as well.

Pharmacological studies exploring the influence of age on the reactivity of the myocardium to drugs have not been extensive. The literature that is available deals primarily with investigations aimed at characterizing the direction (increases, decreases) of age-related physiological or biochemical changes in the heart following administration or use of pharmacological agents. Some reported studies have as their main objective a more therapeutically oriented approach. Furthermore, it is not always possible to compare or relate the effects obtained with pharmacological agents in one species of animals to the effects in another species. Although certain generalizations may be drawn from previous studies, for example, that with increasing age there is greater sensitivity to drugs and that toxic manifestations occur with greater frequency, it is not possible in many cases to elucidate fundamental principles of aging and their influence on drug action and sensitivity.

The agents discussed in this chapter will be limited to those for which there is more than just fragmentary information regarding the effects of aging on pharmacological action. Each class of substances for which age-related studies have been carried out will be treated separately, since the nature of drug effects and the factors responsible for altered myocardial sensitivity owing to age may differ in each case. Most of the studies to be described pertain to changes in responsiveness of the effector organ (the heart) per se and the cardiovascular system as a whole, as opposed to studies describing changes in the disposition of the substance by an organism (pharmacokinetic factors affecting the concentration of the drug in the biophase of the effector organ, Fig. 1). Investigations characterizing effects of aging during

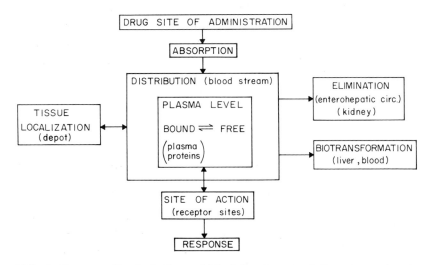

FIG. 1. Pharmacokinetic factors which determine circulating plasma levels of drug and the concentration of drug at its site of action. Since these pharmacokinetic factors are altered by increasing age, the concentration of drug in the biophase of an effector organ is also altered by increasing age, irrespective of alterations in effector organ sensitivity. See text for further explanation.

early development or maturation will not be considered unless they have a direct bearing on the point under consideration. With respect to species variability and age-related alterations in drug action, it was thought important to identify those changes which occur in experimental animals and those changes which occur in man, highlighting the findings common to both. The biological and therapeutic significance for future directions in research will be indicated. In this regard, special attention will be directed to drug classes whose actions and effects deserve additional study to extend our current understanding of the underlying mechanisms responsible for age-related differences. Cardiovascular agents used experimentally or clinically whose effects on the myocardium have not been investigated in relation to age will be identified for the purpose of suggesting directions for future investigation in this area.

DIGITALIS GLYCOSIDES

Of the pharmacological agents which have been used and studied for their actions on the cardiovascular system, the digitalis glycosides represent one of the most important classes of drugs. Indeed, it is not surprising when age is considered as a factor influencing drug action that digitalis represents one of the few drugs on which a large number of investigations have been performed.

In clinical medicine, the most widely employed glycoside is digoxin; whereas in laboratory animal work, ouabain has been extensively studied. The discussions that follow are primarily concerned with these agents. "Digitalis" is used to designate generically the family of cardioactive glycosides.

Clinical Studies

In the elderly, it is well recognized that the dosage range for effective digitalis therapeutic action is limited, and that the probability of untoward and toxic reactions is high as compared to the incidence of digitalis toxicity in the average younger patient (7,28,30,31,63,79,89,109) (Table 1). Indeed, it has been stated frequently that the elderly patient is particularly prone to the toxic manifestations of digitalis therapy (6,19,20,96). It is estimated that of all the patients on digitalis therapy, 20 to 25% exhibit some form of toxicity (6,58). The proportion of toxic manifestations increases with age (20). Contributing to the development of digitalis toxicity may be such age-independent factors as excessive dosage, incorrect indications, missing early signs of toxicity, insufficient supervision of patients, and concomitant existence of anemia, hypoxia, electrolyte imbalance, and use of other drugs. However, ignoring any of the above factors, digitalis is reported to become more toxic in the elderly even when taken in minimal doses (103). Furthermore, the toxic reactions to digitalis are subtly different in the elderly than in other age groups. For example, in the elderly, instead of the usual nausea and vomiting, there is anorexia; instead of color vision, there is muddy or hazy vision; and cardiac arrhythmias may appear without other signs of toxicity and may be the first evidence of overdosage (7,35). It should be noted that the myocardium of the elderly patient may have suffered previous ischemic events. If these resulted in scars, the myocardium may have centers for the emergence of ectopic excitation. Therefore, one should be aware that following digitalis therapy ventricular fibrillation may be more likely to occur in the elderly than in the young patient (31).

Since 5% of old people at home are on some form of digitalis (102), and since toxicity in the elderly is a major hazard, it is essential to practice great care in digitalizing an elderly patient. Indeed, unless there is great urgency, the wisdom of using loading doses in the elderly appears very doubtful (12). Furthermore, it has been suggested that great care be taken to establish whether digitalis therapy is required at all (21,63). A review of 80 elderly patients (74.3 to 78.9 years of age) receiving digoxin in a maintenance dose, some of whom had toxic effects, showed that in almost 75% of the group digoxin could be stopped without detriment (21). In another group of 22 patients ranging from 78 to

TABLE 1. *Effects of increasing age on sensitivity to digitalis glycosides*

Species	Drug	Effect	Effect of increasing age	Ref.
Guinea pig	Ouabain	Lethal dose	Decrease between birth and maturity (5.5–7.5 months)	110
	Ouabain	Myocardial sensitivity	No change during adult life (up to 5–6.5 years)	110
Rat	Digitoxin Proscillaridin	Toxicity	Decreases during development (7 d) to adult (200 g)	91
	Ouabain	Increase contractile tension of ventricular trabeculae carnaea	Decrease between 6–24 months	41
		Production of contracture of ventricular trabeculae carnaea	Decrease between 6–24 months	41
		Inhibition of $Na^+ + K^+$-sensitive ATPase of spinal cord	Increase during aging from 3–28 months	4
Rabbit	Ouabain	Toxicity	Increase between 3–24 months and 3–5 years	15
		Arrhythmia	Increase between development (1–6 weeks) and maturity (12 weeks)	61
Man	Digitalis Digoxin	Toxicity Absorption Plasma concentration and $t_{1/2}$	Increase No change Increase	20,103 12,102 30,63

92 years of age (average age 86 years) who were on long term digitalis therapy and free of failure and cardiac arrhythmias, 18 remained free of congestive failure during a 6- or 9-month trial without digoxin. Such findings suggest that periodic review should be made of aged individuals on digoxin therapy.

Several patient-related factors contribute to the development of toxicity in the elderly on digitalis therapy. Of particular importance are pharmacokinetic factors, which determine the level and time course of drugs in the circulation (Fig. 1). Pharmacokinetic factors are particularly relevant to the use of digoxin, since 67 to 77% of this agent is present in the blood stream in the free (protein-unbound), pharmacologically active state (29,74). Digoxin absorption is reported to be normal in the elderly patient (12,102), and peak serum concentrations are observed within 1 to 2 hr. In spite of these findings, there is a tendency for elderly patients to require smaller doses of digoxin to achieve adequate therapeutic blood levels (5,14,20,26,30). Baylis et al. (5) found that elderly ambulatory patients taking digoxin frequently had moderate to severe impairment of renal function. Since digoxin is eliminated primarily through the kidneys, renal function would be a major determinant of circulating levels as well as of the duration of action of digoxin.

The importance of assessing renal function in the elderly is revealed in several clinical studies. In one study, serum digoxin concentrations were measured by radioimmunoassay in seven elderly patients during digitalization with digoxin, 0.25 mg daily, without a loading dose (12,102). Serum concentrations in the therapeutic range (1 to 2 ng/ml) were reached in 4 days in five patients with normal renal function, while toxic levels (3 ng/ml) were reached in the same time in two patients with renal impairment. Similar low and high levels of digoxin have been associated with therapeutic and toxic effects, respectively, in other patients (12,14,96). Furthermore, Ewy et al. (30) indicated that since creatinine clearance is decreased in the elderly and since digoxin is predominantly excreted by the kidney, the apparent sensitivity of the elderly patients to digitalis might be related in part to decreased renal excretion. Tritiated digoxin (0.5 mg) was given intravenously to five elderly men (average age 77 years) and nine younger men (average age 27 years). The patients were not in congestive failure. The creatinine clearance averaged 56 ml/min/1.73 m² in the old and 122 ml/min/1.73 m² in the young men. The concentration and the half-life in the circulation of tritiated digoxin was higher in the older group throughout the study. This was attributed to smaller body size and diminished urinary excretion of digoxin in the elderly (53 ml/min/1.73 m² in the elderly versus 83 ml/min/1.73 m² in the young) (30,63). Indeed, administration of the same dose to both groups resulted in blood concentrations nearly twice as high in the elderly as compared to the young. It should also be noted that the 0.25 to 0.5 mg/day recommended oral maintenance dose of digoxin represents an average for adult patients without renal or hepatic impairment.

There is evidence to suggest that the myocardial tissue concentration of digoxin may be directly related to the blood concentration of digoxin. Marcus and associates (75) showed that in nephrectomized dogs there is a higher plasma level of digoxin than in control dogs and that this is associated with higher myocardial levels. Adjustment of digoxin dosage based on individual creatinine clearance often results in a reduction of the daily oral maintenance dose to about 0.125 mg for the elderly patient (95). Furthermore, in patients over 65 years of age, the dose should be further adjusted to account for body size and cardiac status.

Hypokalemia resulting from diuretic therapy (30,53,63), laxative abuse, or increased sensitivity of the aged heart to digitalis may contribute to the development of toxicity in the elderly. Other factors to be considered in relation to digitalis toxicity, especially in the aged, are coexisting pathological conditions and altered cation balance in the tissues or the circulation. For example, altered thyroid states (26) and the presence of severe heart disease or chronic pulmonary disease may predispose an elderly patient to the development of digitalis toxicity. Regarding the role of electrolytes in digitalis toxicity, it has been shown that serum potassium levels are often normal or near normal in patients with advanced congestive heart failure during digitalization, although myocardial or total body potassium stores are markedly depleted (17). It has been noted that serum potassium levels are not reliable prognosticators of digitalis toxicity (6,17,48,94,97,98). Electrocardiographic findings, in addition to serum potassium levels, should be used in assessing intracardiac hypokalemia (17). In addition to low potassium levels, it has been well established that high calcium levels act synergistically with digitalis (17). The synergistic effects of digitalis and calcium have been associated with induction of sudden death (80,92,99). Magnesium deficiencies also predispose patients to digitalis intoxication (62,64). However, there is no evidence that levels of these ions change with increasing age, nor is there conclusive evidence that increased toxicity is due to such changes in the aged (5,6).

Another clinically useful glycoside is digitoxin. This glycoside is approximately 90% protein bound in the circulation and its total serum concentration is much higher than that of digoxin. The half-life in serum for digitoxin is 40 to 50 hr, as compared to a half-life in serum for digoxin of 30 to 33 hr. The half-life for digitoxin in all body compartments is 9 days, in contrast to that for digoxin, which is 1.6 days. Digitoxin is extensively metabolized in the body, in part to digoxin (12,26). The effect of age on digitoxin serum binding or biotransformation has not been determined.

In the aged, there do not appear to be differences in the capacity of various glycosides to produce toxicity (6). In the elderly using digitoxin (0.10 to 0.11 mg), digitalis leaf (0.096 to 0.119 mg, of which 30% is digitoxin), or digoxin (0.25 to 0.26 mg), it has been reported that there was no differential propensity for the development of toxicity with any particular preparation (6). Other studies have also shown no differences in the mean daily doses of digitoxin or digoxin that produced therapeutic effects or toxic manifestations, respectively, in adult patients (96,97). Based on a retrospective study, Herrmann (53) reported that in 202 patients on digitalis therapy (between 1955 and 1966), the occurrence of cardiac dysfunction was attributable to the glycoside rather than the underlying disease. Several digitalis materials were involved in the production of toxicities in this study: digitalis leaf in 119 cases; Gitaligin® in 31 cases; Acylanid® in 17 cases; digitoxin in 20 cases; digoxin in 19 cases; and Cedilanid-D® in one case. In another study of patients 60 to 86 years of age, acetyldigoxin was administered to 27 patients suffering from heart failure (3). The criteria for effectiveness of drug therapy in this study were reduction of heart rate and elimination of congestive phenomena. It was found that the elderly needed doses of acetyldigoxin equal to those in younger patients to produce therapeutic effects. Toxicity was not evaluated in this study. The author concluded that it is not necessary to reduce digitalis doses for the elderly, as had been suggested by earlier studies (77,79). However, based on the total body of evidence regarding the incidence of toxic manifestations in the elderly and their propensity for reduced renal function, as outlined above, it seems prudent to conclude that greater caution and perhaps lower doses of digitalis glycosides should be used in the elderly.

Animal Studies

As in the case of clinical studies, there are a number of reported animal studies noting changes in the sensitivity to digitalis effects as a function of age (Table 1). In cats, Dearing et al. (24) found that digitalis administration was more likely to lead to the development of myocardial lesions in older animals than in young ones. Wollenberger et al. (110) found no change in the sensitivity of the guinea pig myocardium to ouabain during adult life, that is, up to 5 to 6.5 years of age (maximum life span for guinea pigs is 7.5 years) (1). However, the lethal dose of ouabain decreased by about 25% from birth to maturity (5.5 to 7.5 months). Scott et al. (91) showed that toxic effects of digitoxin and proscillaridin were 200 to 1,000 times greater in developing rats (7 days old) than in adult rats (200 g). It should be noted that the toxicity of digitalis glycosides in rats is related to the development of convulsions rather than to direct cardiotoxicity (66). With respect to central nervous system effects of digitalis, it has been observed that the capacity of ouabain to inhibit the activity of $Na^+ + K^+$-sensitive ATPase isolated from spinal cord increases with age in rats (4) and parallels the propensity for toxic reactions. Chen and Robbins (15) showed that rabbits 3 to 5 years of age were more susceptible to ouabain-induced toxicity than were animals 3 to 24 months of age. Interestingly, Kelliher and Roberts (61) showed that adult rabbits (12 weeks or older) were more sensitive to the arrhythmogenic effects of ouabain than young rabbits (1 to 6 weeks). They suggested that this was owing to the development of the sympathetic innervation of the heart during this period of life, and the toxic effects of ouabain were partially because of an action on the sympathetic nerve terminals. To date, experimental evidence indicates that sympathetic control of the heart diminishes with age (see section on autonomic drugs). If future studies should show that digitalis is more toxic to the heart with increasing age to late stages in life, it would suggest that the cardiotoxic effects in old age are manifested more through a direct action on the heart, and less through an indirect action on sympathetic nerve terminals, that is, the mode of toxicity changes with age.

Other studies, using isolated ventricular trabeculae of Wistar rats, have shown that the inotropic effect of ouabain was age related (41). Ouabain produced considerably lower increases of active tension in ventricular muscles from older animals (24 months) than in ventricular muscles from young animals (6 months). In these studies, contracture was observed more frequently in muscles from young animals than old animals following ouabain (41). It appears, therefore, that with increasing age the inotropic effects of digitalis compounds become less prominent, whereas the toxic effects become more prominent (although some species variability may exist), thus narrowing the therapeutic index for a group of drugs with an already narrow therapeutic dosage range.

Since there is evidence suggesting that the changes in the cardiac actions of digitalis associated with age may result not only from altered pharmacokinetic factors (see above), but also from modification of its action on the heart itself, it would be of interest to determine the effect of age on the action of digitalis at the cellular level. It has been noted that unless the glycoside produces a net loss of cellular potassium and an equivalent net gain of cellular sodium, no inotropism is produced (69). There are at least two systems involved in sodium efflux. One system is the classical Na^+-K^+-coupled transport system regulated by $Na^+ + K^+$-activated ATPase (sodium pump). Hokin and associates (56), Kyte (65), and Lane et al. (68) have presented evidence that the $Na^+ + K^+$-activated ATPase is associated with a receptor for digitalis glycosides. The receptor for the drug is probably on the external surface of the cell membrane, since digitalis inhibits the sodium pump of intact cells (13,54,108). Schwartz et al. (90) postulated that the inhibition of the sodium pump by digitalis glycosides is an allosteric event. Since age-associated changes in other receptors have been identified, it will be of importance to study the effects of age on both the receptors and the receptor-induced modification of transmembrane electrolyte movement.

Another system regulating sodium efflux is one that is thought to be coupled to calcium influx (69). This mechanism is increasingly activated as $[Na^+]_i$ increases. Administration of glycoside inhibits the Na^+-K^+-coupled transport system, leading to intracellular accumulation of sodium. Increased $[Na^+]_i$ stimulates the $Na^+ + Ca^{2+}$-coupled system, thereby reestablishing steady state sodium exchange at a higher level of $[Na^+]_i$. The increased Ca^{2+} influx results in the development of increased contractile force (69). As discussed in Chapter 4, there is considerable evidence of age-associated changes in the intracellular handling of the calcium involved in electromechanical coupling. Primary (70) or secondary effects of the glycoside on these control mechanisms may help to explain age-associated differences in toxic and/or inotropic effects.

In addition to the evidence for a direct cardiotoxic action for digitalis (76,100), there are many observations suggesting that digitalis may produce cardiotoxic effects indirectly through an action on the central and autonomic nervous systems (42). Roberts and his co-workers (83–85) have suggested that digitalis compounds may act on multiple sites in the sympathetic–adrenal axis, leading to the development of cardiac rhythm disturbances. Cardiac glycosides may cause the release of catecholamines from the adrenal medulla of the cat, which in turn may sensitize the heart to the toxic effects of digitalis (60). Birks and Cohen (9) and Donaldson et al. (27) have suggested that cardiac sympathetic nerve terminals may be more reactive to digitalis glycosides than other areas of the nerve (e.g., axons). Saunders and Jenkins (88) have postulated that simultaneous parasympathetic and sympathetic activation is necessary for the production of arrhythmias. Since changes in neural function, both central and peripheral, have been observed during aging (81), it is possible that such alterations are involved in the changes of digitalis effects associated with aging.

AUTONOMIC DRUGS

One of the most widely studied groups of pharmacological agents which act on the heart are the autonomic drugs. Pharmacologically, this is by no means a homogeneous group of substances. Sympathomimetic, parasympathomimetic, and ganglionic agonists and their respective antagonists can have chronotropic and inotropic effects on the heart. Specific receptors for these substances are present in many organs in addition to the heart, especially in those which receive autonomic innervation. Thus, the effects of autonomic drugs on cardiac function in an intact organism may be the result of a complex series of interactions. First, there may be an effect of the agent through direct interaction with the heart. Second, there may be an effect on the heart indirectly through autonomic reflex mechanisms because of interaction with other organs (e.g., constriction of the vasculature initiating reflex vagal slowing of the heart). Third, an indirect effect on the heart may result from an action of the drug to liberate a cardioactive substance into the general circulation (e.g., release of catecholamines from the adrenal medulla). Fourth, the heart may be affected via its autonomic innervation because of a central or ganglionic site of action for the drug. In the intact organism, the effect of an autonomic agonist or antagonist on the heart is the net expression of a direct and all the indirect actions of the drug.

Within a framework such as described above, it becomes difficult, if not impossible, to identify a mechanism that might be responsible for alterations in responsiveness of cardiac tissue per se to autonomic drugs in relation to aging. More appropriately, the heart and other organs subject to the effects of autonomic drugs should be studied *in vitro* as well as in the whole animal. Furthermore, efforts should be made to perform such studies on hearts that have been chronically denervated. Although *in vivo* and *in vitro* studies on cardiac responsiveness to some autonomic drugs have been reported in relation to aging, in the majority of cases these studies had different objectives, so that complementarity of findings is rare. The limited number of studies on the effects of increasing age on cardiac sensitivity to several autonomic drugs in reality pose more questions than they answer, and serve mainly as a guideline for future research directions.

The specific autonomic substances whose effects on the heart have been studied as a function of age can be divided into several subcategories. Information is available for some sympathomimetic amines (e.g., epinephrine, norepinephrine), for parasympathomimetic agonists (e.g., acetylcholine), and for parasympathetic antagonists (e.g., atropine) (Table 2). Other substances in some of these categories (e.g., tyramine, which acts through release of norepinephrine from prejunctional sympathetic nerve terminals) have been studied either as pharmacological tools (Table 2) or not at all in relation to aging. Autonomic drugs whose study could provide insight into mechanisms of aging will be discussed at the closing of this section.

TABLE 2. *Effect of increasing age on cardiovascular sensitivity to autonomic and antiarrhythmic drugs*

Drug	Species	Effect studied	Effect of increasing age	Ref.
Sympathetic				
Epinephrine	Mouse	LD$_{50}$	Decrease	36
	Rat	Increase blood pressure	Increase	57
	Rabbit	Increase blood pressure	Increase	37
	Man	Increase heart rate	Increase	55
Norepinephrine	Rat	Increase blood pressure	Increase	57
		Increase ventricular active tension	Decrease	67
		Increase ventricular maximum rate of tension development	Decrease	67
		Decrease ventricular contraction duration	Decrease	67
		Relax aortic smooth muscle	Decrease	106; Yin (this volume)
	Rabbit	Increase blood pressure	Increase	37
Isoproterenol	Rat	Increase ventricular active tension	Decrease	67
		Increase ventricular maximum rate of tension development	Decrease	67
		Decrease ventricular contraction duration	Decrease	67
		Relax aortic smooth muscle	Decrease	35,36
	Rabbit	Relax aortic smooth muscle	Decrease	35,36
	Dog	Increase heart rate	Decrease	111
	Man	Increase heart rate	Decrease	111
Phenylephrine	Rat	Reflex decrease heart rate	Decrease	87
	Man	Reflex decrease heart rate	Decrease	51
Ephedrine	Rat	LD$_{50}$	Decrease, young to adult, increase adult to old	16

Reserpine	Cat	Deplete cardiac catecholamines	Decrease, young to adult	23
Tyramine	Rabbit	Increase heart rate *(in vitro)* due to release of cardiac neuronal catecholamines	Decrease, young to adult	10
Propranolol	Man	Decrease systolic and diastolic blood pressure	Increase	18
		Decrease cardiac index	Increase	18
Parasympathetic				
Acetylcholine	Rabbit	Decrease blood pressure	Increase	37,38
		Decrease cardiac output	Increase	38
		Decrease atrial rate *(in vitro)*	Decrease, neonatal to adult	10,105
Methacholine	Man	Decrease blood pressure	Increase	78
Atropine	Man	Increase heart rate	Decrease	22
Antiarrhythmic				
Quinidine	Rat	Depress atrial pacemakers *(in vitro)*	Decrease	45,81
		Depress ventricular pacemakers *(in vitro)*	Decrease	45,81
		Depress atrial membrane responsiveness *(in vitro)*	Decrease	43,44
Lidocaine	Rat	Depress atrial pacemakers *(in vitro)*	Increase	43,81
		Depress ventricular pacemakers *(in vitro)*	Decrease	43,81
		Decrease atrial action potential overshoot *(in vitro)*	Increase	43,44,81
		Increase atrial action potential duration and plateau duration *(in vitro)*	Increase	43,44,81

Sympathetic Agonists and Antagonists

In the whole animal, sensitivity to sympathomimetics has generally been found to increase with increasing age (8,46), although there are many opposite findings and there is confusion between maturational and senescent changes. For example, the LD_{50} for epinephrine was found to decrease significantly with increasing age in mice (36). In contrast, the LD_{50} for ephedrine was found to decrease significantly during maturation between young (4 months old) and adult (12 months old) rats, then to increase somewhat in old (24 months) rats (16). If it is assumed that cardiac toxicity of the substance contributes to its lethality, then it is evident that cardiac sensitivity to the substance has changed as a function of age. Other evidence of increased sensitivity is obtained from measurements of blood pressure and heart rate changes. Thus, it has been shown that old rabbits require lower intravenous doses of epinephrine and norepinephrine than do adult rabbits to evoke equivalent changes in arterial blood pressure (37). In rats, it was found that for a given dose of epinephrine and norepinephrine, greater blood pressure changes were evoked in adult (14 months) than in young adult rats (3 months) (57). Similar results have been obtained in humans, where it was found that infusion of a standard dose of catecholamines increased heart rate in older individuals (67.5 years mean age) to a greater extent than in young individuals (25.5 years mean age) (55). Opposite results have been found in aging dogs (111). Propranolol, a β-adrenergic receptor antagonist, in comparable doses was found to produce significant decreases in systolic and diastolic blood pressure, as well as in cardiac index, in humans 50 to 65 years of age, whereas it failed to bring about similar changes in humans 18 to 35 years of age (18).

The above observations indicate that alterations of the pharmacological effects of sympathetic agonists and antagonists occur as aging progresses. However, because of the complexity of the *in vivo* situation, it cannot be ascertained whether the changes occur in the heart per se or in other structures, e.g., the vasculature, the cardiovascular reflex mechanisms, or all three. Indeed, it has been shown that the baroreceptor reflex is more reactive in young animals (87) and man (51) than in old individuals, indicating that reflex influences and autonomic regulation of cardiac function diminishes with increasing age. In these studies, phenylephrine was used as the pressor agent. Since it has negligible direct effects on the heart, the observed changes in heart rate can reasonably be assumed to result from reflex pathway activation. The study of Rothbaum et al. (87) further pursued the question of whether the diminished baroreceptor reflex in the old animals was owing to a differential aging effect on sympathetic or parasympathetic control of the heart. This was accomplished by the use of a β-adrenergic receptor antagonist (propranolol) and a parasympathetic antagonist (atropine). They found that with increasing age both sympathetic and parasympathetic influences on the heart decreased, but that the latter decreased to a greater extent. However, this conclusion was based on the assumption that the antagonists have similar blocking potentials in young and old hearts (i.e., the affinity and the number of cardiac receptors for these antagonists do not change with increasing age). That this is indeed the case is open to question, based on the observations with propranolol discussed above (87). Such questions could better be resolved through studies on the heart *in vitro*.

The number of studies dealing directly with alterations in cardiac responsiveness to sympathetic drugs during aging is very small. Of the *in vitro* studies that have been carried out, only one deals with mechanical responsiveness to catecholamines, and the others deal with myocardial content and metabolism of catecholamines.

The effect of increasing age on direct myocardial contractile responsiveness to catecholamines was studied in rat hearts (67). In the absence of exogenously added drugs, the authors found that contraction duration (for electrically elicited twitches) of rat cardiac ventricular muscle increased with increasing age between 12 and 25 months. Noreprinephrine in this study increased active tension and the maximum rate of tension development and decreased contraction duration in a concentration-related manner. The increase in active tension and the rate of tension rise with norepinephrine were significantly reduced in muscles from old rat hearts (25 months) as compared to muscles from younger rat hearts (6 and 12 months). No change in the degree of shortening of contraction duration was found with age. The effects of high concentrations of isoproterenol were similar; however, no differences were observed in contractile responsiveness to calcium. It may be concluded from these observations that the ability of the cell to respond to calcium as an inotropic agent is unimpaired by aging. However, increasing age seems to impair the positive inotropic response to catecholamines. The authors suggest that this could be owing to a decreased ability of catecholamines to make calcium available to the contractile machinery. Since the catecholamines bring about their cellular effects (e.g., membrane depolarization, increased levels of cyclic AMP, increased calcium concentration, increased contractility, etc.) by interacting with β-adrenergic receptors on the plasma membrane surface, it may be that aging results in a decreased affinity of these receptors for catecholamines or that the total number of receptors is decreased. Indeed, where β-adrenergic receptors have been studied in other tissues [e.g., vascular smooth muscle (32,33,106); cerebellum, corpus striatum, and pineal gland (50)], it has been found that the number of functional receptors decreases with increasing age. If this is the case for the heart as well, then it can be anticipated that responsiveness to β-adrenergic agonists would decrease as a function of age, whereas responsiveness to β-adrenergic antagonists would increase with age. The study of Conway (18) described above, indeed showed an increased effectiveness of β-adrenergic antagonists in older humans. An approach to study cardiac muscle by means of drug-receptor interaction techniques (39,40,59,72) could prove fruitful in elucidating the underlying mechanisms responsible for altered sensitivity to catecholamines and their antagonists brought on by increasing age.

A number of reports have described the effects of increasing age on cardiac catecholamine content and metabolism (for references, see refs. 47 and 82). Although a review of this literature is more appropriate in a discussion of cardiac innervation, it is included here in order to gain a better understanding of the *in vivo* effects of sympathetic agonists and antagonists on the heart and to speculate about possible development of postsynaptic receptor sensitivity changes.

Cardiac catecholamine content has been shown to undergo age-related changes. From birth through early development, catecholamines in the heart appear to increase with increasing age (71). The increase in catecholamines during development is associated with the elaboration of sympathetic innervation to the heart. During development, it has been found that reserpine, a catecholamine-depleting agent, is more effective in reducing catecholamine content in hearts from young cats than in hearts from older cats (23). The indirectly acting sympathomimetic tyramine appears to be more effective in releasing neuronal catecholamines in young rabbits than in adult rabbits, as indicated by the concentration of this agent necessary to produce half-maximal and maximal increases of heart rate *in vitro* (10). However, the absolute maximal response to tyramine in these studies was greater in the adult rabbits. It appears, therefore, that although the intraneuronal pools of catecholamines are more labile in the young animals (i.e., more completely depleted by reserpine and more readily released by tyramine), the responsiveness of the heart to catecholamines is greater in the adults (the adults being capable of attaining a greater increase in heart rate response than the young). Increased cardiac responsiveness during this phase of life may be owing to the development of cardiac receptors in parallel with innervation or to a general development of physiological and biochemical function. Studies aimed at understanding and resolving such questions would be most productive.

During later phases of aging, that is, with increasing age from maturity through old age, catecholamine content in the heart decreases (2,82). For this later phase of the life span, neurotransmitter regulating enzymes, such as DOPA decarboxylase in the synthetic pathway and monoamine oxydase in the degradation pathway, decrease in activity (47,104). Obviously, the net effect of all the catecholamine metabolic changes is a decreased neurotransmitter content. In addition, it appears that with increasing age, cardiac sympathetic nerve terminals become increasingly less efficient in storing catecholamines in the granular compartment, and eventually begin to lose catecholamines from the nongranular compartment (73). The overall pattern of decreasing catecholamine availability in sympathetic nerve terminals of the heart explains, at least in part, the decreasing sympathetic control of the heart as aging progresses, observed in the studies on the baroreceptor reflex (51,87) discussed above. Furthermore, within the framework of decreasing nervous input to the heart, postsynaptic receptor sensitivity (receptor density and/or affinity for drugs) changes may also take place. Early on, the change may be a compensatory supersensitivity of the heart, whereas later it is conceivable that homeostatic mechanisms may fail and subsensitivity might result. Such receptor sensitivity changes, initiated by a failing innervation, would be consistent with the results of Lakatta et al. (67), who showed that the inotropic response of cardiac muscle to exogenously applied catecholamines decreased with increasing age (see above). This aspect of the problem needs further investigation.

Parasympathetic Agonists and Antagonists

Work on pharmacological effects of parasympathetic agonists and antagonists on the heart in relation to aging is less extensive than that of sympathetic agonists and antagonists. Following is a summary of the salient work in this area.

The pharmacological effects of parasympathomimetics in whole animal studies have been shown to increase with increasing age (37,78) (see Table 2). In old rabbits (4.5 to 5 years), a lower intravenous dose of acetylcholine was required to produce a hypotensive response than in adult rabbits (1 to 1.5 years) (37). A uniform dose of acetylcholine (0.05 μg/kg) produced a greater decrease in blood pressure and cardiac output in old rabbits than in adults (38). Similarly, a study in humans has shown that methacholine elicited greater hypotensive responses in older subjects (over 45 years) than in young subjects (under 45 years) (78). The effects of parasympathomimetics in the whole animal result from a direct negative chronotropic action on the heart and a direct vasodilator effect on vascular smooth muscle. Depending on the dose of acetylcholine, its direct parasympathetic effects on the heart may be attenuated by cardiovascular reflexes and its ability to release catecholamines from the adrenal medulla and sympathetic postganglionic nerve fibers. The role of reflex control of cardiac function has been discussed above, where it was suggested that parasympathetic control of the heart very likely decreases with increasing age (87). It has also been shown by Dauchot and Gravenstein (22) that in humans, atropine, a parasympathetic antagonist, elicits progressively smaller increases in heart rate with age, further supporting the hypothesis of diminishing parasympathetic control. It is possible that supersensitivity to acetylcholine may develop during aging, which would account for the reduced effect of atropine. However, there is no experimental evidence as yet documenting the development of supersensitivity of parasympathetic receptors in older animals.

In vitro studies on the effects of increasing age on cardiac responsiveness to parasympathetic drugs are very few indeed. During early growth and development, it appears that acetylcholine activity decreases. For example, Brus and Jacobowitz (10) have shown that in rabbit atria, the ED_{50} of acetylcholine in producing bradycardia increased approximately 100-fold from the neonatal to the adult (3 months) phase. Another study indicates that the ED_{50} for acetylcholine-induced bradycardia in rabbit atria increased approximately four- to fivefold during development from neonate to adult (6 months) (105). In the latter study, initial atrial rate decreased during this time period, so that the actual change (beats per minute) in atrial rate was greater in the young animals than in the old. The manner of expressing data notwithstanding, the results of these studies are somewhat ambiguous, since cholinesterases were not inhibited in either study. Since acetylcholine is highly susceptible to hydrolysis by tissue cholinesterases, it cannot be said with certainty whether the decreased effectiveness of acetylcholine was owing to altered cholinesterase activity, to altered sensitivity of cardiac parasympathetic receptors, or to both phenomena. Indeed, in rat hearts (atria and ventricles), it has been reported that both choline-acetyl transferase activity and cholinesterase activity decrease with aging between 1 and 26 to 28 months of age (38).

The above summary of the effects of increasing age on cardiac responsiveness to sympathetic and parasympathetic drugs clearly points to possible mechanisms for age-associated changes. Doubtless, autonomic nervous control of the heart decreases with increasing age. Postsynaptic changes in cardiac tissue per se most likely also occur; however, the nature of these changes is as yet unclear. It would be most interesting to define the reciprocal nature of interaction between nerve and cardiac membranes during aging. Does the innervation begin to deteriorate first? What compensatory mechanisms, if any, is the heart capable of? How long can the heart compensate for diminishing nervous input? Are the interactions the same or different for the sympathetic and parasympathetic components? What is the pharmacological significance of age-related changes? How, and at what point in time can pharmacological interventions be effectively instituted? Autonomic agonists and antagonists would be invaluable experimental tools in elucidating the mechanisms of physiological and pharmacological changes with age.

ANTIARRHYTHMIC DRUGS

Studies have shown that cardiovascular abnormalities, including disorders of cardiac rhythm, are prevalent among the elderly (11). Substances in the category of antiarrhythmic therapeutic agents act by modifying some aspect of cardiac electrical activity. Antiarrhythmic drugs are absorbed through the gastrointestinal tract and are therefore generally effective by the oral route of administration. However, some antiarrhythmic agents are extremely fat soluble (e.g., lidocaine) or have a great capacity for binding to plasma proteins (e.g., phenytoin). Because of these properties, long periods of time are required to saturate the storage pools, thus making these agents less effective by the oral route and more effective by the intravenous route. Antiarrhythmic substances distribute to all body compartments and undergo extensive biotransformation in the liver. Metabolites, as well as the small fraction of unmetabolized drugs, are excreted by the kidney. In the general adult population, undesirable reactions to antiarrhythmic agents are usually dose related. Toxic manifestations include cardiovascular, central nervous system, and gastrointestinal disturbances. Although there is little direct experimental evidence that aging produces alterations in sensitivity to antiarrhythmic agents, cautionary statements appear in the literature regarding the use of these drugs, particularly quinidine, in the elderly (25,31,34,49,107). It should be anticipated that alterations of pharmacokinetic factors, such as absorption, biotransformation, plasma binding, tissue storage, and excretion during aging would affect drug availability to the myocardium and other tissues, thus affecting sensitivity in the elderly (25,112).

In our laboratories, several antiarrhythmic drugs (e.g., quinidine, lidocaine) have been studied for their effectiveness on the myocardium at different stages in the life span of rats (Fisher 344 males, 1 to 28 months of age) (Table 2). The studies were carried out with the heart *in vitro,* allowing us to observe the effects of aging on sensitivity to drugs at the effector organ level. Rat hearts were perfused by the method of Langendorff, and atrioventricular blockade was produced surgically in order to observe atrial and ventricular pacemaker activities independently in the same preparation. Under these conditions, it was observed that the antiarrhythmic agents quinidine and lidocaine depressed both the atrial and ventricular pacemakers of hearts from animals at all ages studied (45,81). Both drugs produced a greater decrease in ventricular rate than in atrial rate. However, the important observation was that the effect of quinidine to depress atrial and ventricular pacemakers decreased with increasing age; that is, the hearts from the young animals were depressed to a greater degree than the hearts of old animals. Lidocaine had a similar effect with respect to increasing age on the ventricles; however, on atria the effect of lidocaine to decrease pacemaker activity increased with increasing age. In this study, then, sensitivity to a drug was found not only to change with age, but also to increase in one case and decrease in another. This indicates that particular attention must be paid to investigations of the action of each drug on a given organ, and that generalizations regarding the effects of age on responsiveness to drugs should not be made indiscriminately.

In order to investigate the electrophysiological basis for the observed differences in sensitivity with increasing age to the anti-arrhythmic agents discussed above, the effects of quinidine and lidocaine on transmembrane electrical activity were studied in atria from rats over the same life span range. It was found that quinidine decreased membrane responsiveness[1] to a greater extent in atria from young rats than in atria from old rats (43,44). Since in cardiac tissue membrane responsiveness determines such properties as return of excitability and conduction velocity, the observations that quinidine produces less of an effect on membrane responsiveness of atria from old rats are consistent with the observations of decreasing effectiveness of quinidine in depressing atrial pacemakers with age.

Lidocaine was found to decrease action potential overshoot and maximum rate of rise of phase 0 and to increase action

---

[1] Membrane responsiveness is a property relating the ability of an excitable cell to propagate a normal action potential at different levels of membrane polarization. It is customarily measured by the size of the maximum rate of rise of phase 0 of an action potential interposed at a time before complete repolarization of a cell occurs from a previous action potential, so that the membrane potential is less negative than resting potential.

potential duration and plateau duration (43,44,81). The effects of lidocaine on atrial action potential overshoot, action potential duration, and plateau duration increased with increasing age, in a manner similar to the increasing depressant effect of lidocaine on atrial pacemakers as a function of age. Since these drugs are thought to bring about changes in electrical activity by interacting with some membrane receptors, which then leads to interference with cation movement across excitable membranes, it seems reasonable to conclude that with increasing age, either the drug–receptor interaction is altered or the transmembrane cation movement mechanisms are altered. More definitive work in this direction is being carried out.

CONCLUDING REMARKS

The gerontological literature on the pharmacology of the heart has been reviewed with the aim in mind of summarizing available information and evolving a broad picture of the effects of aging on the heart and its responsiveness to drugs. A search of the literature revealed that in only several areas, i.e., digitalis glycosides, autonomic drugs, and antiarrhythmic drugs, was there any information available, and that it was diverse and fragmented in experimental approach. To extend our knowledge of these drugs as they relate to gerontology, directions for systematic studies have been suggested.

Our search revealed a lack of information of many pharmacological agents which are used for their effects on the heart, or which are used for their effects on other tissues but have important actions on the heart as well. For example, coronary vasodilators, anesthetic agents, hormones, polypeptides, prostaglandins, electrolytes, and antibiotics, to name but a few categories of pharmacological agents, have not been studied in any meaningful way in relation to aging. Since these agents are used or have potential use in the elderly, they should be investigated for their actions in relation to aging, both at the organ and cellular levels and in the whole organism.

Another area for fruitful research is the innervation of the heart and its relation to drug action. For drugs known to have multiple sites of action, for example, on the central and autonomic nervous systems, as well as on the heart per se, studies should be carried out on the innervated heart, on the acutely denervated heart, and on the chronically denervated heart. These studies would address such important questions as: (a) Does cardiac sensitivity change as nervous influences change during aging? (b) How are such changes manifested? and (c) If the pharmacological agent acts directly on the heart and indirectly through the innervation, which component is more important with regard to alterations in action brought on by aging?

Finally, one aspect of the pharmacology of the aging heart that requires elucidation is the effect of various forms of stress (e.g., hypoxia, hypertension, exercise, etc.) on sensitivity to drugs. It has become almost axiomatic that the older an organism becomes, the less it is able to invoke homeostatic mechanisms to cope with stress. Within such a framework, do drugs help alleviate various forms of stress in the elderly as efficiently as they do in younger populations, or do they in fact provide another form of stress?

REFERENCES

1. Altman, P. L., and Dittmer, D. S., editors (1972): *Biology Data Book,* Vol. 1, 2nd ed., p. 230. FASEB, Bethesda, Maryland.
2. Angelakos, E. T., King, M. P., and Millard, R. W. (1969): Regional distribution of catecholamines in the hearts of various species. *Ann. N.Y. Acad. Sci.,* 156:219–240.
3. Aravanis, C. (1969): The use of acetyldigoxin in the aged with congestive heart failure. *Geriatrics,* 24:75–81.
4. Baskin, S. I., Roberts, J., and DeSousa, B. N. (1977): $Na^+ + K^+$ ATPase and age dependent toxicity. *Pharmacologist,* 19:132.
5. Baylis, E. M., Hall, M. S., Lewis, G., and Marks, V. (1972): Effects of renal function on plasma digoxin levels in elderly ambulant patients in domiciliary practice. *Br. Med. J.,* 1:338–341.
6. Beller, G., Smith, T. W., Abelman, W. H., Haber, E., and Hood, W. (1971): Digitalis intoxication; a prospective clinical study and serum level correlations. *N. Engl. J. Med.,* 284:989–997.
7. Bender, A. D. (1964): Pharmacologic aspects of aging: A survey of the

effect of increasing age on drug activity in adults. *J. Am. Geriatr. Soc.,* 12:114–134.

8. Bender, A. D. (1970): The influence of age on the activity of catecholamines and related therapeutic agents. *J. Am. Geriatr. Soc.,* 18(3):220–232.

9. Birks, R. I., and Cohen, M. W. (1968): The influence of internal sodium on the behavior of motor nerve endings. *Proc. Roy. Soc. (Lond.), Series B.* 170:401–421.

10. Brus, R., and Jacobowitz, D. (1972): The influence of norepinephrine tyramine and acetylcholine upon isolated perfused hearts of immature and adult rabbits. *Arch. Pharmacodyn. Ther.,* 200:266–272.

11. Burch G. E., and DePasquale, N. P. (1969): Geriatric cardiology. *Am. Heart J.,* 78:700–708.

12. Caird, F. I. (1972): Metabolism of digoxin in relation to therapy in the elderly. *Gerontol. Clin.,* 16:68–74.

13. Caldwell, P. C. (1960): The phosphorus metabolism of squid axons and its relationships to the active transport of sodium. *J. Physiol. (Lond.),* 152:545–560.

14. Chamberlain, D. A., White, R. J., Howard, M. R., and Smith, T. W. (1970): Plasma digoxin concentrations in patients with atrial fibrillation. *Br. Med. J.,* 3:429–432.

15. Chen, K. K., and Robbins, E. B., (1944): Influence of age of rabbits on the toxicity of ouabain. *J. Am. Pharm. Assoc.,* 33:61–62.

16. Chen, K. K., and Robbins, E. B. (1944): Age of animals and drug action. *J. Am. Pharm. Assoc.,* 33:80–82.

17. Chung, E. K. (1971): The current status of digitalis therapy. *Mod. Treatment,* 8:643–714.

18. Conway, J. (1970): Effect of age on the response to propranolol. *Int. J. Clin. Pharmacol.,* 4:148–150.

19. Crouch, R. B., Hermann, G. R., and Hejtmanik, M. R. (1956): Digitalis intoxication. *Tex. J. Med.,* 52:714–718.

20. Dall, J. L. C. (1965): Digitalis intoxication in elderly patients. *Lancet,* 1:194–195.

21. Dall, J. L. C. (1970): Maintenance digoxin in elderly patients. *Br. Med. J.,* 2:705–706.

22. Dauchot, P., and Gravenstein, J. S. (1971): Effects of atropine on the electrocardiogram in different age groups. *Clin. Pharmacol. Ther.,* 12:274–280.

23. Davidson, W. J., and Innes, I. R. (1972): Increased depletion of catecholamines by reserpine in immature cats. *Can. J. Physiol. Pharmacol.,* 50(6):612–613.

24. Dearing, W. H., Barnes, A. R., and Essex, H. E. (1943): Experiments with calculated therapeutic and toxic doses of digitalis; effects on the myocardial cellular structure. *Am. Heart J.,* 25:648–664.

25. DeGroff, A. C. (1974): Drug therapy of cardiovascular disease. *Geriatrics,* 29(6):51–54.

26. Doherty, J. E. (1968): The clinical pharmacology of digitalis glycosides: A review. *Am. J. Med. Sci.,* 255:382–414.
27. Donaldson, J., Minnich, J. L., and Barbeau, A. (1972): Ouabain-induced seizures in rats: Regional and subcellular localization of 3H-ouabain associated with Na⁺,K⁺,ATPase in brain. *Can. J. Biochem.* 50:888–896.
28. Evered, D. C., and Chapman, C. (1971): Plasma digoxin concentrations and digoxin toxicity in hospital patients. *Br. Heart J.,* 33:540–545.
29. Evered, D. C., Chapman, C., and Hayter, C. J. (1970): Measurement of plasma digoxin concentration by radioimmunoassay. *Br. Med. J.,* 3:427–428.
30. Ewy, G. A., Kapadia, G. G., Yao, L., Lullin, M., and Marcus, F. I. (1969): Digoxin metabolism in the elderly. *Circulation,* 39:449–453.
31. Fine, W. (1959): The effects of drugs on old people. *Med. Press (Lond.),* 242:4–8.
32. Fleisch, J. H. (1974): Pharmacology of the aorta. A brief review. *Blood Vessels,* 11:(4)193–211.
33. Fleisch, J. H., Maling, H. M., and Brodie, B. B. (1970): Beta-receptor activity in aorta. Variations with age and species. *Circ. Res.,* 24:151–162.
34. Freeman, J. T. (1963): Some common cardiovascular agents. In: *Clinical Principles and Drugs in the Aging,* edited by J. T. Freeman, pp. 383–404. Charles C Thomas, Springfield, Illinois.
35. Friend, D. (1961): Drug therapy and the geriatric patient. *J. Pharmacol. Exp. Ther.,* 2:832–836.
36. Frolkis, V. V. (1965): The sensitivity to and the endurance of pharmacological substances in aging of the organism. *Farmakol. Toksikol.,* 28:612–616.
37. Frolkis, V. V. (1969): The autonomic nervous system in the aging organism. *Triangle,* 8:322–328.
38. Frolkis, V. V., Berzrukov, V. V., Duplenko, Y. K., Shchegoleva, I. V., Shevtchuk, V. G., and Verkhrotsky, N. S. (1973): Acetycholine metabolism and cholinergic regulation of functions in aging. *Gerontologia,* 19:45–57.
39. Furchgott, R. F. (1978): Pharmacological characterization of receptors: Its relation to radioligand-binding studies. *Fed. Proc.,* 37(2):115–120.
40. Furchgott, R. F., and Bursztyn, P. (1967): Comparison of dissociation constants and of relative efficacies of selected agonists acting on parasympathetic receptors. *Ann. N.Y. Acad. Sci.,* 144(2):882–889.
41. Gerstenblith, G., Lakatta, E. G., Spurgeon, H., Shock, N. W., and Weisfeldt, M. L. (1975): Diminished ouabain sensitivity in aged myocardium. *Fed. Proc.,* 34(3):365.
42. Gillis, R. A., Raines, A., Sohn, Y. J., Levitt, B., and Standaert, G. (1972): Neuroexcitatory effects of digitalis and their role in the development of cardiac arrhythmias. *J. Pharmacol. Exp. Ther.,* 183:154–168.
43. Goldberg, P. B., Cavato, F. V., and Roberts, J. (1975): Age-related changes in sensitivity to antiarrhythmic drugs. *Fed. Proc.,* 34:277.

44. Goldberg, P. B., Cavoto, F. V., and Roberts, J. (1975): Alterations in reactivity to antiarrhythmic agents produced by age. *Clin. Res.,* 23:185.
45. Goldberg, P. B., and Roberts, J. (1975): Age effects on atrial and ventribular sensitivity to quinidince and lidocaine. *Gerontologist,* 15(5):II24.
46. Goldberg, P. B., and Roberts, J. (1976): Influence of age on the pharmacology and physiology of the cardiovascular system. In: *Special Review of Experimental Aging Research, Progress in Biology,* edited by M. F. Elias, B. F. Eleftheriou, and P. K. Elias, pp. 71–103. Experimental Aging Research, Bar Harbor, Maine.
47. Goldberg, P. B., and Roberts, J. (1976): Changes in the biochemistry of the rat heart with increasing age. *Exp. Aging Res.,* 2(6):519–529.
48. Gotsman, M. S., and Schrire, V. (1966): Toxicity—a frequent complication of digitalis therapy. *S. Afr. Med. J.,* 40:590–592.
49. Gotthold, E. (1961): Quinidine therapy of the heart in old age. *Med. Monatsschr.,* 15:396–398.
50. Greenberg, L. H., and Weiss, B. (1978): Beta-adrenergic receptors in aged rat brain: Reduced number and capacity of pineal gland to develop supersensitivity. *Science,* 201:61–63.
51. Gribbin, B., Pickering, T. G., Sleight, P., and Peto, R. (1971): Effect of age and high blood pressure on baroreflex sensitivity in man. *Circ. Res.,* 29:424–431.
52. Heller, L. J., and Whitehorn, W. V. (1972): Age-associated alterations in myocardial contractile properties. *Am. J. Physiol.,* 222:1613–1619.
53. Herrmann, G. R. (1966): Digitoxicity in the aged. *Geriatrics,* 21:109–122.
54. Hoffman, J. F. (1966): The red cell membrane and the transport of sodium and potassium. *Am. J. Med.,* 41:666–680.
55. Hoffman, V. H., Kiesewetter, R., Krohs, G., and Schmitz, C. (1975): Dependence on age of the effects of catecholamines in man I. Effect of noradrenaline, adrenaline and isoprenaline on blood pressure and heart rate. *Z. Gesamte Inn. Med.,* 30(3):89–95.
56. Hokin, L. E., Dahl, J. L., Deupree, J. D., Dixon, J. F., Hackney, J. F., and Perdue, J. F. (1973): Studies on the characterization of the sodium–potassium transport adenosine triphosphatase. *J. Biol. Chem.,* 248(7):2593–2605.
57. Hrůza, Z., and Zweifach, B. W. (1967): Effect of age on vascular reactivity to catecholamines in rats. *J. Gerontol.,* 22:469–473.
58. Hurwitz, N., and Wade, O. L. (1969): Intensive hospital monitoring of adverse reactions to drugs. *Br. Med. J.,* 1:531–536.
59. Karlin, A., Damle, V., Valderrama, R., Hamilton, S., Wise, D., and McLaughlin, M. (1978): Interactions among binding sites on acetylcholine receptors in membrane and in detergent solution. *Fed. Proc.,* 37(2):121–122.
60. Kelliher, G. J., and Roberts, J. (1974): A study of the antiarrhythmic action of certain beta-blocking agents. *Am. Heart J.,* 87(4):458–467.
61. Kelliher, G. J., and Roberts, J. (1976): Effect of age on the cardiotoxic action of digitalis. *J. Pharmacol. Exp. Ther.,* 197(1):10–18.

62. Kim, Y. W., Andrews, C. E., and Ruth, W. E. (1961): Serum magnesium and cardiac arrhythmias with special references to digitalis intoxication. *Am. J. Med. Sci.,* 242:87–92.

63. Kirsten, E., Rodstein, M., and Duster, Z. (1973): Digoxin in the aged. *Geriatrics,* 28:95–101.

64. Kleiber, E. E. (1949): Wolff-Parkinson-White syndrome with congenital heart disease. *Pediatrics,* 4:210–213.

65. Kyte, J. (1974): The reactions of sodium and potassium ion-activated adenosine triphosphatase with specific antibodies. Implications for the mechanism of active transport. *J. Biol. Chem.,* 249:3652–3660.

66. Lage, G. L., and Spratt, J. L. (1966): Structure–activity correlation of the lethality and central effects of selected cardiac glycosides. *J. Pharmacol. Exp. Ther.,* 152(3):501–508.

67. Lakatta, E. G., Gerstenblith, G., Angell, C. S., Shock, N. W., and Weisfeldt, M. L. (1975): Diminished inotropic response of aged myocardium to catecholamines. *Circ. Res.,* 36:262–269.

68. Lane, L. K., Copenhaver, J. H., Lindenmayer, G. E., and Schwartz, A. (1973): Purification and characterization of a 3H ouabain binding to transport adenosine triphosphatase from outer medulla of canine kidney. *J. Biol. Chem.,* 248:7197–7200.

69. Langer, G. A., and Serena, S. D. (1974): Glycoside effects on ionic exchange in perfused mammalian heart. *Ann. N.Y. Acad. Sci.,* 242:688–692.

70. Lee, K. S., Hong, S. A., and Kang, D. H. (1970): Effect of cardiac glycosides on interaction of Ca^{++} with mitochondria. *J. Pharmacol. Exp. Ther.,* 172:180–187.

71. Lee, W. C., Lew, J. M., and Yoo, C. S. (1970): Studies on myocardial catecholamines related to species ages and sex. *Arch. Int. Pharmacodyn. Ther.,* 185:259–268.

72. Lefkowitz, R. J. (1978): Indentification and regulation of alpha- and beta-adrenergic receptors. *Fed. Proc.,* 37(2):123–129.

73. Limas, C. J. (1975): Comparison of the handling of norepinephrine in the myocardium of adult and old rats. *Circ. Res.,* 9:664–668.

74. Lullman, H., and van Zwieten, P. A. (1969): The kinetic behavior of cardiac glycosides *in vivo,* measured by isotope techniques. *J. Pharm. Pharmacol.,* 21:1–8.

75. Marcus, F. I., Peterson, A., Salel, A., Scully, J., and Kapadia, G. G. (1966): Metabolism of tritiated digoxin in renal insufficiency in dogs and man. *J. Pharmacol. Exp. Ther.,* 152:372–382.

76. Mason, D. T., Spann, J. F., Jr., and Zelis, R. (1969): New developments in the understanding of the actions of the digitalis glycosides. *Prog. Cardiovasc. Dis.,* 11:443–478.

77. Master, A. M. (1955): Practical consideration of digitalis administration. *N.Y. State J. Med.,* 55(5):619–627.

78. Nelson, R., and Gellhorn, E. (1957): The action of autonomic drugs on normal persons and neurophychiatric patients. The role of age. *Psychosom. Med.,* 19:486–494.

79. Raisbeck, M. J. (1952): The use of digitalis in the aged. *Geriatrics,* 7(1):12–19.

80. Resnick, N. (1964): Digitalis: A double edged sword. *Med. Sci.,* 4:31–38.

81. Roberts, J., and Goldberg, P. B. (1975): Changes in cardiac membranes as a function of age with particular emphasis on reactivity to drugs. In: *Explorations in Aging, Vol. 61: Advances in Experimental Medicine and Biology,* edited by V. J. Cristofalo, J. Roberts, and R. C. Adelman, pp. 119–148. Plenum Press, New York.

82. Roberts, J., and Goldberg, P. B. (1976): Changes in basic cardiovascular activities during the lifetime of the rat. *Exp. Aging Res.,* 2(6):487–517.

83. Roberts, J., and Kelliher, G. J. (1972): The mechanisms of digitalis at the subcellular level. *Semin. Drug Treat.,* 2(2):203–220.

84. Roberts, J., Kelliher, G. J., and Lathers, C. M. (1976): Minireview: Role of adrenergic influences in digitalis-induced ventricular arrhythmia. *Life Sci.,* 18(7):665–678.

85. Roberts, J., and Modell, W. (1961): Pharmacologic evidence for the importance of catecholamines in cardiac rhythmicity. *Circ. Res.,* 9:171–176.

86. Rothbaum, D. A., Shaw, D. J., Angell, C. S., and Shock, N. W. (1973): Cardiac performance in the unanesthetized senescent male rat. *J. Gerontol.,* 28:287–292.

87. Rothbaum, D. A., Shaw, D. J., Angell, C. S., and Shock, N. W. (1974): Age differences in the baroreceptor response of rats. *J. Gerontol.,* 29:488–492.

88. Saunders, B. A., and Jenkins, L. G. (1973): Cardiac arrhythmias of central nervous system origin, possible mechanism and suppression. *Can. Anaesth. Soc. J.,* 20:617–628.

89. Schott, A. (1964): Observations on digitalis intoxication—A plea. *Postgrad. Med. J.,* 40:628–643.

90. Schwartz, A., Lindenmayer, G. E., and Allen, J. C. (1975): The sodium potassium adenosine triphosphatase: Pharmacological, physiological and biochemical aspects. *Pharmacol. Rev.,* 27(1):3–134.

91. Scott, W. J., Beliles, R. P., and Silverman, H. I. (1971): The comparative acute toxicity of two cardiac glycosides in adult and newborn rats. *Toxicol. Appl. Pharmacol.,* 20:599–601.

92. Shrager, M. W. (1957): Digitalis intoxication. *Arch. Intern. Med.,* 100:881–893.

93. Shreiner, D. P., Weisfeldt, M. L., and Shock, N. W. (1969): Effects of age, sex, and breeding status on the rat heart. *Am. J. Physiol.,* 217:176–180.

94. Smith, T. W. (1970): Radioimmunoassay for serum digoxin concentration: Methodology and clinical experience. *J. Pharmacol. Exp. Ther.,* 175:352–360.

95. Smith, T. W. (1973): Letter to the editor: Effect of digoxin. *N. Engl. J. Med.,* 288(3):1356.

96. Smith, T. W., and Haber, E. (1970): Digoxin intoxication: The relation-

ship of clinical presentation to serum digoxin concentration. *J. Clin. Invest.,* 49:2377–2386.

97. Smith, T. W., and Haber, E. (1971): The clinical value of serum digitalis glycoside concentration in the evaluation of drug toxicity. *Ann. N.Y. Acad. Sci.,* 179:322–337.

98. Soffer, A. L. (1962): The importance of atrio-ventricular dissociation in the diagnosis of digitalis intoxication. *Dis. Chest,* 41(4):422–424.

99. Somlyo, A. P. (1960): The toxiocology of digitalis. *Am. J. Cardiol.,* 5:523–533.

100. Spann, J. F., Jr., Sonnenblick, E. H., Cooper, T., Chidsey, C. A., Willman, V. L., and Braunwald, E. (1967): The intrinsic contractile state of heart muscle and its response to digitalis: Two properties independent of cardiac norepinephrine stores. In: *Factors Influencing Myocardial Contractility,* edited by R. D. Tanz, F. Kavaler, and J. Roberts, pp. 579–589. Academic Press, New York.

101. Task Force on Prescription Drugs (1969): Final Report, p. 2. U.S. Department of Health, Education and Welfare, Washington, D.C.

102. Taylor, B. B., Kennedy, R. D., and Caird, F. I. (1974): Digoxin studies in the elderly. *Age Aging,* 3:79–84.

103. Thomas, J. H. (1971): The use and abuse of digitalis in the elderly. *Gerontol. Clin.,* 13:285–295.

104. Thompson, J. H., Su, C., Shik, J. C., Aures, D., Choi, L., Butcher, S., Loskota, W. S., Simon, M., and Silva, D. (1974): Effects of chronic nicotine administration and age on various neurotransmitters and associated enzymes in male Fisher 344 rats. *Toxicol. Appl. Pharmacol.,* 27:41–59.

105. Toda, N., Ju, W. L. H., and Osumi, Y. (1976): Age-dependence of the chronotropic response to noradrenaline, acetylcholine and transmural stimulation in isolated rabbit atria. *Jpn. J. Pharmacol.,* 26:359–366.

106. Tuttle, R. S. (1966): Age related changes in the sensitivity of rat aortic strips to norepinephrine and associated chemical structural alterations. *J. Gerontol.,* 21:510–516.

107. Weisman, S. A. (1949): Quinidine in geriatrics. *Geriatrics.,* 4(2):85–89.

108. Whittam, R. (1962): The asymmetrical stimulation of a membrane adenosine triphosphatase in relation to active cation transport. *Biochem. J.,* 84:110–118.

109. Wilson, G. M. (1957): Therapeutics in the elderly. In: *Modern Trend in Geriatrics,* edited by W. Hobson, and Paul B. Hoeber, pp. 272–302. Harper Bros., New York.

110. Wollenberger, A., Jehl, J., and Karsh, M. L. (1953). The influence of age on the sensitivity of the guinea pig and its myocardium to ouabain. *J. Pharmacol. Exp. Ther.,* 108:52–60.

111. Yin, F. C., Spurgeon, H. A., Raizes, G. S., Greene, H. L., Weisfeldt, M. L., and Shock, N. W. (1976): Age-associated decrease in chronotropic response to isoproterenol. *Circulation,* 54(4):II167.

112. Yount, E. H., Rosenblum, M., and McMillan, R. L. (1953): Quinidine for chronic auricular fibrillation in the patient over 60. *Geriatrics,* 8(1): 19–22.

The Aging Heart (Aging, Vol. 12),
edited by Myron L. Weisfeldt.
Raven Press, New York © 1980.

Chapter 9

Noninvasive Assessment of Cardiac Function in the Elderly

Gary Gerstenblith

Cardiology Division, Department of Medicine, Johns Hopkins Medical Institutions, Baltimore, Maryland 21205

The number and proportion of aged individuals in the American population is ever increasing. It is expected that by the year 1980 there will be 24 million Americans 65 years of age or older (63,64). Although this number will be just over 10% of the population, the elderly utilize medical care more than any other age group. Cardiovascular disease is the most frequent reason for hospitalization of the elderly population and cardiac disease is responsible for more than 40% of the deaths in this age group (65). The detection and treatment of cardiac disease in an individual, however, is dependent on the determination that a particular person's cardiovascular status differs from normal. It is important, therefore, to define age-adjusted criteria for clinically important variables of cardiac function. Thus, an understanding of the changes in the cardiovascular system which occur with normal aging are important because they aid in the management of disease states. Such an understanding is also important because, although age-associated changes may be "normal," they may nevertheless be clinically important. Aging of the myocardium has been likened by Dock to aging of the eye, an organ which shows its most pronounced aging change when stressed (11). Although not striking at rest, age changes in the cardiovascular system may become apparent and assume clinical importance during the stress of an intercurrent illness, a tachycardia, or a more chronic illness such as hyperthyroidism. Age changes may also decrease the reserve capacity of the heart, so that in the setting of certain forms of heart disease, an aged heart may show more evidence of deterioration than a younger one.

The noninvasive evaluation of the effect of age on cardiovascular function is often stressed. One reason for this is the increased risk of performing invasive studies on healthy, aged individuals in order to obtain information concerning the effect of the aging process itself. Another is that normal parameters of noninvasive measurements of cardiovascular function in the aged are needed because the clinician relies more on noninvasive methods in the ill elderly population since they often have more advanced or multisystem disease, which makes an invasive evaluation difficult to perform. However, characterization of the effect of age on cardiovascular structure and function in man by noninvasive or invasive studies is difficult for several reasons (2). In cross-sectional studies it is most important to be certain that the aged individuals studied are free of cardiovascular disease. If one compares healthy, young adult individuals with aged individuals suffering from hypertension or latent coronary artery disease, differences found between the two groups cannot be attributed solely to the aging process. In addition, the elderly group represents a select, long-lived subset of the population and therefore is a biased sample. Furthermore, it is impossible to eliminate genetic or environmental differences between the two groups. Longitudinal studies eliminate these differences but have certain disadvantages as well (21). The vast majority of studies discussed in this chapter are cross-sectional; therefore, an important consideration in their evaluation must be the methods taken, if any, to insure that the comparison groups were free of cardiovascular disease (see Chapter 1).

HISTORY

The first stage in the noninvasive evaluation of the elderly is the taking of the history. Symptoms in the elderly population can be misleading and unreliable. It may be more difficult to communicate with an aged than a young patient, the patient's understanding of medical terms may be less, and cerebral changes resulting in memory loss and confusion may be present. A negative history does not necessarily indicate lack of disease in the elderly as compared with the younger population, as the sedentary individual with heart disease may not exercise sufficiently to be aware of anginal or failure symptoms. Furthermore, symptoms of heart disease, e.g., dyspnea, are often due to disease in other organ systems.

PHYSICAL EXAMINATION

There are certain aspects of the clinical examination as well which are peculiar to the aged population. It is generally agreed that at rest heart rate does not vary with age (59). However, blood pressure, primarily the peak systolic pressure, increases (20,39,58). Pickering (38,39) noted that arterial pressure tends to rise more and faster in some subjects than in others. He noted (38) that "what is inherited seems to be a tendency for a given pressure at a given age; the rate of rise of pressure with age seems to be . . . due to the impact of environmental influences." One of the factors he believed most likely to account for the initial rise in pressure with age was the Western way of life. He wrote, ". . . it would seem that the difference between the way of life in a primitive tribe and that in 'civilized' society provides the key to the rise of arterial pressure with age that is the outstanding feature of essential hypertension." He believed that transient episodes of hypertension associated with everyday stresses eventually result in permanent arterial changes which in turn are responsible for sustained elevation in arterial pressure.

Brown and associates (5) believed that "essential hypertension is an exaggeration of the tendency for blood pressure to increase with age" and that it resulted from transient episodes of autonomic nervous overactivity which produced permanent changes in the kidney which, in turn, became the basis for sustained hypertension.

In considering whether a person's blood pressure is elevated, the age, sex, and activity of the individual at the time of measurement must be considered. There is no number which serves as a dividing line between what is normal and what is abnormal. Controlled trials have shown that in men and women patients with diastolic pressures above 110 and in male patients with diastolic pressure between 90 and 114, treatment reduces morbidity and mortality (16,17,23). The mean ages in the latter study were 52.0 and 50.5 years in the control and treatment groups, respectively. Studies in an elderly population with asymptomatic hypertension have not been performed.

Neck veins are one of the more reliable signs to search for in the diagnosis of right heart failure. The liver edge may be palpable because of a low diaphragm or abnormalities in the thoracic cage. Peripheral edema is often due to poor venous drainage or reduction in skin tone and pressure rather than right heart failure. Rales may be present in many elderly patients because of chronic lung disease from previous infections or exposure to toxins. The examination of the heart is also associated with certain unusual features. Abnormalities of the thoracic cage may make palpation of the apex difficult. An S4 gallop is often heard in older individuals regardless of whether they do or do not have cardiac disease. Spodick and Quarry (55) examined 246 subjects aged 50 to 82 years in sinus rhythm and found that an S4 gallop was present in 73% of the 93 subjects without heart disease and in 74% of the 153 subjects with heart disease. They concluded that "an S4 gallop in older persons appears to be a normal phenomenon." This area was further examined in another study by Kino and associates (26). They found that 32 subjects with an S4 gallop as defined by phonocardiography could be divided into two groups by auscultation; those with an easily heard S4 gallop and those whose S4 gallops were often not heard. Those whose gallops were easily heard were significantly older (50 ± 4.0 years) than the other group, whose average age was 31.2 ± 2.8 years. The two groups did not differ in regard to the PR interval, P wave to onset of S4, P wave to peak of S4, relative S4 amplitude as compared to the amplitude of S1, or the duration of S1 vibrations. However, the S4 to S1 interval was significantly shorter in the older group and it was postulated that this resulted from an age-associated decrease in left ventricular compliance. The authors suggested that the short interval between S4 and the low-frequency vibratory components of S1 permitted both vibrations to behave as one sound of longer duration which would, therefore, be easier to hear.

Respiratory splitting of the second heart sound may be less marked in elderly subjects. Resistance of the pulmonary vascular bed, which in part determines the time of P2 (47), probably increases with advancing age (12). This would tend to narrow the A2–P2 interval, making splitting less prominent. Slodki (54) reported that of 17 patients without heart disease, relative variation in the Q–A2 and Q–P2 intervals gave rise to reverse-type splitting in 25% of the group, a single S2 in 38% of the group, and normal splitting in 37%. Neither diastolic hypertension nor ischemia were known to be present in the group with reverse splitting. The authors postulated that these findings were secondary to systolic hypertension, myocardial fibrosis, or the normal aging process. It has been estimated that a systole ejection murmur at the base is present in 60% or more of patients 70 years of age or older (7). This may originate in the aortic area and be secondary to calcification of the aortic valve ring, sclerosis of the aortic cusps, or changes in the aorta itself, or may originate from the mitral area secondary to calcification of the ventricular leaflet, papillary muscle dysfunction, or age changes in the chordae tendineae.

ELECTROCARDIOGRAM

The electrocardiogram shows some small but significant age-associated changes in healthy adults. These changes are more pronounced in men than in women (33,50). As previously mentioned, heart rate does not vary with age. An increase in the PR interval of about 10 msec (49) in one study and 8 msec in another (40), and an increase in the QT interval corrected for heart rate of 10 msec (51) have been reported from the third to the sixth and seventh decades. The amplitude of the QRS complexes decreases as well (50). The QRS axis shifts toward the left, in one study from a mean of 62.0° in men at ages 20 to 29 to 36.2° at ages 50 to 59 (49). The spatial vectorcardiogram shows a decrease in the QRS vector, especially in the initial 20-msec vector, distortion of the QRS sE loop, a more superior orientation of the QRS vector in the frontal plane, and a leftward orientation of the same vector in the horizontal plane (6,52). These changes may be due to latent coronary artery disease, age-associated fibrosis of the conducting system or of the myocardium itself, or age-associated alterations in the orientation of the heart because of changes in the AP diameter of the chest, the position of the diaphragm, or a change in the resistance of the tissues surrounding the heart.

In an interesting study it was found that changes in body position resulted in a much greater change in the electrocardiogram in older as compared with younger patients (37). The authors suggested that there may be greater freedom of movement of the heart in the thorax of elderly individuals because of decreased elasticity and atrophy of lung tissue. Okajima et al. (36) compared the frequency of premature beats in two groups of 715 subjects who were free of cardiovascular disease as judged by blood pressure, X-ray, electrocardiogram, and physical examination. The frequency of ventricular premature beats observed in the group aged 50 to 59 years, 1.32%, was significantly greater than the 0.75% frequency observed in the group aged 40 to 49 years. Because of these age-associated changes in the electrocardiogram, Simonson (50) has suggested that the normal upper limit of the PR interval be 220 msec, that the normal limit of the QRS axis be $-30°$ in the group aged 50 years or older, that the upper normal limit be 5% for premature supraventricular bears and 10% for premature ventricular beats in the group aged greater than 60 years, and that poor progression of the R wave in the anterior chest leads be considered a normal age trend in this population.

PHONOCARDIOGRAM AND APEXCARDIOGRAM

Most noninvasive studies of cardiac function have tended to confirm the clinical impression of Dock that the aged heart relaxes slowly (10). In 1966, Dock particularly stressed the increased susceptibility of the aged heart to fail in the face of tachycardiac stress. He stated (10) that it was his "clinical impression that [one of] . . . the greatest changes caused by the aging of the myocardium is delay in the recovery of contractility." In a comparison between stress-induced bradycardia and tachycardia, he stated (10) that, ". . . In people over 60, heart failure is rare with complete heart block or in fevers with bradycardia, such as typhoid. The rates of 120–150, due to paroxysmal tachycardia or to fever, frequently precipitate failure in older people. It would therefore appear that the old myocardium has a slow rate of recovery, but contracts well as long as there is an adequate period for rest between beats."

In addition to prolonged relaxation, which appears to be confined primarily to isovolumic diastole, some studies have shown prolongation of mechanical systole. Strandell (60) found that the average value for the interval between the first and second heart sounds in a group of men 61 to 83 years of age, 345 msec, was 11 msec longer than that of the group 21 to 25 years of age. However, this difference was not statistically significant. Willems and associates (68) measured left ventricular ejection time from carotid artery pulse tracings in 512 elderly subjects, some of whom had cardiovascular disease, and compared the results with previous studies on young and middle-aged adults. The authors reported an age-associated increase in left ventricular ejection time which by multiple regression analysis could not be attributed to heart rate or blood pressure. Harrison et al. (24) examined the effect of age on the duration of contraction, ejection, and relaxation as determined by the electrocardiogram, carotid pulse tracing, and apexcardiogram. He reported a slight decrease in the interval between the Q wave and the start of the carotid upstroke which he attributed to an increased pulse wave velocity with increasing age. There was also a trend toward a slight increase in isovolumic contraction time. Ejection time increased slightly but this was attributed to a slower heart rate in the older subjects. The most striking change was an increase in isovolumic relaxation time measured as the interval between the carotid incisural notch and the onset of filling as judged on the apexcardiogram. It was determined that left ventricular isovolumic relaxation increased by an average of about 40% between the third and ninth decades. The authors (24) compared the older normal heart to a used tennis ball which "having been compressed many times, has a diminished capacity to rebound."

Other studies (18,24,48,53), however, have shown no change in ejection time with age, but have described an increase in the pre-ejection period and in the Q–S1 and the Q–S2 intervals. Friedman and Davison (18) reported an age-associated increase in the Q–S1 interval from an average of 55 msec in a group with a mean age of 34 years to 75 msec in a group of 17 patients without evidence of heart disease and whose mean age was 76 years. Slodki et al. (54) studied the intervals between the onset of the QRS and the aortic and pulmonic components of the second heart sound. A tendency to a prolongation of both intervals was found. Shaw et al. (48) reported that plots of systolic time intervals versus age by decade revealed an increase in the pre-ejection period and in the Q–S2 interval as well as an increase in those indices corrected for heart rate up to age 60 and a decline thereafter. There was an increase of approximately 25 msec in the Q–S2 interval and 13 msec in the pre-ejection period from the third to the sixth decade in individuals free of cardiac disease. The pre-ejection period divided by the left ventricular ejection time fraction also increased significantly with age. Montoye et al. (34) examined subjects without heart disease and also found an increase in the pre-ejection period in these healthy subjects of approximately 4 msec a decade from the third to the seventh decade. In Shaw's study, the pre-ejection period and the Q–S2 interval declined after age 60, and in the Montoye study these values declined after age 70. The authors suggested that these declines were the result of selective mortality.

BALLISTOCARDIOGRAM

The ballistocardiogram has also been used to examine age-associated changes in cardiac function (35,57). Moss (35), using a modification of the ultralow-frequency model originally described by Reeves et al. (43), performed a cross-sectional study on 307 healthy men aged 18 to 54 years. He described a decrease in the HI and HJ forces with increasing age. This was attributed to latent coronary artery disease, a change in the resistance of the supporting structures of the body, or a change in the direction of the cardiac force vector. Since only longitudinal forces are recorded, it was postulated that the ballistic systolic forces are directed more longitudinally in younger persons and more laterally in older age groups. Starr and Hildreth (57) repeated ballistocardiogram examinations in 1951 and 1952 on 65 healthy adults who were initially studied in 1937 to 1939. The amplitudes of the H, I, J, and K waves, adjusted for body surface area, were recorded. A cross-sectional analysis disclosed that although the mean amplitude of the H and K waves did not change with age, there was a continued decrease in the mean amplitude of the I and J waves. The mean depth of the I wave was 5.0 ± 1.1 mm (SD) in the 20- to 29-year age range and 2.2 ± 1.2 mm in the group aged 60 or over. There was no significant effect of aging on the duration of any of the waves. A longitudinal analysis performed by comparing the change in wave amplitude in the same volunteers over the 10- to 14-year period disclosed that there was not a progressive diminution over the entire age range, but rather that the diminution occurred primarily in the advanced age range. The authors had previously performed experiments in which cardiac action was simulated in cadavers and it was found that the amplitudes of the I and J waves reflect the early acceleration of blood leaving the heart. Therefore, it was concluded (57) that "as the heart grows older it lifts its load more slowly."

Although the above studies indicate increased contraction and relaxation time in aged individuals at rest, it is unclear whether these findings reflect intrinsic differences in myocardial function or changes in work load, impedance, or properties of other tissues. Changes in the degree of fibrosis or relative stiffness of the mitral and aortic valves with age could alter the timing of valve motion and, therefore, the phonocardiographic assessment of mechanical systole. The recording of the carotid pulse is dependent on a pressure-induced lateral displacement of the arterial wall. Since the arterial wall stiffens with age (30), the rate of transmission of the pulse to the carotid would be expected to be more rapid in the older individual with stiffer central arteries. Since the apex-cardiogram records low-frequency chest wall movements, it would be influenced by the characteristics of the cartilage, bone, muscle, and skin layers between the sensor and the moving ventricle. The ballistocardiogram would be altered by any age changes in the compliance of the vessel walls and body tissues. Therefore, although these noninvasive techniques provide useful information in an individual patient of any age group with cardiac pathology, they are not likely to provide an adequate assessment of age changes in cardiac structure, function, and contractility in large groups of participants.

ECHOCARDIOGRAM

The echocardiogram is a tool particularly suited for studying the effect of age on the heart and evaluating cardiovascular function in elderly patients with possible cardiac disease. This is because it is noninvasive and it enables the investigator to obtain direct and accurate information on certain indices of cardiac function. It also provides structural information which is unobtainable by any other technique in living individuals. For these reasons, echocardiograms were performed on 105 male participants in the National Institute on Aging Longitudinal Study Program (20). The individuals studied were all physically active and had complete examinations at approximately 18-month intervals. All subjects studied showed no evidence of chest wall abnormalities or coronary artery, valvular, or hypertensive disease. Hypertension was defined as blood pressure greater than 140/90 mm Hg on repeated baseline determinations over a 48-hour period. None was taking medication known to influence cardiac function. In addition, all subjects had negative submaximal treadmill stress tests to a heart rate of 90% of the mean age-specific heart rate. Measurements were obtained of the initial portion of the E–F slope of the anterior mitral valve leaflet, the aortic root and left ventricular cavity dimensions, and the thickness of the posterior left ventricular wall. Diastolic cavity and wall thickness measurements were made at the time of the Q wave inscription. The systolic cavity was measured at the time of the most anterior motion of the posterior endocardial echo. Fractional shortening of the minor semiaxis was calculated as (diastolic dimension minus systolic dimension) divided by diastolic dimension. Velocity of circumferential fiber (VCF) shortening was calculated as mean VCF equal to (diastolic dimension minus systolic dimension) divided by (diastolic dimension times ejection time). Measurements were made to the nearest millimeter. The coefficient of beat-to-beat variation in each parameter was as follows: mitral valve slope, 6%; aortic root dimension, 4%; left ventricular diastolic wall thickness, 6%; left ventricular systolic wall thickness, 2%; left ventricular diastolic dimension, 2%; and left ventricular systolic dimension, 2%. The relationship between the obtained echocardiographic parameters and age was analyzed using linear regression analysis. The regression equation, standard error of estimate, coefficient correlation, and significance of the correlation coefficient were determined. These parameters and those derived from them were also expressed per square meter of body surface area, since cardiac dimension measurements may be related to body size. The participants were also divided into three 20-year age brackets: group 1, age 25 to 44 years; group 2, 45 to 64 years; and group 3, age 65 to 84 years.

Satisfactory mitral valve recordings were obtained in 105 subjects. The E–F slope was found to decrease with increasing age. The mean slope of group 1 was 102.3 mm/sec; for group 2, 79.0 mm/sec ($p < 0.001$); and for group 3, 67.1 mm/sec ($p < 0.001$ versus group 1). The aortic root diastolic dimension was obtained from 89 participants and increased slightly with increasing age. The mean dimension for group 1 was 30.9 mm; for group 2, 32.0 mm; and for group 3, 32.9 mm ($p < 0.05$ versus group 1). Left ventricular systolic and diastolic wall thickness per square meter body surface area also increased with advancing age. The average diastolic wall thickness was 4.3 mm/m² for group 1, 5.0 mm/m² for group 2 ($p < 0.01$), and 5.7 mm/m² for group 3 ($p < 0.001$ versus group 1). Systolic wall thickness was 7.6 mm/m² in group 1, 9.2 mm/m² in group 2 ($p < 0.001$), and 10 mm/m² in group 3 ($p < 0.001$ versus group 1). Although systolic blood pressure increased with age, averaging 118 ± 2 mm Hg for group 1 and 132 ± 3 mm Hg for group 3, there was no correlation between systolic blood pressure and wall thickness per square meter by multivariant analysis. Heart rate, left ventricular systolic and diastolic cavity dimensions, left ventricular ejection time, calculated velocity of circumferential fiber shortening, and fractional shortening of the minor semiaxis did not vary with age.

Similar findings have been reported by other investigators who have examined some of these parameters (9,19,31,53,66,69). Derman (9) performed mitral echograms on 80 volunteers who had a normal ECG, blood sugar, and cholesterol level and a blood pressure less than 150/90. He described a decrease in the angle formed at the E point with advanced age. Luisada and associates (31) recorded the echocardiogram of the mitral valve while the

ECG, phonocardiogram, and carotid and jugular pulse tracings were simultaneously obtained in 42 young and middle-aged adults and 15 aged persons without evidence of heart disease. He reported an increase in the interval between the aortic component of the second sound and the peak of the E wave from 122 ± 21.4 msec in the group aged 18 to 59 years to 142 ± 18.5 msec in the group aged 62 to 84 years. In the same study the E–F diastolic closure interval increased from 103 ± 15.8 msec in the young adults to 124 ± 29.9 msec in the aged adults.

Sjögren (53) measured left ventricular wall thickness in systole and diastole in 100 subjects with no heart disease as judged by clinical findings, ECG, or chest X-ray. He reported that left ventricular systolic thickness increased from a mean of 12.3 ± 1.61 mm in men aged 17 to 29 to 15.08 ± 1.05 mm in men aged 50 to 69 years. Left ventricular diastolic thickness increased from 6.92 ± 1.08 mm to 9.08 ± 1.38 in the same two groups. Valdez et al. (66) reported that mitral valve diastolic excursion and early diastolic slope decreased with increasing age.

Gardin et al. (19) compared echocardiographic findings in 105 individuals ranging in age from 40 to 93 years with the findings in 27 individuals aged 18 to 23 years. Increases in mean left atrial dimension, aortic root dimension, and left ventricular wall thickness and a significant decrease in the mean mitral E–F slope were noted in the older subjects. No significant differences were found in left ventricular internal dimension or ejection fraction. Yin and associates (69) also found no age difference in left ventricular diastolic or systolic dimension or velocity of circumferential fiber shortening between 17 young men with a mean age of 29 years and 11 aged men of mean age 68 years.

The decrease in E–F slope probably reflects a limitation in mitral valve motion in early diastole, imposed by age-associated changes in either the mitral valve or the left ventricle. Age-associated sclerosis and thickening of the valve leaflets (32,41,46) have been described in pathological studies and, hence, an age-associated change in the leaflets themselves may account for the decrease in the E–F slope.

Alternatively, an age-associated decline in the ability of the left ventricule to accommodate large amounts of blood in early diastole could also result in the same findings. Such a change could be secondary to delayed left ventricular relaxation or increased left ventricular stiffness in early diastole. Delayed ventricular relaxation is also suggested by noninvasive studies discussed above which indicate prolonged diastolic time periods in aged myocardium. Animal studies also have indicated prolonged relaxation time (1,27,67) as well as increased myocardial (56) and chamber stiffness (61) with increasing age. The increased diastolic aortic root dimension reported in the two studies discussed above correlates well with pathological studies which have also reported an increase with age in aortic diameter and volume (3). This would tend to compensate for the increased aortic stiffness associated with aging (22,30,45), since a larger aorta undergoes a smaller radius change for a given volume injected into it.

Although aortic diameter may increase with aging, other age-associated changes in the amount or composition of collagen (29), the ability of the aorta to relax in response to catecholamines (13,14,62), and age-associated changes in the size, stiffness, and arterial tone of the peripheral vascular bed probably result in an increased impedance to ejection both during rest and exercise with increasing age. This increased impedance over a period of time would be expected to result in the age-associated increase in wall thickness with unchanged cavity dimension observed in the above studies. Left ventricular hypertrophy which would decrease stress may therefore represent an adaptation to a chronic state of increased impedance to left ventricular ejection. The lack of an age-associated change in fractional shortening of the minor semiaxis and in the velocity of circumferential fiber shortening indicate the lack of a decline in cardiac performance with age in the resting state.

MEASUREMENTS OF CARDIAC OUTPUT

Studies utilizing resting cardiac output and stroke volume to indicate ventricular performance have shown conflicting results.

Invasive studies have shown that resting cardiac output and stroke volume determined by Fick or dye dilution techniques decline with age (4,8,25,58). In a group of 67 male subjects between the ages of 19 and 86 years, cardiac output was estimated to fall an average of 1% a year from a mean of 6.49 liters/min in the third decade to 3.87 liters/min in the ninth (4). The authors attributed the decline in part to a smaller body surface area and in part to a lower heart rate. Stroke volume index nevertheless declined by 0.49% a year, a change which was attributed solely to aging. Another study compared a mean cardiac output of 7.89 liters/min in 10 young adult healthy males (average age 23 years) with 5.85 liters/min in 17 healthy male subjects 60 to 83 years of age. Heart rate did not vary between the two groups. It is clear, however, that the lower cardiac output at rest in the aged population is not imposed by a limitation in the functional capacity of the heart. Cardiac output in aged individuals can increase considerably above the resting level with stress owing to increases in both stroke volume and heart rate (8,25,58). In addition, the mean pulmonary artery pressure was less in the older group; therefore, a difference in preload resulting from differences in peripheral factors, rather than an intrinsic alteration in cardiac performance, may account for this age difference. Furthermore, there was no age difference in resting cardiac output or stroke volume in this same study when the subjects were in the sitting position, indicating that changes imposed by the pericardium rather than intrinsic cardiac muscle changes may account for part of the age difference as well. However, it is unclear whether all of the older individuals studied were free of cardiovascular or hypertensive disease and were physically active. It is probably also true that the performance of an echocardiographic examination in a darkened room would represent less of a stress than measurement of cardiac output with pulmonary or brachial artery catheters in place. This is an important consideration since it is generally agreed that the perception of stress and/or the capacity of the cardiovascular system to react to a catecholamine-mediated response to stress is diminished with advancing age. Cardiac output determinations have also been made by precordial counters following intravenous injection of labeled material (28,42). In a study of normal male volunteers a decline in cardiac output from 3.97 liters/min/m² in 37 subjects aged 21 to 30 years to 2.92 liters/min/m² in 4 subjects aged 41 to 50 years was found (28). However, in a much larger sample of subjects, Proper and Wall (42) reported no significant correlation between age and cardiac output, cardiac index, stroke volume, or stroke index by precordial counting in a group of 500 healthy men aged 20 to 70 years.

Until the advent of the echocardiogram, precise details concerning the effect of age on cardiac structure and function were impossible to obtain because of the invasiveness such studies would require. The echocardiogram provides a noninvasive, reproducible and sensitive technique for the measurement of left ventricular structure and function during rest and also during exercise. However, the determination of dimensional changes by one-dimensional echocardiography is dependent on a distance measurement between the interventricular septum and one area of the left ventricular posterior wall. Movement along this line may not be as representative of the entire left ventricle in some age groups as it is in others. Lateral resolution problems caused by an inability to focus ultrasonic waves over the entire depth range of the beam may also cause distortion (44). Some of these problems are overcome by utilization of two-dimensional echocardiography, which makes it possible to obtain quantitative data concerning age-associated changes in left ventricular mass and chamber size, age changes in global and regional function, mean and maximum velocity of fiber shortening, rates of left ventricular wall thickening and thinning, and direct measurement of time intervals in the cardiac cycle.

Latent or manifest coronary artery disease has been invoked as a possible mechanism to explain nearly all of the age-associated cardiac changes which have been reported. However, the incidence, severity, and rate of progression of coronary artery disease in a normal, asymptomatic population is unknown because until recently noninvasive techniques for the measurement of myocardial blood flow have been unavailable. Although stress electrocardiography has been used, it has a low predictive value when applied to an asymptomatic population (15). This limitation is particularly marked in women because of the high incidence of false-positive tests in this group. Myocardial imaging after the intravenous injection of the radioactive tracer thallium 201 is a noninvasive method of measuring myocardial perfusion since thallium 201 is taken up by the myocardium in proportion to blood flow. Longitudinal studies utilizing two-dimensional echocardiogram and myocardial scanning techniques will enable one to define precisely and accurately which age-associated changes in left ventricular structure and function are accompanied by abnormalities in left ventricular perfusion and which are related to a more "normal" intrinsic aging process of the heart muscle itself.

SUMMARY

Several conclusions can be drawn from noninvasive aging studies in man. Measurements of systolic time intervals have indicated prolonged isovolumic, diastolic, and systolic time periods and possibly delayed relaxation. There are some minor changes in the electrocardiogram. Measurements of cardiac output which indicate a decline at rest do not appear to reflect a limitation in cardiac contractile function. Technically satisfactory, reproducible measurements of echocardiographic parameters of left ventricular structure and function can be obtained in a normal aging population. Decreased early diastolic mitral valve slope and increased left ventricular systolic and diastolic posterior wall thickness with unchanged systolic and diastolic cavity dimension appear to be associated with normal aging in man.

REFERENCES

1. Alpert, N. R., Gale, H. H., and Taylor, N. (1967): The effect of age on contractile protein ATPase activity and the velocity of shortening. In:

Factors Influencing Myocardial Contractility, edited by R. D. Tanz, R. Kavaler, and J. Roberts, pp. 127–133. Academic Press, New York.

2. Andres, R. (1969): Physiological factors of aging significant to the clinician. *J. Am. Geriatr. Soc.,* 17:274–277.

3. Bader, H. (1967): Dependent of wall stress in the human thoracic aorta on age and pressure. *Circ. Res.,* 20:354–361.

4. Brandfonbrener, M., Landowne, M., and Shock, N. W. (1955): Changes in cardiac output with age. *Circulation,* 12:557–566.

5. Brown, J. J., Laser, A. F., and Robertson, J. I. S. (1976): Pathogenesis of essential hypertension. *Lancet,* 1:1217–1219.

6. Burch, G. E., and DePasquale, N. P. (1969): Geriatric cardiology, *Am. Heart J.,* 78:700–708.

7. Burch, G. E., Golder, L. H., and Cronvich, J. A. (1958): An analysis of changes in the spatial vectorcardiogram with aging. *Am. Heart J.,* 55:582–590.

8. Conway, J., Wheeler, R., and Sannerstedt, R. (1971): Sympathetic nervous activity during exercise in relation to age. *Cardiovasc. Res.,* 5:577–581.

9. Derman, U. (1972): Changes of the mitral echocardiogram with aging and the influence of atherosclerotic risk factors. *Atherosclerosis,* 15:349–357.

10. Dock, W. (1966): How some hearts age. *JAMA,* 195:148–150.

11. Dock, W. (1972): Cardiomyopathies of the senescent and senile. *Cardiovasc. Clin.,* 4:362–373.

12. Emirgil, C., Sobol, B. J., Campodonico, S., Herbert, W. H., and Mechkati, R. Pulmonary circulation in the aged. *J. Appl. Physiol.,* 23:631–640.

13. Fleisch, J. H. (1971): Further studies on the effect of aging on beta-adrenoceptor activity of rat aorta. *Br. J. Pharmacol.,* 42:311–313.

14. Fleisch, J. H., Maling, H. M., and Brodie, B. B. (1970): Beta-receptor activity in aorta. Variations with age and species. *Circ. Res.,* 26:151–162.

15. Fortuin, N. J., and Weiss, J. L. (1977): Exercise stress testing. *Circulation,* 56:699–712.

16. Freis, E. D. (1967): Effects of treatment on morbidity in hypertension: Results in patients with diastolic blood pressure averaging 11.5 through 129 mm Hg. Veterans Administration Cooperative Study Groups on Antihypertensive Agents. *JAMA,* 202:1028–1034.

17. Freis, E. D. (1970): Effects of treatment on morbidity in hypertension. II. Results in patients with diastolic blood pressure averaging 90 through 114 mm Hg. Veterans Administration Cooperative Study Group on Antihypertensive Agents. *JAMA,* 213:1143–1152.

18. Friedman, S. A., and Davison, E. T. (1969): The phonocardiographic assessment of myocardial function in the aged. *Am. Heart J.,* 78:752–756.

19. Gardin, J. M., Henry, W. L., Savage, D. D., and Epstein, S. E. (1977): Echocardiographic evaluation of an older population without clinically apparent heart disease. *Am. J. Cardiol.,* 39:277.

20. Gerstenblith, G., Frederiksen, J., Yin, F. C. P., Fortuin, N. J., Lakatta,

E. G., and Weisfeldt, M. L. (1977): Echocardiographic assessment of a normal adult aging population. *Circulation,* 56:273–278.

21. Gerstenblith, G., Lakatta, E. G., and Weisfeldt, M. L. (1976): Age changes in myocardial function and exercise response. *Prog. Cardiovasc. Dis.,* 19:1–21.

22. Gozna, E. R., Marble, A. E., Shaw, A., and Holland, J. G. (1974): Age-related changes in the mechanics of the aorta and pulmonary artery of man. *J. Appl. Physiol.,* 36:407–411.

23. Hamilton, M., Thompson, E. N., and Wisniewski, T. K. M. (1964): The role of blood pressure control in preventing complications of hypertension. *Lancet,* 1:235–238.

24. Harrison, T. R., Dixon, K., Russell, R. O., Bidwai, P. S., and Coleman, H. N. (1964): The relation of age to the duration of contraction, ejection, relaxation of the normal heart. *Am. Heart J.,* 67:189–199.

25. Julius, S., Amery, A., Whitlock, L. S., and Conway, J. (1967): Influence of age on the hemodynamic response to exercise. *Circulation,* 36:222–230.

26. Kino, M., Shahamatpour, A., and Spodick, D. (1976): Auscultatory perception of the fourth heart sound. *Am. J. Cardiol.,* 37:848–852.

27. Lakatta, E. G., Gerstenblith, G., Angell, C. S., Shoel, N. W., and Weisfeldt, M. L. (1975): Prolonged contraction duration in aged myocardium. *J. Clin. Invest.,* 55:61–68.

28. Lammerant, J., Veall, N., and DeVisscher, M. (1961): Observations of cardiac output and "pulmonary blood volume" in normal man by external recording of the intracardiac flow of ^{131}I labelled albumin. *Nucl. Med.,* 1:353–379.

29. Lansin, A. I. (1959): *The Arterial Wall: Aging, Structure, and Chemistry.* pp. 136–160. Williams & Wilkins, Baltimore.

30. Learoyd, B. M., and Taylor, M. G. (1966): Alterations with age in the viscoelastic properties of human arterial walls. *Cir. Res.,* 18:278–292.

31. Luisada, A. A., Watanabe, K., Bhat, P. K., and Rao, D. B. (1975): Correlates of the echocardiographic waves of the mitral valve in normal subjects of various ages. *J. Am. Geriatr. Soc.,* 23:216–223.

32. McMillian, J. B., and Lev, M. (1964): The aging heart. II. The valves. *J. Gerontol.,* 19:1–14.

33. Mihalick, M., and Fisch, C. (1974): Electrocardiographic findings in the aged. *Am. Heart J.,* 87:117–128.

34. Montoye, J. H., Willis, P. W., Howard, G. E., and Keller, J. B. (1971): Cardiac preejection period: Age and sex comparisons. *J. Gerontol.,* 26:208–216.

35. Moss, A. J. (1961): Ballistocardiographic evaluation of the cardiovascular aging process. *Circulation,* 23:434–451.

36. Okajima, M., Scholmerich, P., and Simonson, E. (1960): Frequency of premature beats. *Minn. Med.,* 43:751–753.

37. Olbrich, O., and Woodford-Williams, E. (1953): The effect of change of body position on the precordial electrocardiogram in young and aged subjects. *J. Gerontol.,* 8:56–62.

38. Pickering, G. (1976): Blood pressure, *Lancet,* 1:1403–1404.
39. Pickering, G. (1974): *Hypertension: Causes, Consequences, and Management,* 2nd ed. Churchill Livingstone, Edinburgh.
40. Pipberger, H. V., Goldman, M. J., Littmann, D., Murphy, G. P., Cosma, J., and Synder, J. R. (1967): Correlations of the orthogonal electrocardiogram and vectorcardiogram with constitutional variables in 518 normal men. *Circulation,* 35:536–551.
41. Pomerance, A. (1973): The many facets of cardiac pathology. *Geriatrics,* 28:110–115.
42. Proper, R., and Wall, F. (1972): Left ventricular stroke volume measurements not affected by chronologic aging. *Am. Heart J.,* 83:843–845.
43. Reeves, T. J., Hefner, L. L., Jones, W. B., and Sparks, J. E. (1957): Wide frequency range force ballistocardiogram: Its correlation with cardiovascular dynamics. *Circulation,* 16:43–53.
44. Roelandt, J., Van Dorp, W. G., Bom, N., Laird, J. D., and Hugenholtz, P. G. (1976): Resolution problems in echocardiography: A source of interpretation errors. *Am. J. Cardiol.,* 37:256–262.
45. Roy, C. S. (1880–1882): The elastic properties of the arterial wall. *J. Physiol. (Lond.),* 3:125.
46. Sell, S., and Scully, R. E. (1965): Aging changes in the aortic and mitral valves. *Am. J. Pathol.,* 46:345–355.
47. Shaver, J. A., Nadolny, R. A., O'Toole, J. D., Thompson, M. E., Reddy, P. S., Leon, D. F., and Curtiss, E. I. (1974): Sound pressure correlates of the second heart sound. *Circulation,* 49:316–325.
48. Shaw, D. J., Rothbaum, D. A., Angell, C. S., and Shock, N. W. (1973): The effect of age and blood pressure upon the systolic time intervals in males aged 20–89 years. *J. Gerontol.,* 28:133–139.
49. Simonson, E. (1958): The normal variability of the electrocardiogram as a basis for differentiation between "normal" and "abnormal" in clinical electrocardiography. *Am. Heart J.,* 55:80–103.
50. Simonson, E. (1972): The effect of age on the electrocardiogram. *Am. J. Cardiol.,* 29:64–73.
51. Simonson, E., Cady, L. D., and Woodbury, M. (1962): The normal Q-T interval. *Am. Heart J.,* 63:747–753.
52. Simonson, E., and Keys, A. (1956): The effect of age on mean spatial QRS and T vectors. *Circulation,* 14:100–104.
53. Sjögren, A. L. (1971): Left ventricular wall thickness determined by ultrasound in 100 subjects without heart disease. *Chest,* 60:341–346.
54. Slodki, S. J., Hussain, A. T., and Luisada, A. A. (1969): The Q–H interval. III. A study of the second heart sound in old age. *J. Am. Geriatr. Soc.,* 17:673–679.
55. Spodick, D. H., and Quarry, V. M. (1974): Prevalence of the fourth heart sound by phonocardiography in the absence of heart disease. *Am. Heart J.,* 87:11–14.
56. Spurgeon, H. A., Thorne, P. R., Yin, F. C. P., Shock, N. W., and Weisfeldt, M. L. (1977): Increased dynamic stiffness of trabecula carneae from senescent rats. *Am. J. Physiol.,* 232:H373–H380.

57. Starr, I., and Hildreth, E. A. (1952): The effect of aging and of the development of disease on the ballistocardiogram. *Circulation,* 5:481–495.
58. Strandell, T. (1964): Circulatory studies on healthy old men. *Acta Med. Scand. [Suppl.],* 175(414):1–44.
59. Strandell, T. (1964): Heart rate, arterial lactate concentration and oxygen uptake during exercise in old men compared with young men. *Acta Physiol. Scand.,* 60:197–216.
60. Strandell, T. (1964): Mechanical systole at rest, during and after exercise in supine and sitting position in young and old men. *Acta Physiol. Scand.,* 61:279–298.
61. Templeton, G. H., Willerson, J. T., and Weisfeldt, M. L. (1975): Influence of aging on left ventricular stiffness. *Clin. Res.,* 23:210A.
62. Tuttle, R. S. (1966): Age-related changes in the sensitivity of rat aortic strips to norepinephrine and associated chemical and structural abnormalities. *J. Gerontol.,* 21:510–516.
63. U. S. Bureaus of the Census (1973): Some demographic aspects of aging in the United States. Current Population Reports, Ser. P-23, No. 43. U. S. Government Printing Office, Washington, D. C.
64. U. S. Congress Senate Special Committee on Aging (1974): Developments in aging 1973 and January–March 1974. Report No. 93–846, pp. 1–400. U. S. Government Printing Office, Washington, D. C.
65. U. S. Department of Health, Education and Welfare. National Center for Health Statistics (1971): Health in the later years in life. DHEW Publication No. (HSM) 72–1207, pp. 1–60. U. S. Government Printing Office, Washington, D. C.
66. Valdez, R., Motta, J., Martin, R., London, E., Haskell, W., Popp, R., and Horlick, L. (1977): Survey of a normal population with the echocardiogram. *Am. J. Cardiol.,* 39:277.
67. Weisfeldt, M. L., Loeven, W. A., and Shock, N. W. (1971): Resting and active mechanical properties of trabeculae carneae from aged male rats. *Am. J. Physiol.,* 220:1921–1927.
68. Willems, J. L., Roelandt, J., De Geest, H., Kesteloot, H., and Joossens, J. V. (1970): The left ventricular ejection time in elderly subjects. *Circulation,* 42:37–42.
69. Yin, F. C. P., Guarnieri, T., Sprugeon, H. A., Lakatta, E. G., Fortuin, N. J., and Weisfeldt, M. L. (1978): Age-associated decrease in ventricular response to hemodynamic stress during beta-adrenergic blockade. *Br. Heart J.,* 40:349–355.

The Aging Heart (Aging, Vol. 12),
edited by Myron L. Weisfeldt.
Raven Press, New York © 1980.

Chapter 10

The Effect of Aging on the Cardiovascular Response to Dynamic and Static Exercise

*Peter B. Raven and **Jere Mitchell

*Department of Physiology, Texas College of Osteopathic Medicine, North Texas State University Health Science Center, Fort Worth, Texas 76107; and **Departments of Medicine and Physiology, University of Texas Southwestern Medical School at Dallas, Dallas, Texas 75235

It is generally accepted that aging, accompanied by a more sedentary lifestyle, produces a linear decline in the functional capacities of the human organism. This is exemplified physiologically by a reduction in the cardiovascular and pulmonary reserves and a decrease in strength and endurance of the skeletal muscular system (7). Some of these changes are seen in Fig. 1A. Heart weight and volume, body weight, and blood volume tend to increase with advancing age, whereas cardiovascular performance and muscle strength tend to decrease with age (6). Despite the large body of literature dealing with physiological aspects of aging, minimal evidence is available to delineate those functional losses attributable to (a) true aging, (b) unrecognized diseases, and (c) the deconditioning associated with the increased sedentary lifestyle of the aged. The primary physiological symptoms of aged populations are noted increases in variability of response within systems and the delayed response of the elderly to physiological stressors (7).

Exercise can be described as a procedure in which the organism shifts from one level of homeostasis (rest) to another (activity).

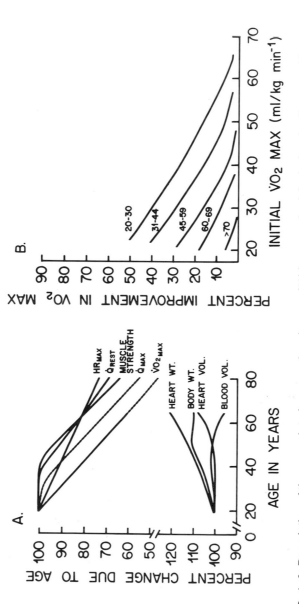

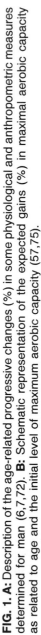

FIG. 1. A: Description of the age-related progressive changes (%) in some physiological and anthropometric measures determined for man (6,7,72). **B:** Schematic representation of the expected gains (%) in maximal aerobic capacity as related to age and the initial level of maximum aerobic capacity (57,75).

Broadly speaking, there are two primary forms of exercise, usually delineated as dynamic (isotonic) and static (isometric) exercise (52). Dynamic exercise may be described as occurring when the skeletal muscles undergo a contraction which principally results in a change in length of the muscle with little or no change in tension within the muscle (i.e., an isotonic contraction). On the other hand, static exercise occurs when the skeletal muscle contracts and principally results in a large change in tension within the muscle with little change in the length of the muscle (i.e., an isometric contraction). Generally, activities such as swimming, bicycling, rowing, and rhythmic calisthenics are described as predominantly dynamic exercise, while activities including lifting or pushing heavy weights, and contracting muscles against fixed objects are described as static exercise. As dynamic exercise is being used increasingly as a preventative modality against diseases of the aged, such as atherosclerotic disease and hypertension, it is important that the normal response of the elderly to exercise be understood. Furthermore, it has been suggested on the basis of minimal evidence that once certain functional losses have occurred within the aged organism, the capability to regain an optimal functional level is reduced as aging progresses (34,41,57,75). This concept is represented schematically in Fig. 1B and indicates that the percent improvement that can be expected from a chronic activity program is limited by the individuals' initial level of fitness (expressed as $\dot{V}O_{2\,max}$) and their chronological age. It is our intention to summarize the cardiovascular response to acute and chronic dynamic exercise of the aged. In addition, we shall briefly outline the acute responses to static exercise as a function of age, but will not discuss the chronic effects of this type of activity even though extensive use has been shown to produce left ventricular hypertrophy (37,53).

ACUTE RESPONSE TO DYNAMIC EXERCISE

The maximal capacity of the cardiovascular system to deliver oxygen to the working muscles is reflected by the level of maximal oxygen uptake ($\dot{V}O_{2\,max}$) expressed in absolute terms (liters O_2/min) and relative to body weight (ml O_2/kg $\times$ min^{-1}) or lean body mass (LBM) (ml O_2/kg $\times$ LBM min^{-1}) (49,50). Cardiovascularly, $\dot{V}O_{2\,max}$ is the product of the maximal cardiac output ($\dot{Q}_{max}$) and the maximal oxygen extraction of the body (or the arteriovenous oxygen difference at maximal levels)

$$\dot{V}O_{2\,max} = \dot{Q}_{max} \times A\text{-}\dot{V}O_{2\,diff\,max} \qquad [1]$$

As cardiac output ($\dot{Q}$) is directly related to heart rate (HR) and stroke volume (SV)

$$\dot{Q} = HR \times SV \qquad [2]$$

it follows that alterations due to age in either the attained HR$_{max}$ or SV$_{max}$ will change both $\dot{Q}_{max}$ and $\dot{V}O_{2max}$. A-$\dot{V}O_{2diff}$ is related to the maximal oxygen content of arterial blood and the capacity of the tissues to extract oxygen from the blood, reflected in the minimal oxygen content of mixed venous blood. Obviously, factors which inhibit hemoglobin saturation at the lung and desaturation at the tissue level will also affect the attained $\dot{V}O_{2\,max}$.

Cross-sectional analysis of available data (5,12,20,67,70) indicates that the rate of decline in aerobic capacity ($\dot{V}O_{2\,max}$) of males between the ages of 20 and 65 years approximates 0.45 ml O_2/kg $\times$ min^{-1} $\times$ year^{-1}, irrespective of the level of activity (20,22,65). In sedentary women the rate of decline appears to be slightly lower, or 0.3 ml O_2/kg $\times$ min^{-1} $\times$ yr^{-1} (33). However, both Hodgson and Buskirk (33), and Dehn and Bruce (22) emphasize the fact that longitudinal approaches are essential in determining the specific effects of age on the rate of decline of functional capacity. In subjects that were inactive over a span of only 2.5 years the rate of decline in $\dot{V}O_{2\,max}$ approaches 0.94 ml O_2/kg $\times$ min^{-1} $\times$ yr^{-1}, nearly double that obtained by the cross-sectional analysis (22). As this rate of decline agreed well with the reported data of Dill et al. (25) and others (33) (1.04 and 0.93 ml O_2/kg $\times$ min^{-1} $\times$ yr^{-1}, respectively), it is likely that cross-sectional samples include a multitude of factors (i.e., different levels of fitness, etc.) that alter the apparent rate of decline in functional capacity from that specifically related to true aging. However, the rate of decline in $\dot{V}O_{2\,max}$ owing to age is markedly less than that observed during 20 days of detraining by bed rest (0.25 l O_2/kg $\times$ min^{-1} $\times$ yr^{-1}) (68). Obviously, when active subjects become sedentary [as described by Dill et al. (25)], the apparent age-related decline in $\dot{V}O_{2\,max}$ is a composite of a rapid decline owing to detraining and the slow decline owing to aging, exemplified by the idealized curve in Fig. 2. The composite factors of this age-related decline in $\dot{V}O_{2\,max}$ have recently been verified by Kanstrup and Ekblom (39). In this investigation of 15 males and 5 females, the authors related the individuals' physical activity levels to age-related alterations in $\dot{V}O_{2\,max}$ and central hemodynamic variables. Further discussion of their findings is carried out below; however, one of their major conclusions is that much

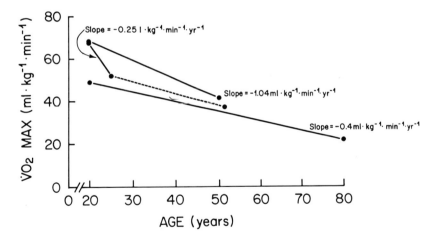

FIG. 2. Solid line regression representing −0.41 ml $\times$ kg $\times$ min^{-1} $\times$ year^{-1} is the average decline in maximal capacity obtained from cross-sectional data (32). The line representing 0.25 liters $\times$ kg^{-1} $\times$ min^{-1} $\times$ year^{-1} is that which would be observed strictly owing to bed rest of active subjects (68). The solid line 1.04 ml $\times$ kg^{-1} $\times$ year^{-1} (25), representing the active subjects becoming inactive and progressing in age, is probably a composite of the other two lines as shown by adjoining the dashed regression line of unknown slope.

of the age-related decline in work capacity is probably because of a process of detraining.

Along with the reduction in maximal aerobic capacity there is significant linear reduction in basal metabolic rate (BMR) from the age of 3 years (3,7,8,13,14,28,42,46,64,73). As BMR is proportionally linked with the surface area (A) to mass (M) ratio of the body, the reduction occurring during the formative years (up to age 20 to 24) can readily be explained by the decreasing A/M ratio brought about by the greater relative increase in mass. However, after the age of 35 the body composition of the sedentary individual alters such that active metabolic tissue, estimated as LBM is reduced, while an increase in body fat occurs (10, 59,60). Hence, even though the A/M ratio may continue to decrease along with the BMR, the primary reason for decreased BMR with age after 35 years is the progressive decrease in active metabolic tissue. Data obtained by Shock and Yiengst (73) suggest that BMR from 30 to 90 years falls some 20%, while Bafitis and Sargent (7) surmise that from the peak measurement available at 3 years of age the decrement in BMR at 85 years is some 48%. Hence, the decreasing A/M ratio occurring due to growth from 3 to 30 years accounts for only 28% of the decrement in BMR, while the remainder is related to loss of active metabolic tissue. Interestingly, the reduced LBM that occurs with age has no effect on the absolute level of oxygen uptake ($\dot{V}O_2$) occurring for a given submaximal workload (Watts) below the maximal level (6,24,32,81), although it does appear that at higher relative levels of work (percent $\dot{V}O_{2\,max}$) a difference in efficiency will be observed (5,6,81). Obviously, because of the age-related decrease in $\dot{V}O_{2\,max}$, the greater the relative level of work (percent $\dot{V}O_{2\,max}$) will be for a given workload with advancing age.

The effect of age on the cardiovascular response to acute dynamic exercise has primarily been investigated by means of cross-sectional evaluation of young and elderly groups of subjects (15,19,30,51,76) and are relatively few in number. Primarily, the work of Granath (30) and Strandell (76,78) form the major basis of our knowledge concerning the untrained healthy elderly individual's circulatory response to exercise. In retrospect, the paucity of information is primarily owing to the researchers' reluctance to use invasive catheterization techniques in the healthy elderly. Perhaps with the present day development and validation of non-invasive cardiovascular techniques more information concerning the response of the elderly to exercise will be forthcoming.

In general, the elderly have lower resting cardiac outputs ($\dot{Q}$) and oxygen uptakes ($\dot{V}O_2$) than younger subjects (15,19,30,54, 76,78) in the supine position. Table 1 summarizes the major central hemodynamic findings of Granath et al. (30) while subjects were at rest in two different positions. It was noted from the data obtained in the supine position that the lower $\dot{Q}$ of the elderly subjects results in an increased oxygen extraction of approximately 7.0 ml/liter of $\dot{Q}$. Therefore, if one assumes a constant rate of tissue oxygen extraction (A-$\dot{V}O_{2\,diff}$) from a young age to an old age, the predicted resting $\dot{V}O_2$ of the elderly based upon the decrement in $\dot{Q}$ would be 214 ml O_2/min, 41 ml O_2/min less than what was obtained. It was concluded from this that the decreased $\dot{Q}$ was related to both an age-related decrease

TABLE 1. *A comparison of resting hemodynamics between young (23.5 years) and elderly (70.8 years) subjects*

	Elderly males		Young males	
	Supine (N = 17)	Sitting (N = 10)	Supine (N = 23)	Sitting (N = 9)
Oxygen uptake (ml/min)	255	353	285	339
Cardiac output (liters/min)	5.8	5.2	7.7	5.7
A–$\dot{V}O_{2\,diff}$ (ml/liter)	44.8	68.6	38.0	60.6
Heart rate (beats/min)	67	79	70	84
Stroke volume (ml/beat)	86	67	111	67

Data from Granath et al., ref. 30.

in the mass of active metabolic tissue (10,59,60) and a hypokinetic circulation reflected in an increased A-$\dot{V}O_2$ difference (30,76,78). Unfortunately, similar conclusions cannot be drawn from the sitting rest data, challenging the concept of a hypokinetic circulation at rest. Perhaps the omission of numerous subjects from the original pool spuriously alters the data obtained during sitting rest and thereby adds to the ambiguity of the data.

The elderly's central circulatory response to exercise is similar to that of the younger adult in that the linear relationship between heart rate (HR) and oxygen uptake for a given submaximal workload is the same for both young and old subjects (4–6,30,63,77,81). In addition, the slope of response of cardiac output with the increasing oxygen uptake of progressive increases in workload is the same (30). However, the absolute level of cardiac output for a given level of work is lower in the elderly than in the young and was shown to be a result of a decreased stroke volume (Fig. 3). Compensatory increases in A-$\dot{V}O_2$ difference enable the elderly to obtain the oxygen required by the working muscles (30). This response to exercise supports the idea of a hypokinetic

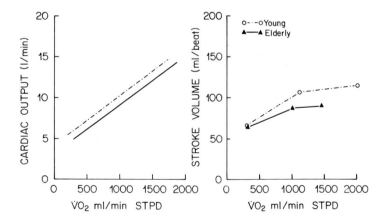

FIG. 3. A comparison of the relationships between oxygen uptake ($\dot{V}O_2$) and cardiac output and stroke volume obtained for young (○) and elderly (▲) subjects. (Adapted from Strandell, ref. 76.)

circulation per unit of oxygen uptake. However, whether the reduced stroke volume (and resultant cardiac output) is a result of central or peripheral modifications has yet to be determined. Granath et al. (30) and Strandell (78) argue that the same increase in $\dot{Q}$ with increasing $\dot{V}O_2$ of young and old men should indicate that the increase of blood flow to the working muscles is identical for both young and old. Yet Wahren et al. (82) have shown by direct catheterization that the rise in leg blood flow during exercise was less in a middle-aged (52 to 59 years) group of subjects than in a young group (25 to 30 years) (Fig. 4). The relative reduction in blood flow was compensated for by an increase in femoral arteriovenous oxygen difference.

To what level this relative hypokinesis continues in later decades of life (60, 70, and 80 years) has not been established. Strandell (78) has recently argued that the ^{133}Xe clearance technique utilized by Wahren et al. (82) may signify lower flows in the trained than in the untrained subject. In addition, other studies with untrained subjects have not verified the age-related reduction in exercise muscle-blood flow. However, Wahren's data (82) sug-

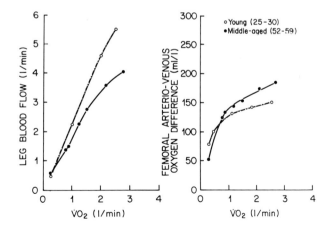

FIG. 4. The alterations in leg blood flow and oxygen extraction of young (○) and middle-aged (●) subjects as related to absolute level of oxygen uptake ($\dot{V}O_2$). (Adapted from Wahren et al., ref. 82.)

gest that the blood flow to the working muscles of the older person does not rise linearly with increasing $\dot{V}O_2$ above 2 to 2.5 liters O_2/min. This indicates that the greater the relative workload (percentage of $\dot{V}O_{2\,max}$), the greater the need for an increased extraction as a compensation for the relative reduction in blood flow to the working muscles. Hence, if this response is related to the relative workload (i.e., the degree of linearity decreases as we approach maximal levels) it would appear that the older one is, the greater will be the degree of hypokinesis in the peripheral circulation. During exercise, the average arterial lactate at a given heart rate or workload was shown to be higher in the elderly compared to the young. This suggests that full compensation of the supposed hypokinetic circulation of the aged was not possible by increasing oxygen extraction within the working muscles. Also, the finding that submaximal arterial lactate concentration of the elderly is more closely related to maximal workload (negatively) than other measures of central function further implies peripheral circulatory limitations within the aged (77).

During maximal work the attained HR_{max} decreases with increasing age regardless of levels of fitness. The average HR_{max} during upright exercise declines from 195 beats/min at 20 years of age to 160 to 165 beats/min at 60 years of age (5,33,65). As the SV is also lower for the elderly, the $\dot{Q}_{max}$ is reduced far more than expected from the reduced HR_{max} (30,76,77).

To date, there have been few studies designed to delineate the mechanisms responsible for the reduced HR_{max} with senescence. Corre et al. (18) measured the heart rates in 5-week-old compared to 19-week-old rats under baseline conditions during atropine blockade, propranolol blockade, and combined blockade both at rest and at maximum exercise. They found a constant difference between the young and mature rats under all conditions. They concluded that the aging decrement in HR was due to alterations in the nonneural component of HR control. However, as correctly pointed out by the authors, their finding may pertain more to development and maturation than senescence since they did not study truly senescent animals. Conway et al. (17) measured the HR and $\dot{Q}$ in 20- to 35-year-old compared with 50- to 65-year-old humans at rest and at maximum exercise both before and after propranolol blockade. After β-blockade they found the same magnitude of reduction in heart rate in the two age groups, but a larger reduction in $\dot{Q}$ in the young group. They concluded that there was an age decline in the amount of sympathetic drive to the heart during exercise, although such a conclusion regarding HR control could not be made from their data. Yin et al. (83) demonstrated a decrease in the maximum chronotropic response to isoproterenol in awake and anesthetized senescent compared to mature beagle dogs. This age-associated decrease in maximum HR persisted during atropine blockade. Since the HRs achieved with the drug were very close to those reported in other studies in dogs exercised to exhaustion, they suggested that part of the mechanism for the age decline in HR_{max} with exercise was a decreased responsiveness to catecholamines (29). Several studies have demonstrated a decreased baroreceptor sensitivity with increasing age (47). How these findings related to the diminished HR_{max} with exercise is not entirely clear. Since HR control is multifactorial, it is clear that further work is necessary to determine the true effect of aging on HR control and its response to exercise.

The marked structural changes occurring in the connective tissue with age result in progressive increases in stiffness of the myocardium and the arteries (see Chapters 1 and 4 and ref. 29). These changes result in the elderly having an increased resistance to filling of the heart and an increased systemic and pulmonary vascular resistance compared to the young both at rest and during exercise (15,30,76) (Fig. 5). Whether the changes in heart wall compliance or arterial wall compliance result in the age-related decrease in SV has yet to be determined. Decrements in left ventricular SV can be related to decreases in end-diastolic volume or increases in end-systolic volume. End-diastolic volume would be diminished if left ventricular filling pressure and/or end-diastolic compliance were decreased. On the other hand, end-systolic

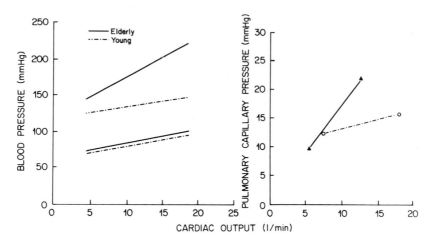

FIG. 5. The relationship between cardiac output and brachial artery pressures (systolic upper lines and diastolic lower lines) and pulmonary capillary wedge pressure in young *(dashed line)* and elderly *(solid line)* subjects. (Data from Granath et al., ref. 30, and Strandell, ref. 76.)

volume would be increased if there were a decrease in myocardial contractility and/or an increase in mean arterial pressure. The data of Strandell et al. (30,76,78) support the conclusion of an age-related increase in mean arterial pressure with an exercise-related increase in left-sided filling pressure (pulmonary capillary venous pressure) (Fig. 5). Hence, from these data it appears that the end-diastolic volume may stay the same or decrease while the end-systolic volume appears to have increased, which probably caused the decreased stroke volume.

Other evidence suggesting an age-related decrease in contractility to a given catecholamine stimulus (Chapters 5 and 8 and ref. 30) implies an increased end-systolic volume as the primary cause of the reduced stroke volume. Also, Granath et al. (30) noted that the individuals with the greatest changes in left-sided filling pressure had the greatest increases in cardiac output and oxygen uptake. In addition, these same elderly individuals also had the largest increase in pulse pressure in both brachial and pulmonary arteries. Thus the higher filling pressures were linked to a higher stroke work (Frank-Starling mechanism). Obviously, the available data are unable to delineate clearly the mechanism behind the age-related decrease in SV, which, in summary, is related to the aging effect on preload (i.e., diastolic stiffness and contraction duration), afterload (i.e., aortic stiffness or arteriolar vasodilating capacity), and the myocardial contractile state (i.e., the intrinsic component and response to inotropic agents).

CHRONIC RESPONSE TO DYNAMIC EXERCISE

Despite the earlier convictions that the elderly person has a reduced capability to adapt to dynamic exercise training (34, 41,57,75), a number of investigations have reported significant improvement in physical performance and functional capacity following a period of exercise training (4,9,23,27,31,55,56,62, 66,68,69,79). Fischer et al. (27), in a cross-sectional evaluation, indicated that life-long activity resulted in significant increases in maximal capacity to perform work and to transport oxygen in individuals in the seventh and eighth decades of life in comparison to their sedentary counterparts. From their data they suggested that the age-related reduction in performance and aerobic capacity is a result of decreased energy production and decreased circulatory delivery of oxygen regardless of activity history.

However, Cantwell and Watt (16) report an extreme case of cardiopulmonary fitness in a 70-year-old subject (following only 10 years of training) who attained a $\dot{V}_{O_2 max}$ of 56.7 liters O_2/kg/min, while Kaman et al. (38) report on a 69-year-old chronic jogger with a $\dot{V}_{O_2 max}$ of 53.4 ml/O_2/kg/min. In a study of champion American track athletes, Pollock et al. (63) report mean levels of $\dot{V}_{O_2 max}$ ranging from 57.5 ml O_2/kg/min at 40 to 49 years of age to 40.0 ml O_2/kg/min at 70 to 75 years of age. However, dramatic reductions in $\dot{V}_{O_2 max}$ did not occur until after the age of 60 years. The decrement in performance of the post-60-year-olds was closely related to the quantity and quality of the training regimen and the actual number of years trained. Undoubtedly, these cross-sectional investigations lead one to suspect that chronic activities delay the age-related reduction in maximal capacity of the circulation to deliver oxygen and increase the ability of the tissues to utilize oxygen. However, there is no definitive evidence to show that longevity is prolonged by physical training.

Relatively few investigators have been able to examine the results of long-term chronic exposure to exercise training of individuals over the age of 60 years in a longitudinal fashion. Barry et al. (9) trained eight subjects (average age, 70 years; range 55 to 78 years) on a bicycle ergometer three times a week for 3 months, utilizing a protocol of intermittent work for 15 min followed by a 6- to 10-min exhaustion ride at a pulse rate of 130 beats/min. This regimen produced a 76% increase in maximal workload and a 38% increase in $\dot{V}_{O_2 max}$. Both pulmonary ventilation (+50%) and pulse rate (+14 beats/min) were increased at exhaustion posttraining, indicating that training greatly improved the subjects' ability to perform work. Additionally, a reduction in the number of exercise EKG abnormalities was also observed. The data of this investigation confirmed some previous work by Benestad (11), who trained 13 individuals within the same age group (70+ years). Unfortunately, this study was limited to a 6-week training period.

DeVries (1,23,24) investigated the effects of a 6- through 42-week rigorous exercise training program on 112 males aged 52 to 87 years ($\overline{X}$ age, 69.5 years) and 17 females aged 52 to 70 years. The exercises consisted of calisthenics, jogging (145 beats/min), and stretching for 1 hr under supervision three times per week. Various subgroups were tested throughout the 42 weeks. Significant increases in transport capacity of oxygen were observed, although $\dot{V}_{O_2 max}$ was unaltered while physical work capacity (load and time) improved. A similar response was observed in a group of seven cardiac-impaired patients placed on a modified program (training HR, 120 beats/min) for 6 weeks. Life history of activity did not appear to correlate with the degree of improvement. The expected changes with long-term training suggested by this investigation were minimal and were probably related to the fact that the bulk of the subjects were tested after 6 weeks of training, while a cohort (ranging from $N = 8$ through 66) was retested at 17 and 42 weeks, with only 8 subjects finally being observed at 42 weeks. The reduction in numbers of trained subjects greatly reduced the impact of the findings of these investigations.

More recently Suominen et al. (79,80) looked at an 8-week endurance program, and Niinimaa and Shephard (55,56) looked at an 11-week endurance program in subjects 56 to 70 and 60 to 76 years old, respectively. Training time was 3 to 5 hr/week and consisted of flexibility, jogging and walking endurance work, and some power work. The average increase in $\dot{V}O_{2\,max}$ was 10%, and in one case (80) it was similar to those reported for younger individuals (26). Some in-depth investigations into the trainability of middle-aged men (31,62,69) have clearly demonstrated that in this age bracket the response to exercise training is not diminished. Training consisted of intermittent 2-mile runs twice a week, while a third 2-mile run was performed continuously once each week. This resulted in a 13% increase in $\dot{V}O_{2\,max}$, while stress EKG abnormalities were reduced.

Pollock et al. (62) have shown that the degree of change in $\dot{V}O_{2\,max}$ of middle-aged men is significantly related to frequency of training and the total amount of work performed. Hence, it may appear that the decreased capacity of the elderly to improve as a result of exercise training is purely a function of absolute amount of work performed. This contention is further supported by the work of Kasch and Wallace (40), who showed that by training middle-aged males ($\overline{X}$ age, 44.6; range, 32 to 56 years) at 60% $\dot{V}O_{2\,max}$ over 15 miles/week for 10 years, the expected aged decline in $\dot{V}O_{2\,max}$ did not occur, although no improvement in $\dot{V}O_{2\,max}$ was effected. Furthermore, earlier work by Siegel et al. (74) showed that a 15-week quantified training program (adjusting training heart rate to be maintained at 20 beats below the maximum) produced a 19% increase in $\dot{V}O_{2\,max}$. The mean age of the group ($N = 9$) was 46 years, with a range of 32 to 59 years. In summary, these early reports suggest that significant cardiovascular benefit can be obtained by the elderly as a result of vigorous dynamic exercise training. In fact, it is possible that the degree of improvement is more related to the absolute amount of work performed rather than the age of the individual.

In the acute responses to exercise, it was observed that the primary difference between young and elderly individuals during exercise was the reduced peripheral circulation (i.e., a hypokinetic circulation) and the increased regional oxygen extraction that occurs as a compensation (4,15,19,30,51,76,77,82). The improvement in maximal capacity in the elderly, documented above, indicates that significant alterations in oxygen delivery and utilization do occur in the elderly. Unfortunately, only a few investigations have attempted to measure the central and peripheral adaptations that occur with exercise training in the elderly (23,24,31,55,56, 69,79). In fact, in-depth evaluations of aging mechanisms have only been attempted on the middle-aged subject (31,69).

Forty-two subjects 35 to 50 years old underwent an 8- to 10-week conditioning program (2 to 3 hr/week of running), which resulted in a mean increase in $\dot{V}O_{2\,max}$ of 14% and an average $\dot{Q}_{max}$ of 13% (18.7 liters/min to 21.1 liters/min) (31,69). Heart rate at maximum was an average 6 beats/min lower, resulting in a calculated increase of 17 ml (16% increase) in SV. Thus, a larger amount of oxygen was transported by a larger $\dot{Q}$, which in turn was due to a larger SV. No change in heart volume or maximal mean blood pressure was observed. During submaximal work for a given oxygen uptake, HR and blood lactate were lower following training; however, when related to the percent of their $\dot{V}O_{2\,max}$ pre- and posttraining, the heart rate-to-$\dot{V}O_2$ and lactate-to-$\dot{V}O_2$ relationship was unchanged by training (69). This finding is similar to that obtained with younger adults and is highly suggestive that the middle-aged person's ability to adapt to chronic training is not reduced because of peripheral or central limitations.

In contrast to this conclusion Hartley et al. (31), from observed A-$\dot{V}O_{2\,diff}$ relationships to $\dot{V}O_2$ found in younger and older subjects following training (see Table 2), suggest that exercise training

TABLE 2. Comparison of some circulatory variables during maximal exercise in young but full-grown subjects and middle-aged men

		$\dot{V}_{O_2}$ (liters/min)	$\dot{Q}$ (liters/min)	HR (beats/min)	SV (ml)	$A-\dot{V}_{O_2\ diff}$ (ml/100 ml)
Training studies in young individuals (N = 17; age = 23 years)	Control	3.11	21.5	196	110	14.4
	Training	3.59	23.2	190	122	15.5
	Diff. (%)	+15	+ 8	− 3	+11	+ 8
Training studies in middle-aged men (N = 13; age = 47 years)	Control	2.68	18.7	182	103	14.4
	Training	3.06	21.1	176	120	14.6
	Diff. (%)	+14	+13	− 3	+16	+ 1

Data from Hartley et al., ref. 31.

will alter the oxygen extraction capability of the younger subjects but is unable to increase oxygen extraction of the middle-aged. They further hypothesize that this inability to increase the maximal A-$\dot{V}O_{2\,diff}$ is the primary reason that the middle-aged and elderly have a less pronounced improvement in $\dot{V}O_{2\,max}$ compared with younger subjects when their initial level of $\dot{V}O_{2\,max}$ is accounted for (31,69). Unfortunately, the cross-comparison of data obtained from younger and older subjects performing different training regimens raises serious questions concerning differences in absolute load and intensity of training. The differences between maintained activity levels and determining effects on the aging response to maximal and submaximal exercise during a longitudinal investigation (39) emphasizes the problems of interpretation of Hartley et al. (31) data. In this study 12 subjects were evaluated over a 13-year period while their physical activity was maintained. $\dot{V}O_{2\,max}$ decreased and was related to a decreased A-$\dot{V}O_{2\,diff}$ (or an increased venous oxygen content), even though $\dot{Q}_{max}$ and SV_{max} were unchanged or increased. In contrast, four subjects that were detrained over an 11-year period showed evidence of decreased $\dot{V}O_{2\,max}$, $\dot{Q}_{max}$, and SV_{max} while C-$\dot{V}O_2$ and A-$\dot{V}O_{2\,diff}$ was unchanged.

In two recent investigations, Niinimaa and Shephard (55,56) have again suggested (on the basis of cross-comparisons) the presence of a relative hypokinetic circulation in elderly subjects (aged 60 to 76 years) of both sexes. Surprisingly, their 11-week training program resulted in a decreased $\dot{Q}$ at a given submaximal level and was related to the decreased heart rate. Training did not alter submaximal levels of stroke volume of A-$\dot{V}O_{2\,diff}$. Although the investigators concluded that training caused an increase in cardiac reserves, the presented data was not supportive of this idea (see Table 3). Unfortunately, this investigation adds to our dilemma. Was the training program stressful enough to produce changes, or have we reached a critical chronological or biological age where functional alterations will not occur?

It can be argued that if local muscular adaptations to exercise training are reduced in the elderly as compared to the young,

TABLE 3. Effects of training on cardiovascular variables of men (N = 8) and women (N = 7) aged 60–70 years old (means and SEM)

	Work load 1		Work load 2		Work load 3	
	Before	After	Before	After	Before	After
Males						
$\dot{V}O_2$ (liters/min STPD)	0.95 ± 0.13	0.98 ± 0.18	1.43 ± 0.34	1.37 ± 0.29	1.97 ± 0.37	1.89 ± 0.33
fh (beats/min)	91.5 ± 13.2	88.8 ± 8.6	110.9 ± 7.1	105.2 ± 6.9[a]	137.3 ± 6.7	129.9 ± 7.8[a]
$\dot{Q}$ (liters/min)	10.2 ± 1.7	10.0 ± 2.2	12.2 ± 2.6	11.3 ± 2.4[b]	14.1 ± 2.5	13.4 ± 2.5
Stroke volume (ml)	112.8 ± 26.0	113.0 ± 27.8	109.5 ± 21.7	107.9 ± 23.0	102.8 ± 17.6	103.4 ± 21.7
CaO_2–CvO_2 (ml/100 ml)	9.4 ± 0.9	10.1 ± 1.9	11.9 ± 1.7	12.3 ± 1.9	14.1 ± 2.4	14.3 ± 2.5
Oxygen pulse (ml)	10.6 ± 2.5	11.1 ± 2.4	12.9 ± 3.2	13.1 ± 2.7	14.4 ± 2.8	14.5 ± 2.4
Females						
$\dot{V}O_2$ (liters/min STPD)	0.80 ± 0.13	0.80 ± 0.14	1.00 ± 0.17	1.00 ± 0.20	1.28 ± 0.10	1.33 ± 0.21
fh (beats/min)	103.2 ± 11.4	99.9 ± 10.3	115.2 ± 18.0	112.6 ± 8.5	136.0 ± 17.8	133.4 ± 11.9
$\dot{Q}$ (liters/min)	9.4 ± 1.8	9.9 ± 2.2	10.3 ± 1.8	10.2 ± 2.0	11.7 ± 1.7	11.5 ± 2.0
Stroke volume (ml)	91.1 ± 12.8	99.0 ± 16.3	91.1 ± 15.0	90.2 ± 15.7	87.2 ± 19.2	86.7 ± 14.6
CaO_2–CvO_2 (ml/100 ml)	8.7 ± 1.7	8.2 ± 0.9	9.9 ± 1.5	9.0 ± 1.0	11.2 ± 1.5	11.6 ± 1.4
Oxygen pulse (ml)	7.9 ± 1.4	8.0 ± 1.3	8.8 ± 1.8	8.9 ± 1.8	9.6 ± 1.6	9.9 ± 1.5

Significance of training effects: [a] $p < 0.05$ (1-tailed t-test) [b] $p < 0.05$ (2-tailed t-test).
Data from Niinimaa and Shephard, refs. 55 and 56.

then the circulatory adaptations will also be reduced. Only a few investigations have looked at the effects of training on the skeletal muscle metabolism of the aged (43,79,80), yet they have demonstrated significant increases in aerobic energy metabolism of previously sedentary middle-aged and elderly men and women. In young adults and animal models (35,36,67) dynamic exercise training resulted in increased activities of oxidative enzymes and increased muscle glycogen content, as well as decreased glycogen consumption and lactate production during submaximal exercise. Suominen et al. (79,80) trained 31 sedentary males aged 56 to 70 years by walking, jogging, swimming, ball games, and gymnastics in three to five 1-hr exercise bouts per week. $\dot{V}O_{2\,max}$ was increased 11%. Using biopsy techniques, muscle glycogen content, aerobic enzymes (malate and succinate dehydrogenase), and anaerobic enzymes (creatine phosphokinase and lactate dehydrogenase) showed increased concentrations within the muscles. Lactate production during submaximal work was reduced following the training. The improvement in oxygen utilization of this group of elderly subjects following training suggests that endurance training has similar effects for both young and old and questions the proposed age-related limitation in adaptation.

In an early evaluation of peripheral circulatory differences between the young (18 to 24 years old) and the elderly (mean age, 72 years), Allwood (2) utilized plethysmographic techniques to determine the subjects' responses to hyperemia. It was found that resting blood flow to the foot and the calf were similar. However, maximal flow during reactive hyperemia was severely attentuated in the elderly in the foot and was slightly lower in the calf when compared to the younger adults. In addition, it was observed that tonic vasomotor variations were diminished in the feet of the elderly compared to the young, while vascular resistance of both the foot and the calf were increased in the elderly. These findings suggest an alteration in autonomic function and/or responsivity to endogenous catecholamines as a function of age, which may play a role in the reduced peripheral flow during exercise of the elderly identified by Wahren et al. (82).

TABLE 4. *The effect of aging on the adaptations of the cardiovascular system to dynamic exercise training[a]*

Measurement	Young	Old
$\dot{V}_{O_2\,max}$	++	+
$\dot{Q}_{max}$	++	+?
HR_{max}	0 or −	−?
SV_{max}	++	+?
LV contractility	++	??
TPR_{max}	− −	+?
Exercise muscle blood flow	++	−?
HR_{rest}	− −	??
Blood pressure	− −	??
End diastolic volume	++	??
End systolic volume	− −	??
Vasomotor response	??	??
Parasympathetic control	++	??
Sympathetic control	− −	??

[a]+, Increase; ++, large increase; −, decrease; − −, large decrease; ?, questionable or unknown.

Evidence of an age-related degeneration in autonomic function is now being obtained (21). However, it is a matter of debate whether autonomic dysfunction can be modified by exercise training. Because of the involvement of the autonomic system in the human's adaptation to acute and chronic exercise (71), it is apparent that the relationship between exercise training, age, and autonomic function must be evaluated further.

Thus, it is seen that the data regarding the effects of age on the adaptation of the cardiovascular system to dynamic exercise training is minimal. A summary of the discussion of the reported findings is given in Table 4.

ACUTE RESPONSE TO STATIC EXERCISE

Static exercise causes a marked increase in mean arterial pressure with a relatively small increase in HR and $\dot{Q}$ as compared to dynamic exercise (51). It is of interest that neither the absolute tension development nor the size of the muscle mass involved is the determining factor; rather, the important parameter seems to be the percentage of maximal contraction by the muscle group.

The few studies concerning the effect of age on the acute cardiovascular response to static exercise have reported somewhat conflicting results. Studies have consistently shown that the heart rate response is greater in young individuals than in the old (44,48,58,61). However, as with dynamic exercise, the mechanism for the diminished heart rate response with aging has not been delineated. Similarly, the response of arterial pressure has not been clearly delineated. McDermott et al. (48) found no difference in the response of systolic and diastolic blood pressure in old and young men. Petrofsky and Lind (61) found greater systolic blood pressure elevations with similar diastolic responses in the old as compared to the young, while Ordway and Wekstein (58) found no difference in the systolic blood pressure response and a greater diastolic pressure in the young. It is difficult to understand these conflicting findings. However, it should be noted that the subjects of Petrofsky and Lind (61) could be described as trained to the static exercise stress by reason of their occupation, whereas those of Ordway and Wekstein (58) were untrained.

The response of the normal left ventricle to the increased afterload of static exercise consists of an increase in the contractile state with only a small rise in end-diastolic pressure (51). This suggests that the Frank-Starling mechanism is not required to meet the imposed stress. Furthermore, studies of plasma catecholamine during sustained static exercise suggest that the hemodynamic responses are due to a powerful activation of the adrenergic nervous system (45). Investigations using systolic time intervals as a measure of contractile state show that the contractile state is markedly reduced or even absent in the older individuals (44). However, it has been reported that the plasma catecholamine response is greater in the elderly compared to the young (48). These findings of a decreased heart rate and contractile state response would support the concept that the change elicited by a given catechol stimulus is less in the elderly than in the young (see Chapters 5 and 7) and is suggestive of receptor dysfunction.

Static exercise causes a marked increase in systolic, diastolic, and mean arterial pressure and a tachycardia with a resultant increase in myocardial oxygen utilization (51). This stress may be especially detrimental to the aged who already demonstrate a reduction in cardiovascular reserve. Whether this danger can be alleviated by a chronic static exercise program performed in a progressive fashion has not been evaluated. Therefore, at this time it would seem judicious to advise the elderly to avoid unsupervised isometric exercise programs.

REFERENCES

1. Adams, G. M., and DeVries, A. A. (1973): Physiological effects of an exercise training regimen upon women aged 52–79. *J. Gerontol.*, 28:50–55.

2. Allwood, M. J. (1958): Blood flow in the foot and calf in the elderly; a comparison with that in young adults. *Clin. Sci.*, 27.331–338.

3. Altman, P. L., and Dittmer, D. S., editors (1974): *Biology Data Book*, 2nd ed. Federation of American Societies for Experimental Biology, Bethesda, Maryland.

4. Asmussen, E., and Mathiasen, P. (1972): Some physiological functions in physical education students reinvestigated after twenty-five years. *J. Am. Geriatr. Soc.*, 20:379–387.

5. Åstrand, I. (1960): Aerobic work capacity in men and women with special reference to age. *Acta. Physiol. Scand. [Suppl.]*, 49(169):1–92.

6. Åstrand, P. O., and Rodahl, K. (1977): *Textbook of Work Physiology*, 2nd ed. McGraw Hill, New York.

7. Bafitis, H., and Sargent, F., II (1977): Human physiological adaptability through the life sequence. *J. Gerontol.*, 32:402–410.

8. Banerjee, S., and Bhatteracharya, A. K. (1964): Basal metabolic rate of boys and young adults of Rajastan. *Indian J. Med. Res.*, 52:1167–1172.

9. Barry, A. M., Daly, J. W., Pruett, E. D. R., Steinmetz, J. R., Page, H. F., Birkhead, N. C., and Rodahl, K. (1966): The effects of physical conditioning on older individuals. I. Work capacity, circulatory-respiratory function and work electrocardiogram. *J. Gerontol.*, 21:182–191.

10. Behnke, A. R. (1953): The relation of lean body weight to metabolism and some consequent systemitizations. *Ann. N. Y. Acad. Sci.*, 56:1025–1053.

11. Benestad, A. M. (1965): Trainability of old men. *Acta Med. Scand.*, 178:321–327.

12. Binkhorst, R. A., Pool, J., VanLeeuwen, P., and Bouhuys, A. (1966): Maximum oxygen uptake in healthy non-athletic males. *Int. Z. Angew. Physiol. Einschl. Arbeitsphysiol.*, 22:10–18.

13. Boothby, W. M., Berkson, J., and Dunn, L. (1936): Studies of the energy

of metabolism of normal individuals: A standard for basal metabolism with a monogram for clinical application. *Am. J. Physiol.,* 116:468–484.

14. Boothby, W. M., and Sandiford, I. (1929): Normal values of basal or standard metabolism. A modification of the Dubois standards. *Am. J. Physiol.,* 90:290–291.

15. Brandfonbrenner, M., Landowne, M., and Shock, N. W. (1955): Changes in cardiac output with age. *Circulation,* 12:557–566.

16. Cantwell, J. D., and Watt, E. O. (1974): Extreme cardiopulmonary fitness in old age. *Chest,* 65:357–359.

17. Conway, J., Wheeler, R., and Sannerstedt, R. A. (1971): Sympathetic nervous activity during exercise in relation to age. *Cardiovasc. Res.,* 5:577–581.

18. Corre, R. A., Cho, H., and Barnard, R. J. (1976): Maximum exercise heart rate reduction with maturation in the rat. *J. Appl. Physiol.,* 40:741–744.

19. Cournand, A., Riley, R. L., Breed, E. S., Baldwin, E. de F., and Richards, D. W. (1945): Measurements of cardiac output in man using the technique of catheterization of the right-auricle or ventricle. *J. Clin. Invest.,* 24:106–118.

20. Dawson, P., and Hellebrandt, F. (1945): The influence of aging in man upon physical work capacity and upon his cardiovascular response to exercise. *Am. J. Physiol.,* 143:420–428.

21. Davies, H. E. F. (1975): Respiratory change in heart rate, sinus arrythmia in the elderly. *Gerontol. Clin.,* 17:96–101.

22. Dehn, M. M., and Bruce, R. A. (1972): Longitudinal variations in maximal oxygen uptake. *J. Appl. Physiol.,* 33:805–807.

23. DeVries, H. A. (1970): Physiological effects of an exercise training regimen upon men aged 52–88. *J. Gerontol.,* 25:325–336.

24. DeVries, H. A., and Adams, G. M. (1972): Comparison of exercise responses in old and young men. I. The cardiac effort/total body effort relationship. *J. Gerontol.,* 27:344–348.

25. Dill, D. B., Robinson, S., and Ross, J. C. (1967): A longitudinal study of 16 champion runners. *J. Sports Med.,* 7:4–27.

26. Ekblom, B. (1969): Effect of physical training on oxygen transport system in man. *Acta Physiol. Scand. [Suppl.],* 328:1–76.

27. Fischer, A., Parizkova, J., and Roth, Z. (1965): The effect of systematic physical activity on maximal performance and functional capacity in senescent man. *Int. Z. Angew. Physiol. Einschl. Arbeitsphysiol.,* 21:269–304.

28. Fleisch, A. (1951): Le metabolisme basal standard et sa determination au moyen du metacalculator. *Helv. Med. Acta,* 18:23–44.

29. Gerstenblith, G., Lakatta, E. G., and Weisfeldt, M. D. (1976): Age changes in myocardial function and exercise response. *Prog. Cardiovasc. Dis.,* 19:1–21.

30. Granath, A., Jonsson, B., and Strandell, T. (1970): Circulation in healthy old men studies by right-heart catheterization at rest and during exercise in supine and sitting position. In: *Medicine and Sport: Physical Activity*

and Aging, edited by D. Brunner and E. Jokl, pp. 48–79. University Park Press, Baltimore.

31. Hartley, L. H., Grimby, G., Kilbom, A., Nilsson, N. J., Astrand, I., Bjure, J., Ekblom, B., and Saltin, B. (1969): Physical training in sedentary middle-aged and older men. III. Cardiac output and gas exchange at submaximal and maximal exercise. *Scand. J. Clin. Lab. Invest.,* 24:335–344.

32. Henschel, A. (1970): Effects of age on work capacity. *Am. Indust. Hyg. Assoc. J.,* 31:430–435.

33. Hodgson, J. L., and Buskirk, E. R. (1977): Physical fitness and age, with emphasis on cardiovascular function in the elderly. *J. Am. Geriatr. Soc.,* 25:385–392.

34. Hollman, W. (1964): Changes in the capacity for maximal and continuous effort in relation to age. In: *International Research in Sport and Physical Education,* edited by E. Jokl and E. Simon, pp. 369–371. Charles C Thomas, Springfield, Illinois.

35. Holloszy, J. O., Molé, P., Baldwin, K. M., and Terjung, R. L. (1975): Exercise induced enzymatic adaptations in muscle. In: *Limiting Factors of Physical Performance,* edited by J. Keul, pp. 66–80. Thieme, Stuttgart.

36. Holm, J., and Schersten, T. (1974): Metabolic changes in skeletal muscles after physical conditioning and in peripheral arterial insufficiency. *Forsvarsmedicin,* 10:71–78.

37. Howald, H., Maire, R., Heirli, B., and Follath, F. (1977): Ecko-kardiographische bepunde hei trainierten Sporttern. *Schweiz. Med. Wochenschr.,* 107:1662–1669.

38. Kaman, R. L., Raven, P. B., Carlisle, C., and Ayres, J. (1978): Age related changes in cardiac enzymes as a result of jogging exercise in man. *Med. Sci. Sports,* 10:46–47.

39. Kanstrup, I. L., and Ekblom, B. (1978): Influence of age and physical activity on central hemodynamics and lung function in active adults. *J. Appl. Physiol.,* 45:709–717.

40. Kasch, F. W., and Wallace, J. P. (1976): Physiological variables during 10 years of endurance exercise. *Med. Sci. Sports,* 8:5–8.

41. Kataski, S., and Masuda, M. (1969): Physical exercise for persons of middle and elder age in relation to their physical ability. *J. Sports Med.,* 9:193–199.

42. Khan, I., and Velvady, B. (1973): Basal metabolism in pregnant and nursing women and children. *Indian J. Med. Res.,* 61:1853–1857.

43. Kiessling, K. H., Pilstrom, L., Bylund, A. C. H., Saltin, B., and Piehl, K. (1974): Enzyme activities and morphometry in skeletal muscle of middle-aged men after training. *Scand. J. Clin. Lab. Invest.,* 33:63–71.

44. Kino, M., Lance, V. Q., Shamatpour, A., and Spodick, D. (1975): Effects of age on response to isometric exercise. *Am. Heart J.,* 90:575–581.

45. Kozlowski, S., Brzezinska, Z., Nazar, K., Kowalski, W., and Franozyk, M. (1973): Plasma catecholamines during sustained isometric exercise. *Clin. Sci. Mol. Med.,* 45:723–729.

46. Lewis, R. D., Duval, A. M., and Iliff, A. (1943): Standards for the basal

metabolism of children from 2 to 15 years of age inclusive. *J. Pedriatr.,* 23:1–18.

47. Lindblad, L. E. (1977): Influence of age on sensitivity and effector mechanisms of the carotid baroreflex. *Acta. Physiol. Scand.* 101:43–49.

48. McDermott, D. J., Steikel, W. J., Barboriak, J. J., Kloth, L. C., and Smith, J. J. (1974): Effect of age on hemodynamic and metabolic response to static exercise. *J. Appl. Physiol.,* 37:923–926.

49. Mitchell, J. H., Sproule, B. J., and Chapman, C. B. (1958): The physiological meaning of the maximal oxygen intake test. *J. Clin. Invest.,* 37:538–547.

50. Mitchell, J. H., and Blomqvist, G. (1971): Maximal oxygen uptake. *N. Engl. J. Med.,* 284:1018–1022.

51. Mitchell, J. H., and Wildenthal, K. (1974): Static (isometric) exercise and the heart: Physiological and clinical considerations. *Annu. Rev. Med.,* 24:369–381.

52. Mitchell, J. H. (1976): Cardiovascular physiology of dynamic and static exercise. *Dallas Med. J.,* 62:502–506.

53. Morganroth, J., Maron, B. J., Henry, W. L., and Epstein, S. E. (1975): Comparative left ventricular dimensions in trained athletes. *Ann. Intern. Med.,* 82:521–524.

54. Nickerson, J. L., Warren, J. N., and Brannon, E. S. (1947): The cardiac output in man, studies with the low frequency, critically damped ballistocardiograph and the method of right atrial catheterization. *J. Clin. Invest.,* 26:1–13.

55. Niinimaa, V., and Shephard, R. J. (1978): Training and oxygen conductance in the elderly. I. The respiratory system. *J. Gerontol.,* 33:354–361.

56. Niinimaa, V., and Shephard, R. J. (1978): Training and oxygen conductance in the elderly. II. The cardiovascular system. *J. Gerontol.,* 33:362–367.

57. Nocker, J. (1965): Die Bedeutung des Sportes fur den abten Mensehen. In: *Handbuch der Praktischen Geriatric,* edited by A. Mittmair, R. Nisser, and F. H. Shultz. F. Enke, Stuttgart.

58. Ordway, G. A., and Wekstein, D. R. (1979): Effect of age on cardiovascular responses to static (isometric) exercise. *Proc. Soc. Exp. Biol. Med.,* 161:189–192.

59. Parizkova, J. (1963): The impact of age, diet and exercise on man's body composition. *Ann. N.Y. Acad. Sci.,* 110:661–673.

60. Parizkova, J. E., Eiselt, J. E., Spaymarova, S., and Wachtlova, M. (1971): Body composition, aerobic capacity and density of muscle capillaries in young and old men. *J. Appl. Physiol.,* 31:323–325.

61. Petrofsky, J. S., and Lind, A. R. (1975): Aging, isometric strength and endurance, and cardiovascular responses to static effort. *J. Appl. Physiol.,* 38:91–95.

62. Pollock, M. L., Miller, H. S., Linnerud, A. C., and Cooper, K. H. (1975): Frequency of training as a determinant for improvement in cardiovascular function and body composition of middle-aged men. *Arch. Phys. Med. Rehabil.,* 56:141–145.

63. Pollock, M. L., Miller, H. S., and Wilmore, J. (1974): Physiological characteristics of champion American track athletes 40 to 75 years of age. *J. Gerontol.,* 29:645–650.
64. Robertson, J. D., and Reid, D. D. (1952): Standards for the basal metabolism of normal people in Britain. *Lancet,* 2:940–943.
65. Robinson, S. (1938): Experimental studies of physical fitness in relation to age. *Arbeitsphysiologie,* 10:251–323.
66. Robinson, S., Dill, D. B., Tzankoff, S. P., Wagner, J. A., and Robinson, R. D. (1975): Longitudinal studies of aging in 37 men. *J. Appl. Physiol.,* 38:263–267.
67. Saltin, B. (1973): Metabolic fundamentals in exercise. *Med. Sci. Sports,* 5:137–145.
68. Saltin, B., Blomqvist, G., Mitchell, H. H., Johnson, R. L., Wildenthal, K., and Chapman, C. B. (1968): Response to exercise after bed rest and after training. *Circulation,* 27/28(Suppl. 7):1–78.
69. Saltin, B., Hartley, L. H., Kilbom, A., and Åstrand, I. (1969): Physical training in sedentary middle-aged and older men. II. Oxygen uptake, heart rate and blood lactate concentration at submaximal and maximal exercise. *Scand. J. Clin. Lab. Invest.,* 24:323–334.
70. Shephard, R. J. (1966): World standards of cardiorespiratory performance. *Arch. Environ. Health,* 13:664–670.
71. Sheuer, J., and Tipton, C. M. (1977): Cardiovascular adaptations to physical training. *Annu. Rev. Physiol.,* 39:221–251.
72. Shock, N. W. (1961): Physiological aspects of aging in man. *Annu. Rev. Physiol.* 23:97–123.
73. Shock, N. W., and Yiengst, M. J. (1955): Age changes in basal respiratory measurements and metabolism in males. *J. Gerontol.,* 10:31–40.
74. Siegel, W., Blomqvist, G., and Mitchell, H. J. (1970): Effects of a quantitated physical training program on middle-aged sedentary men. *Circulation,* 61:19–29.
75. Skinner, J. S. (1973): Age and performance. In: *Limiting Factors of Physical Performance,* edited by J. Keul, pp. 271–282. Thieme, Stuttgart.
76. Strandell, T. (1964): Circulatory studies on healthy old men. *Acta Med. Scand. [Suppl.],* 414:1–43.
77. Strandell, T. (1964): Heart rate, arterial lactate concentration and oxygen uptake during exercise in old men compared to young men. *Acta Physiol. Scand.,* 60:197–201.
78. Strandell, T. (1976): Cardiac output in old age. In: *Cardiology in Old Age,* edited by F. T. Caird, J. L. C. Doll, and R. D. Kennedy, pp. 81–99. Plenum Press, New York.
79. Suominen, H., Heikkinen, E., Liesen, H., Michel, D., and Hollman, W. (1977): Effects of 8 weeks' endurance training on skeletal muscle metabolism in 56–70 year old sedentary men. *Eur. J. Appl. Physiol.,* 37:173–180.
80. Suominen, H., Heikkinen, E., and Parkatti, T. (1977): Effect of eight weeks physical training on muscle and connective tissue of M. vastus lateralis in 69 year old men and women. *J. Gerontol.,* 32:33–37.

81. Trusty, L. (1969): Physical fitness in old age. I. Aerobic capacity and the other parameters of physical fitness followed by means of graded exercise in ergometric examination of elderly individuals. *Respiration,* 26:161–181.

82. Wahren, J., Saltin, B., Jorfeldt, L., and Punow, B. (1974): Influence of age on the local circulatory adaptation to leg exercise. *Scand. J. Clin. Lab. Invest.,* 33:79–86.

83. Yin, F. C., Spurgeon, H. A., Raizes, G. S., Greve, H. L., Weisfeldt, M. L., and Shock, N. W. (1976): Age associated decrease in chronotropic response to isoproterenol. *Circulation,* 54:161–167.

The Aging Heart (Aging, Vol. 12),
edited by Myron L. Weisfeldt.
Raven Press, New York © 1980.

Chapter 11

Left Ventricular Function

Myron L. Weisfeldt

*Cardiology Division, Department of Medicine, Johns Hopkins Medical
Institutions, Baltimore, Maryland 21205*

The present chapter emphasizes integration and evaluation of data related to overall left ventricular function. Much of this material is presented in previous chapters in more detail as individual aspects of cardiovascular structure and function are discussed. In a certain sense, left ventricular function is the final common pathway for assessment of the relative importance of individual observed aging changes in either structure of tissues or functional capabilities of the myocardium and/or pharmacological response to individual hormones or pharmacological agents.

From the physiological point of view there appear to be at least four major factors contributing to age changes in left ventricular function. These four factors are (a) prolonged relaxation or prolonged contraction duration of cardiac muscle; (b) decreased sympathetic responsiveness in terms of chronotropic, inotropic, and vasodilating capacity; (c) decreased left ventricular diastolic compliance; and (d) increased impedance to left ventricular ejection. It is of major importance, as discussed in Chapter 1, to identify those aspects of left ventricular function which appear to show little or no age-associated decline or modification. These relatively unchanging parameters include: (a) ability to develop tension and the rate of tension development in isolated cardiac muslce (1,16,22,28); (b) the inotropic response to specific agents or factors not requiring cell membrane receptors, such as calcium and postextrasystolic potentiation (11,16); and (c) the time course of electrical depolarization and repolarization (5,17).

PROLONGED LEFT VENTRICULAR RELAXATION

Cross-sectional studies in the rat (16,17,28), guinea pig (20), dog (24), and man (6,13) show the presence of delayed or prolonged relaxation of cardiac muscle in the later portions of the life span (Fig. 1). Although, as discussed in Chapter 4, the majority of information related to the mechanism of the prolonged relaxation has been obtained in rats (8), the magnitude of the prolonged relaxation in fact may well be greater in organisms with a longer life span, such as dogs or man. In studies of the rat the prolongation of contraction duration, taken from the time of the onset of electrical depolarization to the return of tension to 50% of its peak value, is 10 to 15% (16,17,28). In the dog (24) contraction duration is defined in a similar fashion for isovolumic beats or is defined as the time from the onset of depolariza-

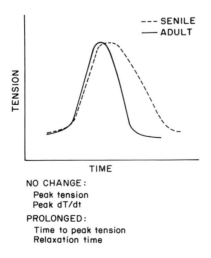

FIG. 1. Representative isometric contraction at the length at which contractile tension is maximal (L_{max}) in muscles from adult and senile rats. The major age changes are in the time course of the twitch rather than the rate of tension development or the maximal tension developed.

tion to return of pressure to half its peak value in a working preparation (the right heart bypass preparation). The prolongation of contraction duration with aging is 20 to 25%. A similar magnitude of change in the time from aortic closure from the phonocardiogram to mitral valve opening time from the echocardiogram has been noted in man.

Studies in the rat suggest that this prolonged contraction duration or delayed relaxation is not the result of abnormalities of sympathetic stimulation or responsiveness even though catecholamines are noted to shorten or accelerate the rate of cardiac muscle relaxation (17). Prolonged relaxation in rats was present even in the presence of sympathetic depletion or sympathetic blockade (17). Some evidence suggests that the prolonged relaxation is owing to specific age-related changes in the relaxing system of the cardiac sarcoplasmic reticulum (8). The difficulty in establishing specific biochemical mechanisms for physiological alterations with age is pointed out in Chapter 1. It may well be that there are more important age-associated changes in the behavior of the contractile proteins or their relationship to stimulation by the mediator (calcium) which account for prolonged contraction duration and delayed relaxation.

There is great similarity between these observations on rat myocardium from aged animals (in terms of prolonged contraction duration and sarcoplasmic reticulum) and observations on myocardium from rats following the onset of left ventricular hypertrophy (3,21). This hypertrophy was induced by higher impedance to left ventricular ejection either by creation of systemic hypertension or by banding of the aorta. Recent observations obtained by Yin and his associates (32) appear to support the notion that the age-associated alteration in relaxation and prolongation of contraction duration may in fact be a secondary phenomenon related to an age-associated increase in left ventricular mass, that is, the age-associated left ventricular hypertrophy. There are other possible causal mechanisms for the age-associated prolongation of relaxation. First, deconditioning or relative inactivity of the animals and humans who have been studied may be responsible (2,19). A number of studies suggest that one of the consequences of physiological conditioning of rats and other animals is an acceleration of the rate of relaxation and a shortening of contraction duration. If this is the case, it is possible that a relative decline in cardiac conditioning in older subjects results in prolonged contraction duration and relaxation. Clearly, this could be tested by examining the extent to which contraction duration can be accelerated through cardiovascular conditioning in aged subjects. Another possibility is that there is an age-associated decrease in effective end-organ thyroid function (4) which may account for prolonged relaxation and contraction duration. In animals it is clear that prolonged contraction duration and delayed relaxation does result from hypothyroidism. With increases in thyroid activity there is shortening of the duration of contraction and acceleration of relaxation in part, related to an increased sensitivity to catecholamines.

The major implications of prolonged or delayed relaxation and prolonged contraction duration relate to the possibility of occurrence of incomplete left ventricular relaxation between beats and the possibility of relative subendocardial myocardial underperfusion as a result of prolonged or delayed relaxation.

We (27) have recently demonstrated that under conditions of sufficiently prolonged relaxation and sufficiently rapid heart rate, incomplete left ventricular relaxation between beats can occur. The process of relaxation appears to go on with a time course that is independent of the rate or extent of left ventricular filling during diastole. Relaxation appears to be an active process that is related perhaps to the time course of uptake of calcium by the sarcoplasmic reticulum and thus is not a passive phenomenon which represents elastic recoil or return of contractile elements to their original resting position as a result of mechanical stretching during the process of filling. Since relaxation appears to be an active process, the rate and time course of relaxation would determine the rate and time course of filling once the mitral valve opens, not vice versa. Left ventricular diastolic pressure remains elevated during the diastolic filling period when relaxation is prolonged. Again, if relaxation is prolonged significantly and the heart rate is rapid enough, the next beat will begin before relaxation is complete. This incomplete left ventricular relaxation will result in an elevated left ventricular end diastolic pressure. The increase in left ventricular end diastolic pressure is not a result of a change in left ventricular contractile function or a change in diastolic stiffness reflecting the actual elastic mechanical properties of the myocardium during diastole in the fully relaxed state.

From the point of view of pulmonary congestion and other secondary effects of acute heart failure, it makes no difference whether the elevation of left ventricular diastolic pressure, particularly end-diastolic pressure, is a result of decreased contractility, increased stiffness of the myocardium during diastole, or incomplete relaxation. Thus, it is possible that during integrated activities such as exercise, where tachycardia is present, incomplete relaxation may, in part, be responsible for any elevation in left ventricular filling pressure, increase in pulmonary venous pressure, and decrease in pulmonary or lung compliance in the elderly. Obviously, this is a distant extrapolation beyond available data, but it is at least a working hypothesis for identifying a potentially important result of an age-associated prolongation of contraction duration or delayed relaxation.

Delayed relaxation results in a prolonged contraction duration or prolonged systole, and there is a shorter period for diastole (29). Thus, there is a shorter period during which the majority of subendocardial–myocardial blood flow occurs. In addition, the pressure gradient for subendocardial flow may be reduced as delayed relaxation continues into the diastolic filling period and results in an elevation in left ventricular diastolic pressure during early and mid diastole. Again, whether this speculation as to the physiological importance of prolonged relaxation is correct is not clear, but it is certainly a reasonable working hypothesis that, under conditions of stress or where the subendocardium is jeopardized through other mechanisms, there would be an additive compromise from these age-related changes. Also, under conditions where maximal left ventricular contractile function is demanded, relatively lower subendocardial flow may limit this maximal capacity.

DECREASED SYMPATHETIC RESPONSIVENESS

Three physiologically important aspects of the cardiovascular response to sympathetic stimulation appear to show a similar pattern of decreased responsiveness: inotrophy, chronotrophy, and vasodilatation.

Inotropic Response

In the isolated isometric left ventricular trabecular preparation of the rat (16), the magnitude of the increase in developed tension and the maximal rate of rise of tension in response to norepinephrine was shown to be depressed in muscles taken from 25-month-old (aged) rats when compared to 6- and 12-month-old rats (Fig. 2). There was no difference in the inotropic response between 6- and 12-month-old rats (both groups are within the mature adult age group for the rat). The lower response was present at all bath levels of norepinephrine studies.

This observation in and of itself might not be of major interest since it can easily be explained in terms of an overall decrease in the ability of the cardiac muscle from the older individual to respond in terms of any inotropic stimulus. That is, the age change may reflect an overall decrease in contractile ability of cardiac muscle from aged animals rather than some alteration in the specific inotropic response to the catecholamine. The former possibility seems unlikely in view of subsequent observations dealing with the inotropic response to noncatecholamine inotropic influence. The inotropic response to increasing bath calcium (Fig. 3) in the same rat trabecular preparation (16) showed no age-associated change.

More recently, we (11) were also able to demonstrate that postextrasystolic potentiation as a result of paired electrical pacing did not show any age-associated decrease. Thus, it appears

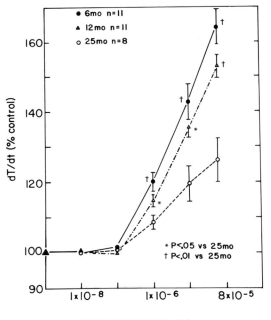

FIG. 2. Inotropic response of trabeculae carneae from the left ventricle of 6-, 12-, and 25-month-old male rats to increasing concentrations of norepinephrine in the muscle bath. A statistically significant age associated decrease in the inotropic response expressed as the maximal rate of tension rise (dP/dt) is seen in the muscles from the oldest group.

that the decreased responsiveness to catecholamines was at least in part related to a specific decrease in catecholamine response mechanism rather than being a reflection of a diffuse or nonspecific inability of the aged cardiac muscle to respond to inotropic influences. The age-associated decrease in catecholamine response was present for both norepinephrine and isoproterenol (16). Isoproterenol is not significantly taken up by storage sites; therefore, one could not account for the decrease in inotropic response to catecholamines on the basis of differential uptake of the mediator by release or storage sites rather than a decrease in responsiveness at the cellular level. Also, there was a similar pattern of age-

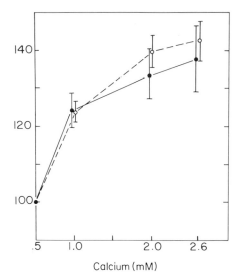

FIG. 3. Inotropic response to increasing amounts of bath calcium in left ventricular trabeculae carneae from (●) 6- and (○) 25-month-old male rats ($N = 6$). There is no age-associated change in the inotropic response expressed in terms of the maximal rate of tension rise (dP/dt).

associated decrease response to stepwise increases in catechol-amines, making differential tachyphylaxis or desensitization an unlikely mechanism for the decreased inotropic response. It remains unclear whether this decrease in inotropic response relates to an alteration in the cell membrane receptor number or binding or to subsequent sequential steps in the action of the agent.

A second inotropic agent, also thought to act through as a cell membrane receptor, ouabain, appears to show an age-associated decrease in inotropic responsiveness in the rat. Clearly, it would be of major importance to identify whether other membrane mediated inotropic agents show depressed inotropic response in aged animals and whether other nonmembrane active inotropic agents show a maintained inotropic response similar to calcium and paired pacing.

Chronotropic Response

Recently, Yin and associates (30) studied the chronotropic response to exogenously administered isoproterenol in adult and senescent purebred beagle dogs. The adult group was 1 to 4 years of age and the senescent group 10 to 12 years of age. Again, in this setting an age-associated decrease in the maximal response to a sympathetic mediator was identified. Baseline heart rate in unanesthetized dogs was similar, whereas at maximal administered dose of isoproterenol there was a lower heart rate in the senescent dogs. The maximum heart rate of the older dogs was approximately 30 beats/min less than in the adult group.

Under pentobarbital anesthesia the entire chronotropic dose-response curve to isoproterenol was examined. The dose-response curves of adult and aged dogs were not significantly different except for the magnitude of the maximal response under anesthesia. Vagal blockade with atropine did not restore the chronotropic response to normal. It is not known if this is a specific decrease in the chronotropic response to catecholamines, since the chronotropic response to other agents was not examined. In terms of physiological implication, this decrease in chronotropic response to catecholamines may account in part for the age-associated decrease in heart rate during maximal exercise in aged individuals.

Vasodilating Response

Most important and generally supportive studies of vasodilating response have been performed by Fleisch and associates (7). The observations in rabbits of varying age seem to identify the most quantitatively dramatic depression in a specific response to a sympathetic mediator. The oldest animals in this study showed a markedly diminished vasodilating response of aortic tissue to isoproterenol. As with the inotropic response, a nonsympathetic vasodilating agent showed a much more similar response in aged and adult animals. Thus again, here there is a specific decrease in the response to catecholamines rather than a nonspecific general decrease in ability of aging vascular tissue to respond. In terms of the integrated response of the organism and in terms of left ventricular function, this decreased vasodilating response may, in fact, be the most important aspect in the diminished response to catecholamines.

In all forms of exercise there is a significant rise in systolic arterial left ventricular pressure. The magnitude of this increase in systolic pressure, as crudely indexed by cuff limb blood pressure, appears to be greater in older individuals at similar levels of work or exercise. Assuming that central arterial pressure is reflected in these measures of peripheral arterial pressure, this would indicate a significantly greater systolic pressure load on the left ventricle as well as an increase in oxygen demands on the left ventricle at any given level of exercise stimulation in the aged individual. Since impedance to left ventricular ejection and peak pressure is, in part, reflective of the properties and state of the arterial vasculature (see Chapter 7), a decreased vasodilatation of major arterial vessels could be the dominant factor here (10). Age-associated decreases in left ventricular function under stress could well reflect a relatively higher left ventricular load rather than diminished contractile ability of the left ventricle. This could result, in part, from this age-associated decrease in vasodilating response to catecholamines.

Thus, in the identification of the factors limiting left ventricular function in aging, there are two general hypotheses. First, that any decrease is owing to cardiac factors, and second, that the age-associated decrease in apparent left ventricular function is owing to noncardiac factors. Among the noncardiac factors which would most likely be responsible in an age-associated increase in left ventricular workload on the basis of increased impedance to left ventricular ejection. In turn, this could be related not only to alterations in primary vascular structure and stiffness, but also quite likely to the ability of the arterial vasculature to dilate in response to physiological stimulation.

Another likely extracardiac factor which might be of importance in terms of the integrated response of the left ventricle to stress is the neurogenic response. The magnitude of the sympathetic nervous system response may be lower in terms of elaboration of mediator. The present discussion will not resolve these issues which are the subjects and direction of future studies.

DIASTOLIC AND SYSTOLIC COMPLIANCE

It is well known that tendinous connective tissue shows an increase in stiffness during the aging process (26). This increase in stiffness is disproportionate to any change in connective tissue mass and thus relates to fine structural details of the tissue as it is modified over the life span. Since a significant portion of the myocardium itself is composed of this type of connective tissue and since the fibrous skeleton of the heart is in series with the contractile elements, it would seem highly likely that there is an increase in passive stiffness of the senescent heart. In addition, since contractile proteins are themselves high-molecular weight proteins, it would not be beyond the bounds of possibility to envision changes in the stiffness properties of these proteins to passive stretch during diastole and even during a contraction cycle.

Changes in stiffness during diastole and systole would have profound implications in terms of functional characteristics of the heart. In terms of systolic function, the greater the stiffness of elastic elements and other elements in series, the less internal shortening; therefore, internal work would be required in the course of generating tension in the left ventricular wall. Thus, an increase in stiffness would probably have a functional advantage during a contraction cycle.

In terms of an increase in diastolic or resting left ventricular stiffness, this would not have a major effect on overall left ventricular function unless the Frank-Starling mechanism were called upon for compensation and the diastolic volume thereby increased significantly. Under conditions in which the diastolic volume is increased significantly and the left ventricle during diastole is stiffer, a greater rise in diastolic left ventricular pressure would occur. Once relaxation was complete all diastolic pressures at any given volume would be higher in the stiffer ventricle than in the ventricle with normal stiffness.

During stress such as exercise, a higher left ventricular diastolic pressure would therefore be anticipated. This higher pressure would be transmitted back into the left atrium and ultimately into the pulmonary venous bed and result in a more rapid appearance of symptoms of dyspnea and perhaps signs of congestive heart failure. Thus, in terms of overall left ventricular function, an increase in systolic stiffness might well be beneficial, whereas an increase in diastolic stiffness is likely to be detrimental.

A number of studies of diastolic or elastic stiffness of anoxic arrested hearts of varying age have been performed and reviewed (14,15,18). Since it is well known that anoxia per se alters resting myocardial length–tension relationships (12), it is difficult to see how these studies provide insight with regard to the elastic characteristics of living cardiac muscle of aged animals.

Within the last several years, methods of measuring dynamic myocardial stiffness in the intact beating heart or in isolated cardiac tissue have been described by Templeton and his associates (23,25). These techniques utilize a sinusoidal forcing function, that is, a volume or length perturbation of a small order of magnitude superimposed on isovolumic or isometric left ventricular or muscle contractions. By computer techniques the component of measured left ventricular pressure or tension which represents the response of the tissue to the sinusoidal forcing function can be identified from the underlying pressure or tension change owing to contraction and can be measured directly during any portion of the cardiac cycle. From such measurements stiffness–tension relationships can be plotted throughout the cardiac or contraction cycle. The relationship between stiffness and systolic pressure or tension during contraction has been shown by a number of investigators under a number of systems to be linear. Therefore, systolic and diastolic stiffness can be characterized in terms of the slope and intercept of the stiffness–developed pressure relationship for the intact heart or stiffness–tension relationship for isolated cardiac muscle.

Templeton and co-workers (24) utilized such forcing functions in isovolumic intact dog left ventricular preparations. These preparations were from eight animals with an average age of 27 months and seven animals with an average age of 128 months. Once the isovolumic preparation was established, 1 ml sinusoidal volume changes were induced by sinusoidal injection and withdrawal of 1 ml of fluid at 20 Hz into and out of the left ventricular balloon. The induced perturbation of the isovolumic pressure curve was measured. As in previous studies, there was a linear relationship during the cardiac cycle between stiffness (derived from this pressure change) and simultaneous pressure without any perturbation. Stiffness at any pressure throughout the cardiac cycle, for both diastole and systole, was higher for the beagles in the older age group. The slope of the stiffness–pressure relationship was not significantly different between the adult and senescent animals (0.086 ± 0.0059 for the younger group and 0.106 ± 0.0093 ml for the older group). The intercept of this stiffness–pressure relationship was highly significantly different: 1.31 ± 0.763 in the younger animals and 4.75 ± 0.647 mm Hg/ml ($p < 0.001$). This means that during both systole and diastole there appears to be an age-associated increase in chamber left ventricular stiffness.

Some support for the general notion of an increase in cardiac muscle stiffness comes from studies performed by Spurgeon and associates (22) in isolated rat trabeculae carneae, again using a forcing function system for assessment of isolated muscle stiffness. These studies demonatrate once more that during contraction there is an age-associated increase in muscle stiffness. In these studies the age-associated increase in stiffness is reflected in an increase in the stiffness coefficient, that is, the slope of the relationship between stiffness and developed tension, rather than a change in the intercept. There was some tendency for this contraction stiffness coefficient to show greater age changes at higher frequencies of perturbation, suggesting a component of the difference in apparent stiffness is accountable on the basis of viscous rather than strictly elastic changes.

Major differences exist between the information obtained in the intact dog ventricles and the isolated rat trabeculae carneae. In the former, we are dealing with not only the cardiac muscle of the intact chamber and the geometric relationships of one myofiber to another; but also the elastic and stiffness properties of the attachments of the muscle. In the rat trabeculae carneae preparation the ends of the muscles are clearly injured, and the attachments lead to unphysiological information.

The fact that age differences during contraction were obtained in the isolated muscle suggests quite strongly that there is a contribution of muscle stiffness to the increase in stiffness noted during the process of contraction. This increased stiffness during contraction may be very important in explaining the apparent discrepancies between decreases in shortening ability of senescent muscle in contrast to maintenance of active tension development and rate of tension development under isometric conditions (see Chapter 4). It may well be that the decrease in internal work required in a stiffer muscle acts in a compensatory fashion to allow tension development and the rate of tension development to be maintained despite decreases in intrinsic cardiac muscle contractility. This remains a hypothesis at the present time.

Increased Impedance to Left Ventricular Ejection

In the previous chapters dealing with the specific determinants of impedance to left ventricular ejection during senescence (Chapter 7) and exercise response of the aging individual (Chapter 10), the nature and importance of an age-associated increase in impedance to left ventricular ejection is discussed more fully. It is quite possible that in terms of what is observed in the intact animal, the age-associated increase in impedance is the dominating factor in the maximal functional capacity of the cardiovascular system. The age-associated increase in myocardial mass observed pathologically and echocardiographically supports the notion that there is an age-associated increase in impedance to ejection. This is at least in part compensated by an increase in muscle mass. With periods of acute stress, where impedance might well be increased to a greater extent in the aged, the maximal capacity of the cardiovascular system may be exceeded.

In terms of experimental design, it will be very difficult to establish whether or not the increase in impedance is in fact determining the capacity of the cardiovascular system. Clearly, maximal cardiac output capacity may be limited by a reduction of maximal cardiac capacity as reflected in maximal heart rate or maximal stroke volume. Also, maximal cardiac output is the same as maximal peripheral blood flow. Maximal peripheral flow may be limited by resistance or impedance outside the heart. Clearly, both cardiac and peripheral factors may be significant components in limiting maximal cardiac output capacity of the aged individual. Within a given individual there may be more limitation placed by peripheral factors, whereas in other individuals the major limitation may be direct cardiac factors.

OVERALL LEFT VENTRICULAR FUNCTIONAL CAPACITY

Throughout this volume, and specifically in this chapter, a number of aspects of left ventricular and cardiac muscle function which appear to show significant age-associated decline or decrease have been identified. However, there is little direct evidence of an overall decrease in left ventricular contractile function (in the absence of disease or severe stress). Available data suggest that the aged heart is not greatly functionally embarrassed. Only on near-maximal exercise is there any likely limitation of the aged organism on a basis of limited cardiac or cardiovascular capacity.

Left ventricular function in man, as in experimental animals, does appear to be characterized by prolonged relaxation. The extent to which there are age-associated alterations in sympathetic responses in man is presently unknown, although the evidence in experimental animals appears to support the possibility of such alterations. In addition, there is every reason to presume that in man there is increased impedance to left ventricular ejection, as discussed previously, but yet there is some hypertrophy (9) which may well compensate for the increased impedance. No measurements of left ventricular diastolic compliance in relationship to age in man have been made.

Echocardiographic studies of left ventricular function utilizing one-dimensional techniques suggest that left ventricular function in man is not greatly diminished. The problems of sampling and of accuracy and reproducibility of this method are of concern. Nonetheless, these are the most extensive pieces of information presently available which include measurements of direct left ventricular functional capability and characteristics.

At rest, ejection (shortening) fraction showed no apparent alteration with age in man. In the same large population it was easily identified that there was an age-associated increase in left ventricular wall thickness, suggesting an increase in left ventricular mass. Thus, the technique was able to identify age-associated alterations in anatomic characteristics, but functional indexes including ejection fraction, velocity of posterior wall motion, and normalized velocity of shortening (Vcf) were unchanged (9).

In a smaller subset of this same normal age population, Yin and colleagues (31) studied left ventricular contractile function in more detail. Eleven normal older male human subjects with an average age of 68.5 years were compared to seventeen younger males with an average age of 29.6 years. At rest, heart rate and systolic blood pressure were not significantly different. There was also no significant difference in left ventricular diastolic dimension, left ventricular systolic dimension, velocity of posterior wall motion, or normalized velocity of contractile element shortening at rest. The same subjects were tested in terms of their response to an increase in afterload stress, utilizing hand grip and phenylephrine to increase afterload. Despite an increase in systolic blood pressure of 28 to 34 mm Hg with these two types of afterload stress, there were no age-associated differences in parameters which might represent functional capabilities of the old versus the young individual. The parameters examined were the same as those listed above. In addition, this entire population was studied after β-adrenergic blockade induced by propranolol. Adequacy of β-blockade was tested by showing similar degrees of obliteration of the heart rate response to small doses of isoproterenol. In the β-adrenergic blockaded state there was no significant age-associated difference in heart rate, systolic blood pressure, left ventricular diastolic or systolic dimension, velocity of posterior wall motion, or contractile element shortening. When hand grip was superimposed on β-adrenergic blockade, again there was no significant age-associated difference. It was only in the presence of β-blockade when phenylephrine was infused to increase blood pressure by an average of 33 and 31 mm Hg in the old and young subjects, respectively, that any age change in these parameters of left ventricular function appeared. Under these conditions left ventricular diastolic dimension increased significantly in the older subject in the presence of the afterload stress, whereas there was no significant change in diastolic dimension with the afterload stress in the young individuals. The older individuals increased the diastolic dimension 2.3 ± 0.6 mm, whereas in the younger individuals the average increase was 0.1 ± 0.05 mm ($p < 0.01$). Other parameters of left ventricular function were not significantly different between the old and young subjects. Thus it appears that in order to maintain shortening ability and left ventricular velocities of wall motion and circumferential shortening, that the older individuals, following β-blockade, must use the Frank-Starling mechanism to compensate for the increase in afterload stress. This was the sole evidence for a relative decrease in maximal functional capability.

Thus it would appear that under stress there is an age-associated decrease in cardiac function, but to reveal this difference one must induce β-blockade and induce a rather significant increase in hemodynamic burden on the left ventricle. Again, it remains to be assessed whether or not under stressful conditions, in which sympathetic responsiveness is an important compensatory mechanism, there is an identifiable decrease in left ventricular systolic function. In this regard, it would be of great interest to examine functional characteristics of normal individuals during stresses such as exercise. The suspicion of this author is that little in the way of functional alterations will be noted until the acute abilities of the sympathetic nervous system to respond are exceeded by long-term and severe exercise or stress or by an increase in load which is far beyond those encountered under usual circumstances in the course of life history.

Certainly, when disease of cardiac muscle or the cardiovascular system is superimposed on aging changes, aging changes may well have a marked additive effect on the deterioration of overall cardiac function. The changes in diastolic compliance, as discussed above, would have profound importance where the left ventricle is unable to deal with the load imposed on it without utilizing the Frank-Starling mechanism or dilating to a significant extent. Under these circumstances there would be more rapid deterioration of apparent function and appearance of symptomatic heart failure. In the presence of disease, symptomatic failure would be likely to be more rapid in appearance, not only because of the age-associated alteration in left ventricular compliance, but also because of any age-associated decrease in sympathetic responsiveness and maximal heart rate and peripheral vasodilating capacities and prolonged relaxation.

REFERENCES

1. Alpert, N. R., Gale, H. H., and Taylor, N. (1967): The effect of age on contractile protein ATPase activity and the velocity of shortening. In: *Factors Influencing Myocardial Contractility,* edited by R. D. Tanz, F. Kavaler, and J. Roberts, pp. 127–133. Academic Press, New York.
2. Bersohn, M. M., and Scheuer, J. (1977): Effects of physical training on end-diastolic volume and myocardial performance of isolated rat hearts. *Circ. Res.,* 40:510–516.
3. Bing, O. H. L., Matsushita, S., Fanburg, B. L., and Levine, H. J. (1971): Mechanical properties of rat cardiac muscle during experimental hypertrophy. *Circ. Res.,* 28:234–245.
4. Buccino, R. A., Sonnenblick, E. H., Spann, Jr., J. F., Friedman, W. F., and Braunwald, E. (1967): Interactions between changes in the intensity and duration of the active state in the characterization of inotropic stimuli on heart muscle. *Circ. Res.,* 21:857–867.
5. Cavoto, F. V., Kelliher, G. J., and Roberts, J. (1974): Electrophysiological changes in the rat atrium with age. *Am. J. Physiol.,* 226:1293–1297.
6. Dock, W. (1966): How some hearts age. *JAMA,* 195:442–444.
7. Fleisch, J. H., Maling, H. M., and Brodie, B. B. (1970): Beta-receptor

activity in aorta: Variations with age and species. *Circ. Res.,* 26:151–162.

8. Froehlich, J. P., Lakatta, E. G., Beard, E., Spurgeon, H. A., Weisfeldt, M. L., and Gerstenblith, G. (1978): Studies of sarcoplasmic reticulum function and contraction duration in young adult and aged rat myocardium. *J. Mol. Cell. Cardiol.,* 10:427–538.

9. Gerstenblith, F., Frederiksen, J., Yin, F. C. P., Fortuin, N. J., Lakatta, E. G., and Weisfeldt, M. L. (1977): Echocardiographic assessment of a normal adult aging population. *Circulation,* 56:273–278.

10. Gerstenblith, G., Lakatta, E. G., and Weisfeldt, M. L. (1976): Age changes in myocardial function and exercise response. *Prog. Cardiovasc. Dis.,* 19: 1–21.

11. Gerstenblith, G., Spurgeon, H. A., Froehlich, J. P., Weisfeldt, M. L., and Lakatta, E. G. (1979): Diminished inotropic responsiveness to ouabain in aged rat myocardium. *Circ. Res.,* 44:517–523.

12. Greene, H. L., and Weisfeldt, M. L. (1977): Determinants of hypoxic and post-hypoxic myocardial contracture. *Am. J. Physiol.,* 232:H526–H533.

13. Harrison, T. R., Dixon, K., Russell, R. O., Bedwai, P. S., and Coleman, H. N. (1964): The relation of age to the duration of contraction, ejection, relaxation of the normal heart. *Am. Heart J.,* 67:189–199.

14. Kane, P. L., McMahon, T. A., Wagner, R. L., and Abelman, W. H. (1976): Ventricular elastic modules as a function of age in the syrian golden hamster. *Circ. Res.,* 28:74–81.

15. Korecky, B., Bernath, P., and Rosengarten, M. (1974): Effects of age on the passive stress–strain relationship of the rat heart. *Fed. Proc.,* 33:321(abstr.).

16. Lakatta, E. G., Gerstenblith, G., Angell, C. S., Shock, N. W., and Weisfeldt, M. L. (1975): Diminished inotropic response of aged myocardium to catecholamines. *Circ. Res.,* 36:262–269.

17. Lakatta, E. G., Gerstenblith, G., Angell, C. S., Shock, N. W., and Weisfeldt, M. L. (1975): Prolonged contraction duration in aged myocardium. *J. Clin. Invest.,* 55:61–68.

18. Mirsky, I. (1976): Assessment of passive elastic stiffness of cardiac muscle: Mathematical concepts, physiologic and clinical considerations, directions of future research. *Prog. Cardiovasc. Dis.,* 18:177–308.

19. Penpargkul, S., Repke, D. I., Katz, A. M., and Scheuer, J. (1977): Effect of physical training on calcium transport by rat cardiac sarcoplasmic reticulum. *Circ. Res.,* 40:134–138.

20. Rumberger, E., and Timmerman, J. (1976): Age-changes of force frequency relationship and the duration of action potential of isolated papillary muscles of guinea pig. *Eur. J. Appl. Physiol.,* 35:277–284.

21. Sordahl, L. A., McCollum, W. B., Wood, W. G., and Schwartz, A. (1973): Mitochondric and sarcoplasmic reticulum function in cardiac hypertrophy and failure. *Am. J. Physiol.,* 224:497–502.

22. Spurgeon, H. A., Thorne, P. A., Yin, F. C. P., Shock, N. W., and Weisfeldt, M. L. (1977): Increased dynamic stiffness of trabeculae carneae from the senescent rat. *Am. J. Physiol.,* 1:H373–H380.

23. Templeton, G. H., Mitchell, J. H., Ecker, R. R., and Blomqvist, G. (1970): A method for measurement of dynamic compliance of the left ventricle in dogs. *J. Appl. Physiol.,* 29:742–745.
24. Templeton, G. H., Platt, M. R., Willerson, J. T., and Weisfeldt, M. L. (1979): Influence of aging on left ventricular hemodynamics and stiffness in beagles. *Circ. Res.,* 44:189–194.
25. Templeton, G. H., Wildenthal, K., Willerson, J. T., and Reardon, W. C. (1974): Influence of temperature on the mechanical properties of cardiac muscle. *Circ. Res.,* 39:624–634.
26. Verzar, F. (1969): The stages and consequences of aging of collagen. *Gerontologia,* 15:233–239.
27. Weisfeldt, M. L., Frederiksen, J. W., Yin, F. C. P., and Weiss, J. L. (1978): Evidence of incomplete left ventricular relaxation in the dog: Prediction from the time constant for isovolumic pressure fall. *J. Clin. Invest.,* 62:1296–1302.
28. Weisfeldt, M. L., Loeven, W. A., and Shock, N. W. (1971): Resting and active mechanical properties of trabeculae carneae from aged male rats. *Am. J. Physiol.,* 220:1921–1927.
29. Weisfeldt, M. L., Scully, H. E., Frederiksen, J., Rubenstein, J. J., Pohost, G. M., Beierholm, E., Bello, A. G., and Daggett, W. M. (1974): Hemodynamic determinants of maximum negative dp/dt and the periods of diastole. *Am. J. Physiol.,* 227:613–621.
30. Yin, F. C., Spurgeon, H. A., Greene, H. L., Lakatta, E. G., and Weisfeldt, M. L. (1979): Age-associated decrease in heart rate response to isoproterenol in dogs. *Mech. Ageing Dev.,* 10:17–25.
31. Yin, F. C. P., Guarnieri, T., Spurgeon, H. A., Lakatta, E. G., Fortuin, N. J., and Weisfeldt, M. L. (1978): Age-associated decrease in ventricular response to hemodynamic stress during beta-adrenergic blockade. *Br. Heart J.,* 40:1349–1355.
32. Yin, F. C. P., Spurgeon, H. A., Lakatta, E. G., Guarnieri, T., Weisfeldt, M. L., and Shock, N. W. (1977): Cardiac hypertrophy indexed by tibial length: Application in the aging rat. *Gerontologist,* 17:135(abstr.)

Subject Index

A

Acetylcholine, influence of on vascular tissue, 181, 277, 229, 235

Action potential, cardiac muscle, 80–83

Acylamid, 223

Acylcarnitine translocase, 44–45, 47–51

Adenosine-3′, 5′-monophosphate, 181, 184–185

Adrenergic response, 181, 182–185, 232, 312–313

Adventita, aging of, 142–146

Aging
  disease contrasted with, 1–2, 12, 19, 269, 270
  maturation contrasted with, 4
  physiological changes with, 4–6

Amyloidosis, age-related, 13–14, 18, 19

Angina equivalence, 201

Angiotensin, 181

Antiarrhythmic drugs, 229, 236–239

Aorta, aging of, 142, 144

Aortic valve, 18

Apexcardiogram, 254–255

Arteriosclerosis, 18, 116–119, 120, 175–176

Atherosclerosis, 116–119, 129

Atrophy, cardiac, 8–9, 13–14

Atropine, 229, 230

Autonomic drugs, 226–236

Autonomic nervous system, 226

B

Ballistocardiogram, 255–256

Baroreceptor sensitivity, 103

Basophilic degeneration, myocardial, 11–12

Blood flow, coronary; *see also* Vasculature
  in ischemic heart disease, 116, 118
  in myocardial microvasculature, 124–127
  oxygen extraction, 127–128

Bradycardia, 103, 235–236

Brown atrophy, cardiac, 9–11

C

Calcification, 18, 118, 130, 144, 148

Calcium
  in digitalis therapy, 225
  in excitation-contraction-relaxation cycle, 78–83, 86, 94–95
  catecholamine influence on, 87–88
  response in aging system, 54, 232, 304

Capillary bed, myocardial, 124–127

Carcinomatosis, 8–9

317